THE SANFORD GUIDE

HIV/AIDS Therapy

2019

26th Edition

Michael S. Saag, M.D.
David N. Gilbert, M.D.
Henry F. Chambers, M.D.
George M. Eliopoulos, M.D.
Andrew T. Pavia, M.D.

Douglas Black, Pharm.D.
David O. Freedman, M.D.
Kami Kim, M.D.
Brian S. Schwartz, M.D.

THE SANFORD GUIDE
To HIV/AIDS Therapy
2019

Editors

David N. Gilbert, M.D.
Chief of Infectious Diseases,
Providence Portland Medical Center, Oregon
Professor of Medicine,
Oregon Health Sciences University

George M. Eliopoulos, M.D.
Beth Israel Deaconess Hospital
Professor of Medicine,
Harvard Medical School, Boston, Massachusetts

Henry F. Chambers, M.D.
San Francisco General Hospital
Professor of Medicine Emeritus
University of California, San Francisco

Michael S. Saag, M.D.
Associate Dean for Global Medicine
Director, UAB Center for AIDS Research
Professor of Medicine and Director,
Division of Infectious Diseases,
University of Alabama, Birmingham

Andrew T. Pavia, M.D.
George & Esther Gross Presidential Professor
Chief, Division of Pediatric Infectious Diseases,
University of Utah, Salt Lake City

Publisher

Antimicrobial Therapy, Inc.

Contributing Editors

Douglas Black, Pharm.D.
Professor of Pharmacy,
University of Washington, Seattle

Brian S. Schwartz, M.D.
Associate Professor of Medicine,
University of California, San Francisco

David O. Freedman, M.D.
Emeritus Professor of Medicine,
University of Alabama, Birmingham

Kami Kim, M.D.
Professor of Internal Medicine,
Division of Infectious Diseases
and International Medicine,
Morsani College of Medicine,
University of South Florida, Tampa

Managing Editor

Jeb C. Sanford

Memoriam

Jay P. Sanford, M.D.
1928-1996

Merle A. Sande, M.D.
1939-2007

Robert C. Moellering, Jr., M.D.
1936-2014

SANFORD GUIDE TO HIV/AIDS & HEPATITIS THERAPY is updated annually and published by:

ANTIMICROBIAL THERAPY, INC.
11771 Lee Highway, P.O. Box 276
Sperryville, VA 22740-0276 USA
Tel 540-987-9480 Fax 540-987-9486
Email: info@sanfordguide.com
www.sanfordguide.com

Acknowledgements
Thanks to Silvina Trapé, Jonatan Bohman and their team for manuscript design and layout of this edition of the SANFORD GUIDE.

Note to Readers
Since 1969, the SANFORD GUIDE has been independently prepared and published. Decisions regarding the content of the SANFORD GUIDE are solely those of the editors and the publisher. We welcome questions, comments and feedback concerning the SANFORD GUIDE. All of your feedback is reviewed and taken into account in updating the content of the SANFORD GUIDE.

Every effort is made to ensure accuracy of the content of this guide. However, current full prescribing information available in the package insert for each drug should be consulted before prescribing any product. The editors and publisher are not responsible for errors or omissions or for any consequences from application of the information in this book and make no warranty, express or implied, with respect to the currency, accuracy, or completeness of the contents of this publication. Application of this information in a particular situation remains the professional responsibility of the practitioner.

For the most current information, subscribe to webedition.sanfordguide.com or Sanford Guide mobile device applications

Printed in the United States of America
ISBN 978-1-944272-12-8
Spiral Edition (English)

— TABLE OF CONTENTS —

— ABBREVIATIONS —

3TC = lamivudine
ABC = abacavir
ABCC = ampho B cholesteryl complex
ABCD = ampho B colloidal dispersion
ABLC = ampho B lipid complex
ACIP = Advisory Committee on Immunization Practices
AD = after dialysis
ADC = AIDS dementia complex
ADV = adefovir
AFB = acid fast bacilli
AIDS = acquired immune deficiency syndrome
AM-CL = Amoxicillin-clavulanate
AM-SB = Ampicillin-sulbactam
AMK = amikacin
Ampho B = amphotericin B
Anidula = anidulafungin
AP = atovaquone proguanil
ART = antiretroviral therapy
ASA = aspirin
ATA = atazanavir
ATS = American Thoracic Society
AUC = area under the curve
Azithro = azithromycin
BIC = bictegravir
bid = twice per day
BW = body weight
C&S = culture & sensitivity
CAPD = continuous ambulatory peritoneal dialysis
Caspo = caspofungin
CD4 = cluster differentiation antigen 4
CIP = ciprofloxacin
Cipro = Ciprofloxacin
Clinda = clindamycin
CLO = clofazamine
CMV = cytomegalovirus
Cobi = cobicistat
CQ = chloroquine phosphate
CrCl = creatinine clearance
CRRT = continuous renal replacement therapy
CSD = cat-scratch disease
CSF = cerebrospinal fluid
CXR = chest x-ray
DAR = darunavir
DBPCT = double blind placebo-controlled trial
dc = discontinue
ddI = didanosine
div = divided
DLV = delavirdine
DOR = Doravirine
DOT = directly observed therapy
DTG = dolutegravir
Doxy = doxycycline
DS = double strength
EBV = Epstein-Barr virus
EFV = efavirenz
EI = entry inhibitor
EIA = enzyme linked immunosorbent assay
ELV = elvitegravir
EMB = ethambutol
ENF = enfuvirtide

ER = Extended release
ERTA = ertapenem
Erythro = erythromycin
ESR = erythrocyte sedimentation rate
ETR = etravirine
ETV = entecavir
FI = fusion inhibitor
Flu = fluconazole
Flucyt = flucytosine
FOS-APV = fosamprenavir
FQ = fluoroquinolone
FTC = emtricitabine
FUO = fever of unknown origin
G = generic
GC = gonorrhea
Gent = gentamicin
gm = gram
HAD = HIV-associated dementia (HIV-D)
Hemo = hemodialysis
HHV = human herpesvirus
HIV = human immunodeficiency virus
HPV = human papilloma virus
HSV = herpes simplex virus
I = investigational
IA = injectable agent
IDP = inflammatory demyelinating polyneuropathy
IDSA = Infectious Diseases Society of America
IDV = indinavir
IMP = Imipenem
INH = isoniazid
IP = intraperitoneal
IRIS = immune reconstitution inflammatory syndrome
IT = intrathecal
Itra = itraconazole
IDU = intravenous drug user
IVIG = intravenous immune globulin
Keto = ketoconazole
KS = Kaposi's sarcoma
LAB = liposomal ampho B
LCM = lymphocytic choriomeningitis virus
LCR = ligase chain reaction
Levo = levofloxacin
LP/R = lopinavir/ritonavir
LPV = Lopinavir
M. TBc = mycobacterium tuberculosis
MAI = mycobacterium avium-intracellulare complex
mcg (or μg) = microgram
MERO = meropenem
Metro = metronidazole
mg = milligram
Mica = micafungin
Mino = minocycline
mL = milliliter
Moxi = moxifloxacin
MQ = mefloquine
MVC = maraviroc
NAAT = nucleic acid amplification test
NAT = nucleic acid test
NB = name brand
NAI = not U.S. FDA approved indication

— ABBREVIATIONS *(continued)* —

NFR = nelfinavir
NRTI = nucleoside reverse transcriptase inhibitor
NSAIDs = non-steroidal anti-inflammatory drugs
NUS = not available in the U.S.
NVP = nevirapine
Oflox = ofloxacin
OI = opportunistic infection
PJP = pneumocystis jirovecii pneumonia
PCR = polymerase chain reaction
Peg-INF = pegylated interferon
PEP = post-exposure prophylaxis
PI = protease inhibitor
PML = progressive multifocal leuko-encephalopathy
po = orally (by mouth)
Posa = posaconazole
PQ = primaquine
Pt = patient
Pyri = pyrimethamine
PZA = pyrazinamide
qam = in the morning
qpm = in the evening
qid = 4 times per day
qow = every other week
qhs = before sleep
QS = quinine sulfate
R = resistant
RAL = raltegravir
RFB = rifabutin
RFP = rifapentine
RIF = rifampin
RPV = rilpivirine
RT-PCR = reverse transcriptase PCR
RTV = ritonavir
Rx/rx = treatment
Sens = sensitive (susceptible)
SM = streptomycin
SQV = saquinavir
STD = sexually transmitted disease
STII = strand transfer integrase inhibitor
TAF = tenofovir alafenamide fumarate
TBc = tuberculosis
TDF = tenofovir disoproxil fumarate
TDM = therapeutic drug monitoring
tid = 3 times per day
TMP-SMX = trimethoprim sulfamethoxazole
Tobra = tobramycin
TPV = tipranavir
TST = tuberculin skin test
UTI = urinary tract infection
Vanco = vancomycin
VL = viral load
Vori = voriconazole
VZV = varicella zoster virus
WB = western blot
WHO = World Health Organization
XR = extended release
ZDV = zidovudine

— JOURNALS AND OTHER REFERENCES —

AAC: Antimicrobial Agents & Chemotherapy
AIDS Res Hum Retrovir: AIDS Research & Human Retroviruses
AJG: American Journal of Gastroenterology
AJM: American Journal of Medicine
AJRCCM: American Journal of Respiratory & Critical Care Medicine
AJTMH: American Journal of Tropical Medicine & Hygiene
AnIM: Annals of Internal Medicine
AnSurg: Annals of Surgery
ArDerm: Archives of Dermatology
Antivir Ther: Antiviral Therapy
ArIM: Archives of Internal Medicine
BMJ: British Medical Journal
Brit J Derm: British Journal of Dermatology
Can JID: Canadian Journal of Infectious Diseases
CCM: Critical Care Medicine
CDC: U.S. Centers for Disease Control
CID: Clinical Infectious Diseases
CROI: Conference on Retroviruses & Opportunistic Infections
DHHS: U.S. Dept of Health and Human Services
DMID: Diagnostic Microbiology and Infectious Disease
EID: Emerging Infectious Diseases
Gastro: Gastroenterology
Hpt: Hepatology
ICAAC: Interscience Conference on Antimicrobial Agents & Chemotherapy
ICHE: Infection Control and Hospital Epidemiology
IDC No Amer: Infectious Diseases Clinics of North America
JAIDS: Journal of Acquired Immune Deficiency Syndrome
J AIDS & HR: Journal of AIDS and Human Retrovirology
JCI: Journal of Clinical Investigation
J Clin Virol: Journal of Clinical Virology
J Hpt: Journal of Hepatology
J Med Micro: Journal of Medical Microbiology
J Ped: Journal of Pediatrics
JAC: Journal of Antimicrobial Chemotherapy
JAMA: Journal of the American Medical Association
JCM: Journal of Clinical Microbiology
JID: Journal of Infectious Diseases
JTMH: Journal of Tropical Medicine and Hygiene
J Viral Hep: Journal of Viral Hepatitis
Ln: Lancet
LnID: Lancet Infectious Disease
Mayo Clin Proc: Mayo Clinic Proceedings
Med Lett: The Medical Letter
Med Mycol: Medical Mycology
MMWR: Morbidity & Mortality Weekly Report
NEJM: New England Journal of Medicine
Peds: Pediatrics
PIDJ: Pediatric Infectious Disease Journal
PLoS Med: Public Library of Science & Medicine
QJM: Quarterly Journal of Medicine
Scand J Inf Dis: Scandinavian Journal of Infectious Diseases
SMJ: Southern Medical Journal

TABLE 1A: ANTIRETROVIRAL THERAPY REDUCES HIV TRANSMISSION RISK

Antiretroviral therapy (ART) prevents infection. Study compared rates of transmission among discordant heterosexual couples in Africa. HIV+ partners randomized to receive early ARV Rx (CD4 >350 cells/ul) vs. Deferred ARV Rx (CD4 <250 cells/ul). There were 27 transmissions in the deferred group (n=882) vs. 1 in the immediate Rx group (n=880); a 96% reduction in transmission from early ARV Rx. First evidence of high level reduction in transmission from ARV Rx alone in a randomized trial *(NEJM 365 (6): 493-505, 2011)*.

In the PARTNERS study, among MSM couples having over 77,000 acts of condomless anal sex, there were no cases of within-couple HIV transmission. The upper end of the 95% CI was 0.23/100 couple years of follow up (CYFU), meaning, at worst, one infection would occur per 433 years of condomless sex *(JAMA 316:171, 2016; 22nd IAC Amsterdam, 2018. Abst WEAX0104LB)*.

Bottom line: HIV transmission is ~ zero risk when the seropositive partner is on ARV therapy and the viral load is <200 c/mL consistently.

Pre-exposure prophylaxis (PrEP) is an effective means of reducing new infections among those at higher risk of infection, such as MSM.

Helpful supplement from CDC: *http://www.cdc.gov/hiv/pdf/PrEPProviderSupplement2014.pdf*

Antiretroviral therapy (ART) use and risk of HIV-1 transmission

	Follow-up during which HIV-1 infected partner had not initiated ART			Follow-up after HIV-1 infected partner initiated ART			Unadjusted incidence rate ratio (95% CI; p value)*	Adjusted incidence rate ratio (95% CI; p value)*
	Number of HIV-1 transmissions	Length of follow-up (person-years)	HIV-1 incidence per 100 person-years (95% CI)	Number of HIV-1 transmissions	Length of follow-up (person-years)	HIV-1 incidence per 100 person-years (95% CI)		
Overall	102	4558	2.24 (1.84-2.72)	1	273	0.37 (0.09-2.04)	0.17 (0.00-0.94; p=0.04)	0.08 (0.00-0.57; p=0.004)
By CD4 cell count[†]								
<200 cells per µL	8	91	8.79 (4.40-17.58)	0	132	0.00 (0.00-2.80)	0.00 (0.00-0.40; p=0.002)	0.00 (0.00-0.38; p=0.001)
200-349 cells per µL	41	1467	2.79 (2.06-3.80)	1	90	1.11 (0.27-6.19)	0.40 (0.01-2.34; p=0.58)	0.65 (0.02-4.00; p=1.0)[‡]
350-499 cells per µL	24	1408	1.7 (1.14-2.54)	0	30	0.00 (0.00-12.30)	0.00 (0.00-8.16; p=1.0)	0.0 (0.0-15.3; p=1.0)[‡]
≥500 cells per µL	29	1592	1.82 (1.27-2.62)	0	21	0.00 (0.00-17.57)	0.00 (0.00-10.29; p=1.0)	0.0 (0.0-15.0; p=1.0)[‡]

* All analyses adjusted for time since study enrolment and, for the overall analysis, CD4 cell count (as ≥200 cells per µL *vs* <200 cells per µL).

† For follow-up before ART initiation, CD4 cell count was lowest than previous value; for follow-up after ART initiation, CD4 cell count at the time of ART initiation was used.

‡ Adjusted incidence rate ratio for combined CD4 cell count strata of 200 cells per µL or more was 0.55 (95% CI 0.01-3.24; p=0.9).

Reference: *Lancet. 2010 Jun 12;375:2092-8*

TABLE 1B: ASSESSMENT OF HIV INFECTION RISKS & RECOMMENDATIONS FOR HIV TESTING

General

HIV risk assessment is an essential component of primary care for all patients. In talking to patients, avoid medical jargon (e.g., "intercourse"), vague terms ("sexually active"), group designations ("homosexual"), or judgmental terms ("promiscuous"). Learn the language & terminology understood & used by patients. Question responses to the depth necessary to elicit risky behavior & define extent of risk of acquisition & transmission. Eliciting risk is particularly difficult but equally important in resource-limited areas of the world, esp. when working through translators. It is essential that the clinician be knowledgeable about cultural sensitivities, customs & traditions relative to HIV risk behavior.

Risk-reduction counseling works to reduce high-risk behavior. *(J Acquir Immune Defic Syndr 2005 Aug 1; 39: 446-53; Ann Intern Med 2008 Oct 7; 149:497. U.S. Preventive Services Task Force).* HIV counseling & testing is a critical component of health care maintenance *[MMWR September 22, 2006 / 55(RR14); 1-17 http://www.cdc.gov/healthyyouth/sexualbehaviors/index.htm].*

Poverty and HIV: Poverty accounts for a large portion of the observed racial and ethnic disparities in the prevalence of HIV in urban areas of the US. 2.8% of heterosexuals living in 23 urban areas with annual income < $10,000 are infected compared to 0.4% infected who earned more than $50,000/yr. 1.5% of those with income between $10,000 and $19,999 were infected with HIV while 1.2% of those earning $20,000 - $49,999 were infected. The overall (urban and non-urban) rate of infection nationally is 0.1% *(MMWR 60 (31): 1045, 2011).*

I. Specific Behaviors Associated With HIV Transmission

A. **Sexual Behaviors.** The CDC recommends ART post-exposure prophylaxis within 72 hrs after high risk sexual, injection-drug use, or other non-occupational exposure to HIV *(MMWR Recom Rep 54:1, 2005)* (See Table 7B, page 56). Not 100% effective; seroconversion still detected in 1% of 702 exposed individuals *(CID 41:1507, 2005).*

1. **High-Risk Sexual Partner(s)**
   - Life-time risk of acquiring HIV in the US is 1 in 64 adults. Among MSM the risk is 1 in 6; for Black MSM, the risk is 1 in 2. *(CROI 2016, abs 52; https://www.cdc.gov/nchhstp/newsroom/2016/croi-press-release-risk.html).*
   - HIV-infected partners [especially those with ↑ HIV-RNA *(NEJM 342:921, 2000, Sex Trans Dis 29:38, 2002)*].
   - Partners who are at risk but have not been HIV tested or do not disclose their HIV status to their partners *(MMWR 52:81, 2003).*
   - Multiple partners: Unsafe sexual activity appears to be ↑ with *MSM MMWR 53(38); 891-894, 2004; PLoS One 6(8): e17502, 2011.*
   - Presence of mucosal ulceration or other STD in either partner *(JID 178:1060, 1998).*

2. **Sexual Practices**
   a. **High infection risk**
      - Unprotected anal receptive intercourse ("barebacking"): popular among gay males
      - Unprotected vaginal receptive intercourse

   b. **Infection risk documented**
      - Unprotected anal insertive intercourse
      - Unprotected vaginal insertive intercourse (risk may be higher during menses)
      - Unprotected oral receptive intercourse [HIV RNA levels in rectal secretions > serum with & without ART use *(JID 190:156, 2004)]*
      - Unprotected oral insertive intercourse rare *(ArIM 159:303, 1999)*

   c. **Lower infection risk**
      - Any of the above with latex/vinyl condom (vaginal or penile) protection. Male condoms are 80–95% effective in ↓ risk of HIV infection *(AmFAR Issue Brief #1, Jan. 2005);* female condoms 94–97% effective.
      - Cunnilingus, esp. with rubber dam, microwaveable plastic food wrap or other water-impervious barrier
      - Circumcision reduced HIV infection by 60% in a prospective randomized study *(PLoS Med e298, 2005).* Two other studies confirmed 50-60% reduction and were stopped early in 2007 *(Ln 369:643, 657, 2007; PLoS Med 4 (7) e223, July 24, 2007).*

   d. **Safer**
      - Deep kissing
      - Protected sex with HIV test negative partner
      - Per act risk from sex with HIV+ person on combined ART for >6 months is <13:100,000 *(CID 59:115, 2014).*
      - Mutual monogamy
      - Mutual masturbation
      - Masturbation or massage

   e. **Safest**
      - Abstinence

Routes of Exposure and HIV

INFECTION ROUTE	RISK OF INFECTION
Sexual Transmission	
a. Female-to-male transmission	1 in 700 to 1 in 3,000
b. Male-to female transmission	1 in 200 to 1 in 2,000
c. Male-to-male transmission	1 in 10 to 1 in 1,600
d. Fellatio??	0 (CDC) or 6% (SF)
Parenteral transmission	
• Transfusion of infected blood	95 in 100
• Needle sharing	1 in 150
• Needle stick	1 in 300
• Needle stick /AZT PEP	1 in 10,000
Transmission from mother to infant	
a. Without ARV treatment	1 in 4

Royce, Sena, Cates and Cohen, NEJM 336:1072-1078, 1997

TABLE 1B (2)

3. **Conditions That Facilitate HIV Sexual Transmission** *(J AIDS 30:73, 2002; JID 191:333, 2005)*

Male-to-Female Transmission	Relative Risk Reported
(a) Oral contraceptives	2.5–4.5
(b) Gonococcal cervicitis	1.8–4.5
(c) Candida vaginitis	3.3–3.6
(d) Genital ulcers	2.0–4.0
(e) Bacterial vaginosis	1.6 *(AIDS 22:1493, 2008)*
(f) HSV-2	2.5
(g) Vitamin A deficiency	2.6–12.9
(h) CD4 count <200	6.1–17.6
(i) Depomedroxyprogesterone acetate (DMPA) subdermal implant use as contraceptive	2.2 *(JID 178:1053, 1998)*
(j) Sharing of HLA-B alleles in discordant couples	2.23 *(Ln 363:2137, 2004)*

Female-to-Male Transmission	
(a) Lack of circumcision	5.4–8.2 risk/coital act ↓ from 1/80 to 1/200 *(Ln 369:643, 2007; MMWR 53:523, 2004; AIDS 23:395, 2009)*
(b) Genital ulcers	2.6–4.7
(c) Sex during menses	3.4
(d) Herpes simplex type 2 (genital herpes)	6–16.8 *(JID 187:1513, 2003 & 189:1209, 2004)*

↑ Titers of viral DNA in vaginal secretions *(JID 175:57, 1997)*

(a) With low CD4 count	9.6 (<200 vs. >500)
(b) Vitamin A deficiency	2.6
(c) Presence of cervical mucopus	2.1
(d) Acute primary HIV infection	↑↑ *(JID 189:1785, 2004; JID 198:687, 2008)*
(e) With ↑ plasma HIV-RNA	↑ *(JID 177:1100, 1998)*
(f) Cervicitis	↑ *(AIDS 15:105, 2001)*
(g) Peak titer just prior to onset of menses	*(JID 189:2192, 2004)*

↑ Titers of viral DNA in semen (ejaculate) *(JID 172:1469, 1995; J AIDS & HR 18:277, 1998)*

(a) Gonococcal urethritis	3.2
(b) Acute primary HIV infection	↑↑ *(Curr Opin HIV AIDS. 5:277, 2010; PLoS One. 2011; 6(5): e19617)*

Not protective:

(a) Nonoxynol-9 intravaginally *(Ln 360:971, 2002; AIDS 18:2191, 2004)*
(b) IUD use

4. **Programs Aimed at Reducing Sexual Transmission**

    The major route of HIV spread worldwide is via heterosexual vaginal intercourse. Efforts to change sexual behavior by reducing number of sexual partners & using safe sex techniques (condoms) have met with varying degrees of success. These are summarized here:

    a. Voluntary counseling & testing (VCT): Prevention based on identifying infected persons & counseling them to prevent transmission to sexual partner(s) *(Am J Public Health. 96:114, 2006)*.

    b. Counseling & controlling STD in female sex workers: ↓ seroincidence of HIV from 16.3 to 6.5/100 person yrs in 500 subjects in Cote d'Ivoire *(AIDS 15:1421, 2000)* & Benin *(AIDS 16:463, 2002; J AIDS 30:69, 2002)*, & U.S. *(JAMA 292:171, 2004)*.

    c. Condom distribution campaigns: Successfully ↓ HIV prevalence in Thailand from 17% in 1992 to 2% in 1999.

    d. Prevention campaign focused on education about AIDS & promotion of safer sexual behavior *(J AIDS 25:77, 2000; JAMA 292:171, 2004)*.

    e. Delivery of message complex. Examples of communication methods used:
        (1) Radio soap opera (Tanzania, *J Health Comm 5(Suppl.): 81, 2000*)
        (2) Combination of drama or video reached >85% in Uganda *(Health Educ Res 16:411, 2001)*
        (3) Traditional healers or theater in Sierra Leone *(J Assoc Nurs AIDS Care 12:48, 2001)*
        (4) Folk media in rural Ghana *(Am J Publ Health 91:1559, 2001)*
        (5) Religion has been shown to reduce protective behaviors toward AIDS & suggest a critical need to work with clergy to embrace the prevention message *(AIDS 14:2027, 2000)*

    f. Circumcision programs for young men are being implemented widely across Africa and other countries with high incidence rates for HIV infection.

    g. Concern regarding increased transmission among older heterosexual adults (>55 years old). Many older adults are sexually active *(NEJM 357: 762, 2007)*, and with increased use of erectile dysfunction drugs, higher rates of STDs, including HIV, expected.

TABLE 1B (3)

h. **Treatment as Prevention (TasP):** Decreasing HIV RNA (viral load) to sustained undetectable levels is associated with ~ zero transmission events *(see Table 1A).*

i. **PrEP (Pre-exposure Prophylaxis):** Use of ARV medication(s) in uninfected high-risk individuals. iPrEx Study showed a 44% reduction in transmission of HIV over one year among high-risk gay men randomized to receive Tenofovir-FTC daily compared to placebo recipients. For those randomized to receive TDF-FTC and who had detectable drug levels, the relative risk reduction was 92% *(NEJM, 363, 2587, 2010).* Using the overall rate of reduction, over 110 uninfected individuals would need to be treated to prevent one infection per year, at an estimated cost of > $1.8M / infection prevented / year. Cost effectiveness studies show, in selected very high risk populations of MSM (estimated risk of 2% seroconversion per year or higher), PrEP is borderline cost-effective (approx. $60,000/QALY. *Ann Int Med 156: 541, 2012).* Helpful supplement from CDC: *http://www.cdc.gov/hiv/pdf/PrEPProviderSupplement2014.pdf*

B. **Injection (intravenous or "skin popping") Drug Use (IDU) or Smoking Crack Cocaine.** Assess injectable anabolic steroid use! Assess sexual behaviors in all drug users! In one study, infection rates in crack cocaine-smoking women are as high as in men who had sex with men (41% vs. 43%). Risk-reduction intervention can ↓ high risk sexual activity in crack cocaine users *(AIDS Edu Prev 15:15, 2003)* & IDUs *(J AIDS 30:573, 2002).*

Drug Use Practices: (Drug abuse treatment & methadone use programs reduce HIV transmission: *AIDS 13:2151 & 1807, 1999)*

1. **Riskiest**
   - Sharing uncleaned needles, syringes, other paraphernalia (works), especially in "shooting galleries." HIV DNA found on 85% of needles/syringes & 1/3–2/3 cottons, cookers, wash waters from shooting galleries.
   - Practicing "registering," "booting," or "back loading"

2. **Less risky**
   - Sharing cleaned needles, syringes, works. (Household bleach is effective, especially after washing & when contact time is greater than 5 minutes. It is important to rinse with water after bleach use)
   - Drug paraphernalia used repeatedly but by single user

3. **Least risky**
   - Single use needles, syringes, works (needle exchange programs reduce HIV transmission, *[see MMWR 54:673, 2005 for update of US programs]*)
   - Sterile needles, syringes, works (needle/syringe exchange appears effective & has not ↑ drug use)

C. **Blood Product Infusion Recipient**

    Blood Product Risks:

1. **Riskiest**
   - Receipt of multiple units of blood products between **1978** and **1985**
   - Receipt of blood products obtained from donors in countries where screening is unreliable or not done

2. **Less risky**
   - Receipt of heterologous blood products in U.S. after 1985 (risk per unit 1:450,000 to 1:660,000 units or 1:28,000 after an average of 5.4 units). [This is because of a window (about 20 days) between infection & seroconversion (18–27 donations/yr are in this window). With widespread use of nucleic acid testing (NAT) procedures, transmission via blood transfusion in the US has been reduced to <1: 2.2 Million transfusions *(MMWR 59:1335-39, 2010)*]. RhoGAM & hepatitis B vaccine (serum-derived) have never been reported to transmit HIV-1.
   - Receipt of donor-selected blood products in U.S. after 1985 (but no safer than random donors)

3. **Safest**
   - Receipt of autologous blood products
   - Receipt of genetically engineered blood product substitutes

D. **Transplant Recipients:** Report of transmission of HIV from HIV infected donor to recipient via kidney transplant *(MMWR: 60: 297-301, 2011).* HIV-to-HIV (donor to recipient) transplants approved via the HOPE (HIV Organ Policy Equity) Act (Nov 2013). Many transplant centers in the US now actively transplanting organs from HIV+ deceased donors into HIV+ recipients, dramatically increasing the number of transplants in HIV+ patients.

E. **Perinatal Infection:** *See Table 8B*

F. **Occupational Exposure** *(See Table 7B) (CDC Guidelines, CDC Guidelines published: Inf Control Hosp Epi 34:875, 2013; see also http://www.hivguidelines.org/clinical-guidelines/post-exposure-prophylaxis/hiv-prophylaxis-following-occupational-exposure/)*

Relative Risk Determinants

1. **Riskiest** (risk may be decreased use and double gloving)
   - Deep parenteral inoculation (RR 16.8) via hollow needle of blood from source with high-titer viremia; seroconversion or advanced HIV disease (RR 7.8)
   - Parenteral inoculation of materials containing high titer virus in research laboratory setting
   - Failure to use ART after inoculation (RR 0.1 when used)

TABLE 1B (4)

2. **Less risky**
   - Small volume exposure via non-hollow needle
   - Mucosal exposure/non-intact skin exposure. Risk is too low to be quantified in prospective studies; not zero but estimated to be at least a log (90%) lower than needlestick risk. Risk may be increased if large volume or prolonged contact occurs.

3. **Risk not identified**
   - **Cutaneous contact** (intact skin)
   - Exposure to urine, saliva, sweat, tears

G. **Donor Organ or Tissue Transplantation**
   1. Test potential donors for HIV (note window between infection & seroconversion (*C.2 above*))
   2. Assess donors for risk factors
   3. Evaluate risk/benefits
      - Risk following artificial insemination with semen from HIV+ donor is 3.5% (*Ln 351: 728, 1998*). HIV testing recommended but not legally required

III. Recommendations for HIV Testing

A. In Sept 2006, the CDC issued guidelines calling for routine universal testing of all persons between ages 13 & 64 yrs (many experts suggest testing ALL sexually active persons regardless of age). Universal HIV testing and linkage to care is a cornerstone of the US National AIDS Policy (*released July, 2010*).

The CDC suggested that signed consent for HIV testing be eliminated and included in the general consent for medical care. Pre-test counseling was not recommended unless pts were from high-risk groups.
Opt-out testing: Pts should be told verbally that they will be tested as part of their medical care and given the opportunity to opt out of testing. This discussion should include an explanation about HIV infection, how it is transmitted, and implications about a positive test. If pt declines, it should be recorded on his/her chart.

The implications of a positive test [screening & confirmatory (*See Table 2*)] can be profound and have the potential for physical & psychological harm, particularly for women. Counseling & referral services for partner notification should be made available.

While the new recommendations indicate a change in direction, they may conflict with established state laws. Clinicians need to be aware of local regulations regarding consent and counseling.

B. **Post-Test Counseling:**

Rapid HIV antibody tests can provide results within 20 minutes. However, a confirmatory test with HIV RNA is still required. It is critically important to offer counseling to those who test positive. Issues to be discussed should include:

1. Emphasize that HIV infection can now be can be managed successfully as a complicated disease like diabetes
2. Stigma & the fear of disclosure HIV status
3. Need to inform previous/current sexual partner
4. Testing of children & partners at potential risk
5. Strict adherence to safe-sex practices (especially consistent use of condoms)
6. Avoidance of drugs that may cause disinhibition (amphetamines, etc.)

FIGURE 1   Natural History of Untreated HIV

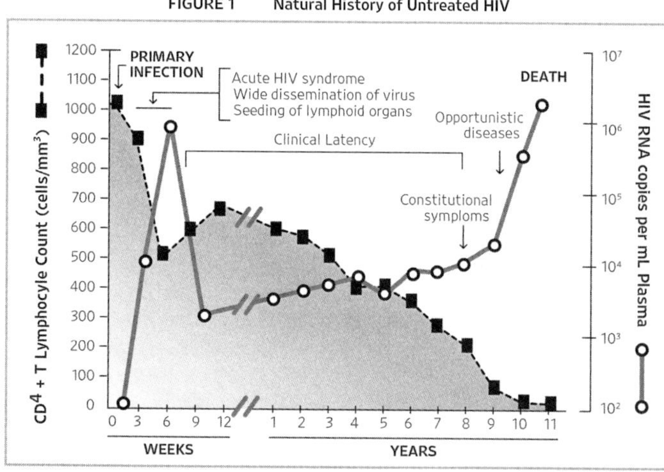

TABLE 2: INITIAL EVALUATION OF HIV-INFECTED ADULT PATIENT

Ref: CID 58: e1, 2014. **Insist on documentation of a positive HIV antibody test: confirm with HIV antigen (part of new testing platforms) or positive plasma viral HIV RNA PCR quantitation**

I. **History, Review of Systems, & Past Medical History**
- A. **General health status**
  1. General well-being; constitutional symptoms
  2. Infectious diseases (TB, leishmaniasis, cocci, histo, etc.): childhood infections, infections in adult life, previous physician visits, hospitalizations (where, when)
  3. Immunization history, e.g., hepatitis A, B, BCG, pneumococcal, HPV
- B. **Drug history**
  1. Medications & dosages
     a. Prescription; non-prescription
     b. Alternative therapies
  2. "Recreational" drug use *(see Table 1B)*
     a. Intravenous/injection; crack cocaine
     b. Other
     c. Identify partners at risk
  3. Smoking & alcohol history
- C. **Sexual history**
  1. Sexual practices *(see Table 1B, page 5)*
  2. Past sexually transmitted diseases
  3. Obstetric/gynecologic history
  4. Contraceptive use
  5. Identify partners at risk
- D. **Past or present HIV-related illness, e.g., candidiasis**
- E. **Risks for opportunistic infections**
  1. Travel history
  2. Geographic location of current/prior residence, e.g., Southwest, Midwest of USA
  3. Occupational history, e.g., poultry worker
  4. Avocational activities
  5. Tuberculosis status: history of BCG vaccination, family members with &/or treated for tuberculosis, contacts (close) with patients with known tuberculosis, results of previous tuberculin tests &/or chest x-rays
  6. Pets, e.g., cats—Bartonella henselae; fish—M. marinum. Cat ownership not associated with toxoplasma antibody seroconversion
- F. **Past history of viral hepatitis, to include type if known, past history of herpes zoster**
- G. **Antiretroviral therapy history**
  1. Prior treatment regimens
  2. CD4 count & viral load responses
  3. Past side effects, toxicities
- H. **Cardiovascular disease risk factors**

II. **Comprehensive Physical Examination**
- A. Document weight & height
- B. Careful funduscopic & oral examination
- C. Complete dermatologic examination
- D. Exam of all lymph node areas: postoccipital, preauricular, cervical, submental, supraclavicular, axillary, epitrochlear, inguinal (measure & record size if palpable, record as negative if not palpable)
- E. Rectal/genital examination, to include pelvic exam with Pap smear in women, inspection for perianal/genital Herpes simplex. Repeat Pap smears every 12 months.
- F. Assess mental status for evidence of dementia.

IV. Laboratory Evaluation
- A. **Baseline**
  1. Complete blood cell count with differential
  2. Electrolytes, blood sugar, BUN, creatinine
  3. Liver enzyme tests: serum bilirubin, aspartate aminotransferase (AST, SGOT), alanine aminotransferase (ALT, SGPT), alkaline phosphatase (indinavir & atazanavir can elevate indirect bilirubin levels)
  4. Creatine kinase
  5. Fasting lipid profile
- B. **HIV staging** (Important for all future care decisions including when to initiate ART & prophylaxis)
  1. CD4 & CD8 T-lymphocyte count every 3-6 mos
  2. Quantitative measurement of plasma HIV RNA *(see page 13)*—"viral load" or plasma "viral burden"
  3. Repeat every 3-6 months.
  4. Genotypic resistance testing
- C. **Additional studies**
  1. **PPD intermediate** (5TU), or blood assay for M. tbc infection (QuantiFERON-TB GOLD),
  2. Chest x-ray (baseline important for future care)
  3. VDRL or RPR (tests for syphilis); repeat annually.
  4. IgG antibody to toxoplasmosis (if + primary prophylaxis indicated when CD4<100
  5. Hepatitis B surface antigen (HBsAg, anti Hep B core antigen), antibody to Hep B surface Ag (anti-HBsAg), antibody to Hep C; IgG antibody to Hepatitis A.
  6. CMV antibody, IgG
  7. G6PD Assay (African-Americans).
  8. Urine nucleic acid amplification test for C. trachomatis & N. gonorrhea.
  9. Type-specific Herpes simplex antibody.
  10. Perhaps serum testosterone level.
  11. Vitamin D serum level.
  12. Screen women for trichomoniasis
  13. HLA-B5701 haplotype test

V. **Initial Health Care Maintenance**
- A. HIV risk reduction education *(see Table 1B)*
- B. Drug rehabilitation/safer needle use/needle exchange
- C. Smoking cessation
- D. Partner notification
- E. Reproductive counseling
- F. Psychosocial support
- G. Immunizations *(see Table 19)*. Immunizations transiently ↑ HIV viral load, clinical significance uncertain
  1. Pneumococcal vaccine (booster every 5 yrs)
  2. Influenza vaccine (annually)
  3. Hepatitis B vaccine, if sexually active or sharing needles; hepatitis A vaccine
- H. Preventive dentistry
- I. If CD4 count <100 cells/mm³, baseline ophthalmologic evaluation
- J. Cervical Pap smear females; anal Pap smear males

VI. **Primary Care of Patients Infected With HIV**
Multiple studies demonstrate that patients cared for by physicians & other health care givers who care for large numbers of HIV-infected persons & who make delivery of this care a major focus of their practice have better outcomes. A team approach with integration of acute & long-term care is the most effective management.

TABLE 3A: LABORATORY DIAGNOSIS OF HIV IN ADULTS AND CHILDREN (AGE >2 YRS)

Overview & references:
- CDC laboratory testing guidance: *www.cdc.gov/hiv/testing/lab/guidelines*
- CDC lab testing algorithm quick reference: *http://www.cdc.gov/hiv/pdf/testingHIValgorithmQuickRef.pdf*
- *See Figure 2* (HIV 1/2 Antigen/Antibody Combined Immunoassay) and *Figure 3* (Temporal Relationships of Circulating HIV RNA)

HIV Immunoassays
- **4 generations of HIV testing** *(CID 2017, 64:53 – complete list).* Examples:
  - 1st generation: Antigen is unpurified viral lysate
    - Example: Western blot
  - 2nd generation: Antigen is synthetic peptide: better sensitivity for HIV-1 grp O & HIV-2
    - Example: HIV enzyme immunoassay & 6 rapid HIV AB tests
  - 3rd generation: Antigen is synthetic peptide which allows detection of HIV IgM & IgG antibodies + HIV-2 antibody
    - Examples: Advia Centaur HIV, GS HIV-1/HIV-2 Plus O EIA (Bio-Rad), Vitros Anti-HIV 1 & 2 (Ortho)
  - 4th generation: Combined synthetic HIV peptides detect both HIV-1 & HIV-2 antibody + monoclonal antibody to detect HIV p24 antigen
    - Examples: Architect HIV Ag/Ab Combo (Abbott), GS HIV Combo Ag/Ab EIA (Bio-Rad), Determine (Alere), Siemens Combo HIV Ag/Ab, BioPlex 2200 HIV Ag/Ab.
- **Sequence of appearance of HIV antigens and antibodies,** *see Figure 3.*
- Approximate **number of days from HIV infection** (exposure) **to positive test result** *(CID 2017, 64:53; JID 2012, 205:521).*

Test Type	Method of Detection	# Days to Positive Test
Enzyme-limited assay		
1st Generation	IgG antibody	35-45
2nd Generation	IgG antibody	25-35
3rd Generation	IgM & IgG antibody	20-30
4th Generation	IgM & IgG antibody; p24 antigen	15-20
Western Blot		35-50
HIV PCR Quantitation		
Sensitivity 50 copies/mL	RNA PCR	10-15
Sensitivity 1-5 copies/mL	RNA PCR	5

- The **ideal HIV test algorithm** would:
  - Identify acute HIV (time window before antibody detection) as early treatment reduces transmission risk
  - Take advantage of increased sensitivity of 3rd& 4th generation assays (positive results days to weeks before Western blot)
  - Increase ability to detect HIV-2 antibody. Note: Most NNRTIs and some PIs are not active against HIV-2.
  - Results available in 30 min
  - Simple point of care testing
  - Rapid detection of acute HIV *(CID 62:501, 2016)*
- **CDC recommended testing algorithm** (2014). *See www.cdc.gov/hiv/testing/lab/guidelines*

FIGURE 2   HIV Testing Algorithm

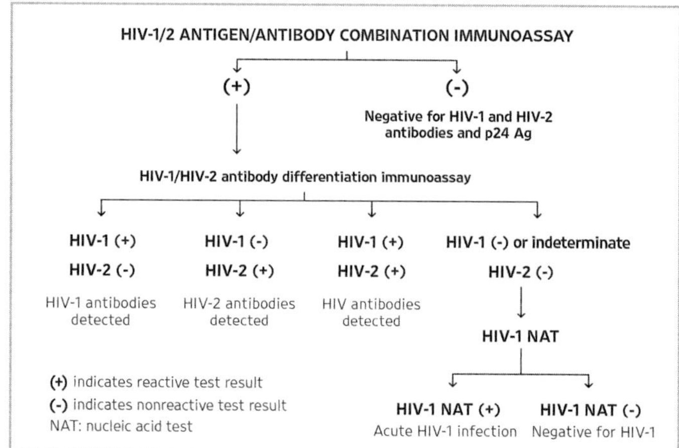

TABLE 3A (2)

- **No further testing needed if blood is negative with an FDA-approved 4th generation assay that detects HIV-1. HIV-2 & HIV-1 p24 antigen.**
  - If positive result with combined assay, next perform FDA-approved immunoassay that differentiates HIV-1 & HIV-2 antibodies, e.g., Multispot HIV-1/HIV-O Rapid (Bio-Rad) or Geenius HIV 1/2 Ab (Bio-Rad).
  - If positive result with combined assay and negative result for presence of HIV-1 and HIV-2 antibody, perform HIV nucleic acid (PCR) test to detect acute HIV.
  - **Note absence of need for Western blot.**
- **False positives reported with 1st, 2nd generation antibody tests:**
  - Multiple myeloma
  - End-stage renal disease
  - Recent immunization
  - Infection with DNA virus
  - Primary biliary cirrhosis
  - Alcoholic hepatitis
  - Malaria
  - Dengue
- **False positive results for initial 4th generation combination test:**
  - Specimen mix-up or mislabeling
  - Infant of HIV+ mother; detect maternal antibody *(See Table 8B, Table 8C)*
  - Autoimmune disease, e.g., SLE
  - If both 4th generation screening and confirmatory tests are positive, false positive rate 0.0004-0.0007%
- **False negative results:**
  - Specimen mix-up or mislabeling
  - Theoretically delayed antibody response and suppressed viral load due to ART for PrEP or PEP
  - Agammaglobulinemia
- **Diagnosis of HIV-2**
  - Only a few hundred patients; most from W. Africa; dual infection with HIV-1 can occur
  - Due to unique pattern of susceptibility to ARVs, accurate diagnosis is important
  - Start with FDA-approved antibody test that differentiates HIV-2 from HIV-1 Geenius HIV 1/2 Supplemental Assay (Bio-Rad); Multispot HIV-1/HIV-2 Rapid Test (Bio Rad)
  - Confirm positive antibody test with RT-PCR. Qualitative PCR from Focus Diagnostics and Quest Laboratories. Quantitative PCR from University of Washington research lab (800-713-5198)
  - Need for expanded access to inexpensive, reliable point of care testing *(CID 62:369, 2016)*
- **Call for expanded access to inexpensive, reliable point of care testing** *(CID 62:369, 2016)*
- **Interpretation of Test Results**
  - **Positive** = positive combination assay & combination confirmatory assay
  - **Negative** = negative screening combination assay or ELISA
  - **Indeterminate** = positive 4th generation combination assay, but indeterminate or negative combination confirmatory assay
    - Could be very recent early only p24 antigen positive
    - HIV-2 infection before detectable HIV-2 antibody
    - Not related to HIV
      - Cross reacting alloantibodies during pregnancy
      - Autoantibodies, e.g., collagen-vascular disease
      - Influenza vaccine
    - Check HIV-1 RNA viral load and maybe HIV-2 viral load
- **Rapid Screening Tests:** Advantages and Comments
  - Results in 20 minutes
  - Can use serum, plasma, whole blood or saliva
    - More false negatives with saliva vs. blood
  - Patient can self-collect specimen to be tested
  - Results are accurate, sensitive & specific but should be considered preliminary
  - May miss acute HIV infection
  - Helpful in resource limited settings
    - Suggest 2 rapid tests
    - If first test is negative, no need for further testing (but note comment above regarding false negatives)
    - If first test is positive, confirm with a second rapid antibody test

TABLE 3B: CD4/CD8 T-LYMPHOCYTE COUNTS IN HIV PATIENTS

I. **Introduction and Definitions**
   - **T-lymphocytes of 2 types:**
     - 1) Helper T-lymphocytes—**CD4 cells;** 2) Cytotoxic T-lymphocytes—**CD8 cells.**
     - Unique surface antigens (cluster determinants) detected by flow cytometry.
     - HIV infects and destroys CD4 cells; CD8 cells cytotoxic for infected CD4 cells.
     - CD4:CD8 ration normally >1. In HIV infection, ratio is <1 due to decrease in CD4 and increase in CD8 cells

II. **CD4**
   - **Normal: 800-1050 cells/mm³**
   - **Clinical Use of CD4 counts in HIV patients:**
     - Marker of the stage of HIV infection
     - Assess risk for opportunistic infections
     - Previously used benchmark for diagnosis of AIDS: CD4 count <200 cells/mm³
     - Previous, but no longer a benchmark for initiating antiretroviral therapy (ART) *(CID 2016, 62:1022)*
     - Benchmark for instituting prophylaxis for opportunistic infections (OIs)
     - Indicator of response to antiretroviral therapy (ART); repeat every 6-12 months
   - **CD4 count by flow cytometry:** perform within 18 hrs of cell collection*. SD = standard deviation

Method	Absolute CD4 Count (cells/mm³)*	Some Prefer % CD4 Cells*	Factors That Can ↑ or ↓ Absolute CD4 Count	Factors That Can Decrease CD4 Counts
Fluoresceniated CD4 antibody added; % CD4 cells counted. Total CD4 count = WBC x % lymphocytes x % CD4 cells	Range 500-1400	≥29% = absolute CD4 count >500	• Variability in test procedure: ↑/↓	• Acute infection other than HIV
	2SD: 500-1400	14-28% = absolute CD4 count of 200-500	• Time of day: ↑/↓	• Acute corticosteroids
			• Season of year: ↑/↓	• Progression of HIV
	≤200 defined as AIDS	<14% = absolute CD4 count <200	• HTLV-1: ↑	• Idiopathic CD4 lymphocytopenia
	Note: cirrhotics have low absolute CD4 counts but normal % CD4 cells *(CID 54:1798 & 1806, 2012).*		• Splenectomy: ↑ • Alpha interferon: ↓	• Alcohol use • Pregnancy

   *** Significant change (2 SD) between 2 tests: 30% change in absolute count or 3% change in % CD4 cells.**
   - There are rapidly evolving less expensive methods designed for use in resource-limited settings *(CID 58:407, 2014).*

   - **Course of CD4 counts (cells/mm³) in untreated HIV-infected gay men:**
     - Mean count prior to seroconversion: 1000/mm³ (mean value)
     - One year after seroconversion: 670/mm³
     - Thereafter, average annual decline: 50/mm³/yr
     - Large variation between patients.
   - **CD4 T-Cell response to antiretroviral therapy (ART)**
     - With viral suppression, expect increase of 100-150 CD4 cells/mm³ after 1 year
     - Then an increase of 20-50 CD4 cells/year over the next 3-5 years
     - If ART is discontinued, expect a drop of 100-150 CD4 cells/mm³ over 3-4 months
   - **Discordant virologic (viral load) & immunologic responses (CD4 count) to ART:**

CD4 Count	Viral Load	Possible Explanations
Increases**	Decreases	Expected response if ART is effective.
Fails to ↑ or decreases	Decreases	CD4 count failure to increase encountered most often in pts with lowest CD4 counts at time of starting ART. One theory: inadequate number of naïve T-cells; associated with increased mortality *(CID 58:1312, 2014).*
Increases	Remains high	Drug-induced defective virus with reduced replicative capacity *(JID 191:1670, 2005; Pediatrics 114:e604, 2004).*
Fails to increase	Increases	Non-adherence to ART or drug-resistant HIV.

   **** *Adequate response = increase of 50-150 cells/mm³/yr.*

   - **Persistent elevation of CD8 counts during ART forecast treatment failure *(JAIDS 57:396, 2011).***

FIGURE 3   Temporal Relationships of Circulating HIV RNA

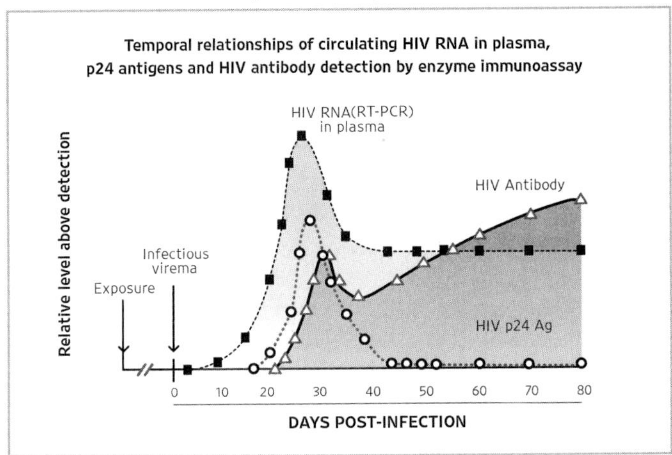

III. **CD8**
- Elevated CD8 counts (cytotoxic T-lymphocytes) linked to ongoing inflammation even when CD4 counts are normalized *(CID 62:392, 2016)*.
- To date, no guideline recommendations on value, or frequency, of checking CD8 counts.

TABLE 3C: ANTIRETROVIRAL DRUG RESISTANCE TESTING IN HIV INFECTION

I. **Genotype and Phenotype Resistance Testing Overview**
Resistance Guidelines: *CID, 2018. https://doi.org/10.1093/cid/ciy463;* Update mutations at:
https://www.iasusa.org/sites/default/files/2017-drug-resistance-mutations-hiv-1-figure.pdf
  - **Genotypic testing is the preferred resistance testing method to guide therapy in treatment-naïve patients, regardless of viral load:**
    o Look for mutations in the reverse transcriptase and protease genes. If considering treatment with integrase inhibitor, look for integrase gene mutations.
    o Acute HIV infection: at time of diagnosis.
    o Chronic HIV:
      - At time of initial evaluation; if ART is delayed, repeat testing prior to initiation of ART.
      - Patients who fail ART if HIV RNA >1000 copies/mL.
      - Pregnancy (HIV+): test prior to initiating ART or when HIV RNA >1000 copies/mL.
  - **Genotypic resistance testing is NOT recommended:**
    o If >4 weeks after stopping ART.
  - **Phenotypic resistance testing is recommended:**
    o In addition to genotypic testing if complex drug resistance mutation patterns are present, especially if genotypic resistance to protease inhibitors.
  - **For resistance testing for integrase inhibitors and CCR5 antagonists,** *see section III.F. of this Table.*

II. **Genotypic vs. phenotypic resistance testing, in general:**

	Genotype Resistance Testing	Phenotype Resistance Testing
Identifies Specific Mutation:	Yes	No
Results Available:	1-2 weeks	2-3 weeks
Cost:	$300-500	$800-1500
Suggested Use:	Either pre-ART or to analyze failure on initial ART regimen	Known/complex resistance mutation patterns

III. **Genotype Resistance Testing**

ARV Drug (by class)	Mechanism of Action	Mechanism of Resistance
Nucleoside Reverse Transcriptase Inhibitors (NRTIs):		
Abacavir Didanosine Emtricitabine/lamivudine Stavudine Zidovudine	Analogues of nucleosides; Active when triphosphorylated; Incorporated into new viral DNA; Prematurely terminate synthesis of HIV DNA	Thymidine analogue (stavudine & zidovudine) mutations promote ATP- & pyrophosphate-mediated **excision** of incorporated chain terminator. Other mutations **impair incorporation** of nucleoside analogues into new HIV DNA.
Nucleotide Reverse Transcriptase Inhibitor (Nucleotide RTI):		
Tenofovir	Same as nucleosides	Specific mutation impairs incorporation into HIV DNA
Non-nucleoside Reverse-transcriptase Inhibitors (NNRTIs):		
Delavirdine Doravirine (DOR) Efavirenz Etravirine (ETR) Nevirapine Rilpivirine (RPV)	Binds to hydrophobic pocket of HIV, type 1 reverse transcriptase IV, type 2 resistant (ETR active vs. HIV-2) Blocks polymerization of viral DNA	Mutations decrease affinity for the enzyme; Single mutation can lead to high-level resistance (except ETR and RPL— usually >1 mutation).
Protease Inhibitors (PIs):		
Atazanavir Darunavir Fosamprenavir Indinavir Lopinavir Nelfinavir Ritonavir Saquinavir Tipranavir	Binds to, and interferes with, the active site of the protease	Mutations reduce affinity of inhibitors for the protease; High level resistance usually requires multiple mutations
Fusion Inhibitor:		
Enfuvirtide	Interferes with glycoprotein 41-dependent membrane fusion	Mutations in a portion of glycoprotein 41
CCR5 Inhibitor:		
Maraviroc	Binds to and interferes with the attachment of HIV to CCR5 co receptor on CD4+ T-lymphocyte	Unmasking of low-level Pre-existent population of dual-mixed trophic virus; Mutations in V3 loop of gp120 not fully characterized yet
Integrase Inhibitor:		
Bictegravir Dolutegravir Elvitegravir Raltegravir	Interferes with integration of HIV into host genome at strand transfer step	Unknown; likely a change in ability of enzyme to function

TABLE 3C (2)

Low Frequency HIV Drug-Resistance Mutations *(JAMA 305:1327, 2011)*

Standard PCR sequencing fails to detect low frequency drug resistance mutations.

With ultra-sensitive methods, low frequency resistance mutations detected in approximately 10% of patients with increased risk of treatment failure (Hazard Ratio 2.3)–especially to NNRTIs (Hazard Ratio 2.6).

What do you need to know to interpret/understand HIV genotype results?

For NRTIs: need to know which drugs are analogs of the same nucleoside. Resistance to one thymidine analog forecasts resistance to all thymidine analogs as exemplified by the thymidine analog mutation (TAM) resistance pattern.

Drug:	Analog Of:
Abacavir	Guanosine
Didanosine	Deoxyadenosine
Emtricitabine	Cytidine
Lamivudine	Cytidine
Stavudine	Thymidine
Tenofovir	Adenosine
Zidovudine	Thymidine

How Are Resistance Mutations Reported?

- Gene (or codon) number is given plus the identified amino acid change.
- Codon number is preceded by letter code indicating the amino acid encoded in wild-type virus.
- M46I = codon (position 46), isoleucine has replaced methionine.
- Amino acid codes:

Code Letter	Amino Acid	Code Letter	Amino Acid
A (Ala)	Alanine	M (Met)	Methionine
C (Cys)	Cytosine	N (Asn)	Asparsgine
D (Asp)	Aspartic acid	P (Pro)	Proline
E (Glu)	Glutamic acid	Q (Glu)	Glutamine
F (Phe)	Phenylalanine	R (Arg)	Arginine
G (Gly)	Glycine	S (Ser)	Serine
H (His)	Histidine	T (Thr)	Threonine
I (Ile)	Isoleucine	V (Val)	Valine
K (Lys)	Lysine	W (Trp)	Tryptophan
L (Leu)	Leucine	Y (Tyr)	Tryosine

Note: Specifics of amino acid substitutions have been deleted in some of the tables below. For full data, *see www.iasusa.org*

Genotype resistance testing comments—detects mutations in resistance-associated target proteins.

- With "ultra-deep" sequencing, **increasing % of treatment-naïve patients harbor resistant virus** *(JAMA 305:1327, 2011)*. Expert advice on interpretation of test results improves virologic response.
- Use PCR to amplify HIV protease & reverse transcriptase genes; some labs do not detect mutations in the envelope gene or integrase gene. Sequence genes, report mutations found, mutations pattern used to predict response to antiretrovirals.
- Genotype resistance patterns change over time. **For current mutation patterns, see http://hivdb.stanford.edu and IAS-USA Resistance:** Resistance Guidelines *(CID, 2018.https://doi.org/10.1093/cid/ciy463).*
  Selected mutations (or combinations) may ↓ replication capacity of HIV clinical isolates.
    - "**Replication capacity**" means number of progeny produced per round of infection per unit of time.
    - "**Fitness**" means relative reproductive success of various subtypes of HIV.
    - "**Virulence**" means ability to destroy CD4 lymphocytes or impair immune system function.

Commercial genotype resistance testing assays:

Testing Assay	Contact	Target Genes	Min Req'd Plasma VL (copies/mL)
GenoSure MG	Monogram Bioscience 800-777-0177	Reverse transcriptase (RT), protease (P) genes	>500
GenoSure PRIme	Monogram Bioscience 800-777-0177	RT, P & Integrase (I) genes	>500
Trugene HIV Genotyping	Siemens Healthcare Malvern, PA	RT & P genes	>1000
Viro Seq. HIV-1 Genotyping	Abbott Molecular 800-553-7042	RT & P genes	>2000
GenoSure Archive	Monogram (part of Lab Corp) 877-436-6243	Uses next generation sequencing to detect cell-associated "archived" resistance mutations in RT, P & I genes	Plasma VL irrelevant. Uses whole blood to probe cell-associated HIV genes

TABLE 3C (3)

IV. **Genotype Resistance Mutations**

There are several data sources for HIV gene mutations associated with antiretroviral drugs. These include the HIV Drug Resistance Database at Stanford University, *http://hivdb.stanford.edu*; the International Antiviral Society-USA, *http://iasusa.org*; and numerous studies and reports in the published literature. The data shown in this table are derived from these sources and adapted for optimal display in the space available. As this data changes, see the *Sanford Guide Web Edition, webedition.sanfordguide.com* and the cited websites for the most current data.

Selected genotype mutations that result in resistance to NRTIs NRTI resistance mutations

Mutation*	Selected By	Mechanism	Effects On Other NRTIs	Comment
M184V	Lamivudine (3TC), Emtricitabine, (FTC), Abacavir	Impairs drug incorporation	Decreased susceptibility to 3TC & FTC. Increased susceptibility to ZDV, d4T & TDF.	Presence delays appearance of TAMs. TAMs + M184V decrease response to ABC.
Thymidine analogue associated mutations - (TAMs), M41L, D67N, K70R, L210W, T215Y/F, K219 Q/E	Zidovudine (ZDV), stavudine (d4T)	Mutation leads to excision of drug from DNA chain terminus	Decreased susceptibility to all NRTIs; the more TAMs, the more resistance.	TAM acquisition slowed by presence of M184V; **TAMs increase susceptibility to NNRTIs.**
Q151 M complex, T69 insertion	(ZDV)/didanosine (ddI)) or (d4T/ddI)	Impairs drug incorporation	**Q151M complex:** resistance to all NRTIs except minimal activity of TDF; **T69 insertion:** resistance to all NRTIs.	
K65R	All NRTIs except zidovudine	Impairs drug incorporation	Variable decreased susceptibility to ABC, ddI, 3TC/FTC & especially TDF	Increases susceptibility to ZDV & d4T
L74V	ABC, ddI		Decreased susceptibility to ABC & ddI	Presented by presence of ZDV in treatment regimen

* *Shows amino acid encoded in wild type virus, number of mutated codons, then code for amino acid encoded in the mutated virus.*

1. **Major mutations that forecast resistance:**
   - **M184V** → Lamivudine, emtricitabine & partial abacavir resistance
   - **K65R** → All NRTIs except zidovudine
   - **Q151M** → All NRTIs except possibly tenofovir

2. Numerous nucleoside (or nucleotide) analog RTI mutations (e.g., M47L, L210W, T215Y) may increase susceptibility to NNRTIs in NNRTI-treatment-naïve patients.

NNRTI resistance mutations. Cross-resistance is the rule with exceptions for etravirine and doravirine (active against most NNRTI mutations except Y188L, and various combination mutations with V106A or E138L).

PI resistance mutations
   - In general, multiple mutations are needed for high-level resistance.
   - Cross-resistance is common, e.g., mutations at codons 82, 84 & 90.
   - Exceptions: no cross-resistance for D30N nelfinavir & I50L atazanavir mutations.

CCR5 Antagonist: Maraviroc

- Activity requires presence of CCR5 co-receptor. HIV enters cells by attachment to CD4 receptor and then binding to either chemokine receptor 5 (CCR5) or chemokine receptor 4 (CXCR4) molecules. **CCR5 inhibitors bind to CCR5 & prevent viral entry.**
- Frequency & rate of emergence of resistance mutations not yet known.
- **Do co-receptor tropism assay prior to use of CCR5 antagonist** (Review: *LnID 11:394, 2011*):
  - Co-receptor assays are phenotypic; tropism assays use lab-generated pseudovirus that expresses gp120 & gp41.
  - **Enhanced Trofile™ assay available from Monogram Biosciences, *www.trofileassay.com*, 800-777-0177:** 1) 2-weeks required, need >1000 HIV RNA copies/mL; 2) detects X4 and dual-mixed (D/M) minor variants with 100% sensitivity down to frequency of 0.3% *(CID 52:925, 2011)*; 3) results reported as: R5 (CCR5-tropic), X4 (CXCR4-tropic), D/M (dual/mixed) or nonphenotypable/non-reportable (NP/NR); 4) **expensive**. Percent positive for CCR5 receptor is only 50-58% in various studies, higher proportion in naïve pts and earlier stage of disease.
  - Trofile DNA Assay: uses viral DNA extracted from cells in a whole blood draw. Can determine tropism from viral DNA in patients with undetectable plasma HIV RNA. Trofile DNA runs on the same clinically validated platform as Trofile.
- Tropism can be detected by **genotypic analysis** with outcomes similar to **phenotype**, especially with 454 (deep) sequencing technologies *(JID 203:146 & 203, 2011)*.

TABLE 3C (4)

Phenotype resistance testing—measures ability of HIV to grow in presence of different concentrations of antiretroviral (ARV) drugs.

- **Indications for testing**: 1) multiple treatment failures; 2) multiple, complex mutation patterns on genotype test, especially resistance to PIs; 3) new drug susceptibility evaluation; 4) patient infected with non-subtype-B HIV.
- **General comments**: 1) methods & interpretation evolving; results reflect: accumulated genetic mutations, variables in assay system, end-point (cutoff) used (see next page); **compared to genotyping, phenotype assays**:
  - Take longer (2-8 weeks), are easier to interpret, provide quantitative degree of resistance, cost more ($800-1500), need minimal viral load of 500-1000 copies/mL of plasma to test.
  - If circulating drug-resistant virus represents <10% of plasma viral load, resistant virus probably non-detectable; **only perform while on ART**.
  - Only detects resistance to single drug, not combinations.
- **Methods comments**:
  - Pertinent genes (reverse transcriptase, protease, integrase, envelope) from pts plasma HIV are inserted into lab strains of HIV. HIV replication in various drug concentrations is measured by expression of a reporter gene and the results are compared to replication of the lab strain of HIV.
  - Results are expressed as **fold increase** (or **fold resistance**). IC_{50} = drug concentration that inhibits viral replication by 50%. IC_{50} patient/virus/IC_{50} reference virus = fold increase (or fold resistance):

FIGURE 4 Phenotypic Resistance Testing

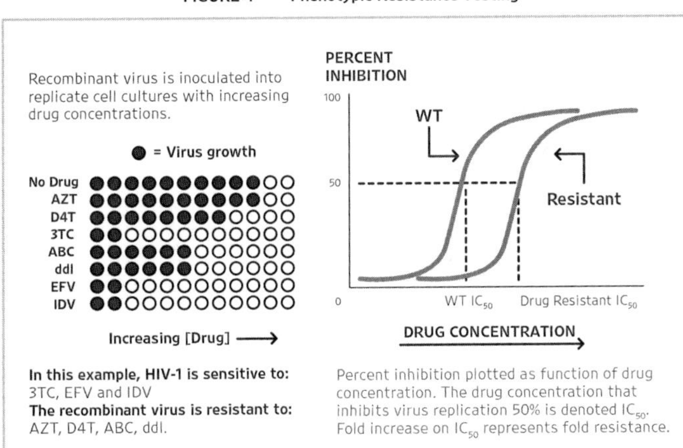

TABLE 3C (5)

- **Defining phenotypic resistance (expert consultation recommended)**

Definition varies depending on cutoff value used. "Cutoff" is dividing point between sensitive and resistant virus. There are 3 levels of cutoff in use: technical/reproducibility; biologic; clinical.

Technical/reproducibility cutoffs (though rarely used):
- Defined as the lowest fold difference for which susceptible isolates are reliably separated from reference HIV strains.
- **Sensitive** means <4-fold increase in IC_{50} patient/virus/IC_{50} reference virus in presence of test drug; **Intermediate** means 4-10-fold increase and **Resistant** means >10-fold increase.

Biologic cutoffs:
- Based on variability of wild-type virus from patients. Determined by study of IC_{50} concentration of test drug vs. HIV from wild-type virus (treatment naïve patients). More relevant but still arbitrary; cutoffs vary depending on assay used.
- Cutoff defined as IC_{50} above mean +250 (99th percentile).

Clinical cutoffs:
- Determined by correlation of in vitro IC_{50} with outcome data (virologic response) in clinical trial. Need large-scale trials. Does not measure influence of multi-drug ART regimens.
- Provides the best definition of phenotypic resistance but is the most difficult to obtain. Some examples of validated clinical cutoffs:

Drug	Clinical Cutoff
Abacavir	4.5-fold increase means resistance (0.5-6.5, some pts may have at least 0.5 log ↓ in viral load) (*Antiviral Ther 9:37, 2004*).
Atazanavir	Decreased virologic response if >3-fold increase in IC_{50} (*AIDS 20:847, 2006*).
Didanosine/ stavudine	1.7-fold increase means reduced susceptibility (*JID 195:392, 2007*).
Etravirine	Clinical cutoff for resistance estimated at >2.9-fold change (*CROI, Abst 687, 2009*).
Indinavir/ ritonavir	>10-fold increase means reduced susceptibility.
Lopinavir	>10-fold increase means reduced susceptibility; >40-fold increase means resistance.
Tenofovir	1.4-fold increase means reduced susceptibility (*JID 189:837, 2004*).
Tipranavir	Decreased virologic response if >3-fold increase in IC_{50} (*AIDS 21:179, 2007*).

Commercial phenotype resistance tests:

Assay	Contact	Target Drugs	Req'd Plasma HIV (copies/mL)
PhenoSense	Monogram Biosciences: www.monogrambio.com 877-777-0177	Reverse transcriptase (RT) & protease inhibitors (PI)	500
PhenoSense Integrase		Strand transfer integrase inhibitors (STII)	500
PhenoSense Entry		Entry inhibitors	500

Combined Phenotype and Genotype Resistance Testing:

Assay	Contact	Target Drugs	Req'd Plasma HIV (copies/mL)
PhenoSense GT	Monogram Biosciences: www.monogrambio.com 877-777-0177	RT, PI	500
PhenoSense GT & Integrase		RT, PI, STII	500

Discordance between genotype and phenotype susceptibility test results:

Genotype Result	Phenotype Result	Cause	Interpretation
Resistant	Susceptible	Mixed HIV subtypes	Resistant
Resistant	Susceptible	Hyper-susceptibility	Resistance mutation, e.g., 184. Mutations in NRTIs increase susceptibility to NNRTIs
Not available	Susceptible or Resistant	New drug	Phenotype result invalid
Susceptible	Resistant	Novel drug	Resistant due to new mechanism of resistance

Failure to respond to ART: percentage of viral population that is drug-resistant; plasma viral load; adherence to ART regimen; low drug potency; poor pharmacokinetics and high plasma protein binding.

TABLE 3D: CO-INFECTION WITH HIV AND HUMAN T-CELL LYMPHOTROPIC VIRUS (HTLV)

- HIV and Human T-cell Lymphotropic Virus (HTLV) co-infection *(ID Cases 2016, 4:53)*
    - Share the same routes of transmission, i.e., blood and sex
    - Share tropism for CD4 T-lymphocytes
    - Frequency of co-infection not documented

- HTLV-1
    - 15 million people infected worldwide
    - 2-5%, after 20 or more years, may develop either:
        - Adult T-cell lymphoma or
        - HTLV-1 associated myelopathy, which is also known as tropical spastic paraparesis

- Why do HIV providers need to know about HIV/HTLV co-infection?
    - HTLV-1 promotes clonal expansion of CD4 lymphocytes
    - Result is artificially elevated CD4 count in patients with HIV/HTLV co-infection *(Frontier Bioscience 2009, 14:3935)*
    - HIV/HTLV-1 co-infection speeds clinical progression of HIV; in contrast, HIV/HTLV-2 co-infection slows progression of HIV
    - Co-infection increases risk of opportunistic infection
    - If co-infection not recognized, there is risk of attributing lymphoma to HIV or myelopathy to drug-induced injury or cytomegalovirus (CMV)

- Diagnosis of HTLV
    - Antibody tests or PCR
    - Blood banks screen blood donors for HTLV

TABLE 4A: 1993 REVISED CDC HIV CLASSIFICATION SYSTEM & EXPANDED AIDS SURVEILLANCE DEFINITION FOR ADOLESCENTS & ADULTS

The revised system emphasizes the importance of CD4 lymphocyte testing in clinical management of HIV infected persons. The system is based on 3 ranges of CD4 counts & 3 clinical categories giving a matrix of 9 exclusive categories. This system is less valuable in clinical decision-making today because of availability of measures of viral RNA.

CRITERIA FOR HIV INFECTION: Persons 13 years or older with a positive combination HIV antibody - antigen test with a confirmatory HIV RNA test.

CLASSIFICATION SYSTEM				Clinical Category A	Clinical Category B	Clinical Category C
	Clinical Category			Asymptomatic HIV infection Persistent generalized lymphadenopathy (PGL)[1] Acute (primary) HIV illness	Symptomatic, not A or C conditions. Examples include but not limited to:	Candidiasis: esophageal, trachea, bronchi Coccidioidomycosis, extrapulmonary Cryptococcosis, extrapulmonary Cervical cancer, invasive
CD4 Cell[§] Category	A	B	C			
(1) ≥500/mm³	A1	B1	C1		• Bacillary angiomatosis	Cryptosporidiosis, chronic intestinal (>1 month)
(2) 200–499/mm³	A2	B2	C2		• Candidiasis, vulvovaginal: persistent >1 month, poorly responsive to rx	CMV retinitis, or CMV in other than liver, spleen, nodes HIV encephalopathy
(3) <200/mm³	A3	B3	C3		• Candidiasis, oropharyngeal • Cervical dysplasia, severe or carcinoma in situ • Constitutional sx, e.g., fever (38.5°) or diarrhea >1 month	Herpes simplex with mucocutaneous ulcer >1 month, bronchitis, pneumonia Histoplasmosis: disseminated, extrapulmonary Isosporiasis, chronic, >1 month Kaposi's sarcoma Lymphoma: Burkitt's, immunoblastic, primary in brain M. avium or M. kansasii, extrapulmonary

See table for clinical definitions. Shaded area indicates expansion of AIDS surveillance definition. Cats. A3, B3 & C require reporting as AIDS.

§ There is a diurnal variation in CD4 counts averaging 60/mm³ higher in the afternoon in HIV+ individuals. Blood for sequential CD4 counts should be drawn at about the same time of day each time (*J AIDS 3:144, 1990*). The equivalence between CD4 counts & CD4 % of total lymphocytes is ≥500 = ≥29%, 200–499 = 14–28%, <200 = <14%.

The above must be attributed to HIV infection or have a clinical course or management complicated by HIV.

M. tuberculosis, pulmonary or extrapulmonary
Pneumocystis jirovecii pneumonia
Pneumonia, recurrent (≥2 episodes in 1 year)
Progressive multifocal leukoencephalopathy
Salmonella bacteremia, recurrent
Toxoplasmosis, cerebral
Wasting syndrome due to HIV

These are the 1987 CDC case definitions (*MMWR 36:15, 1987*). The 1993 *CDC Expanded Surveillance Case Definition* includes all conditions contained in the 1987 definition (*above*) plus persons with documented HIV infection & any of the following: (1) CD4 T-lymphocyte count <200/mm³ (or CD4 <14%), (2) pulmonary tuberculosis, (3) recurrent pneumonia (≥2 episodes within 1 year) or (4) invasive cervical carcinoma. There are no CDC definitions utilizing viral load available to date.

[1] Nodes in 2 or more extrainguinal sites, at least 1 cm in diameter for ≥3 mos.

TABLE 4B: CORRELATION OF COMPLICATIONS WITH CD4 CELL COUNTS/WHO CLINICAL STAGING SYSTEM

CD4 Cell Count*	CORRELATION OF COMPLICATIONS WITH CD4 CELL COUNTS		WHO CLINICAL STAGING SYSTEM		
	Infectious Complications	Noninfectious Complications			
>500/mm³	Acute retroviral syndrome Candidal vaginitis	Persistent generalized lymphadenopathy (PGL) Guillain-Barré syndrome Myopathy Aseptic meningitis	WHO Clinical Stage 1	No clinical symptoms May have persistent generalized lymphadenopathy (PGL) Performance scale 1 * Normal activity	
200-500/mm³	Pneumococcal and other bacterial pneumonia Pulmonary tuberculosis Herpes zoster Oropharyngeal candidiasis (thrush) Cryptosporidiosis, self-limited Kaposi's sarcoma Oral hairy leukoplakia HPV: Cervical intraepithelial neoplasia/Cancer EBV: B-cell lymphoma: HHV-8: Kaposi's sarcoma/Castleman's Disease	Anemia Mononeuritis multiplex Idiopathic thrombocytopenic purpura Hodgkin's lymphoma Lymphocytic interstitial pneumonitis	WHO Clinical Stage 2	Weight loss <10% Minor skin rash Herpes zoster Recurrent oral ulcerations Angular cheilitis Fungal nail infections Recurrent upper respiratory infection Performance scale 2 * Symptomatic but normal activity	

<200/mm³	Pneumocystis jiroveii pneumonia
	Disseminated histoplasmosis and
	  coccidioidomycosis
	Miliary/extrapulmorary TB
	Progressive multifocal leukoencephalopathy
	  (PML)
		Peripheral neuropathy
		HIV-associated dementia
		Cardiomyopathy
		Vacuolar myelopathy
		Progressive polyradiculopathy
		Non-Hodgkin's lymphoma
			WHO Clinical Stage 3	Weight loss >10%
				Chronic diarrhea >1 month
				Recurrent fevers >1 month
				Oral thrush
				Oral hairy leukoplakia
				Severe presumed bacterial infections
				Acute necrotizing ulcerative stomatitis, gingivitis, or periodontitis
				Pulmonary tuberculosis
				Unexplained anemia (<8 gm/dl), neutropenia (<500 cells/ul),
				and/or Chronic thrombocytopenia (<50,000/ul)
				Performance scale 3
				  * Bedridden <50% of the day during the last month	

<100/mm³	Disseminated herpes simplex
	Toxoplasmosis
	Cryptococcosis
	Cryptosporidiosis, chronic
	Microsporidiosis
	Candidal esophagitis
		Wasting	WHO Clinical Stage 4	Cryptococcal meningitis
				Toxoplasmosis of the brain
				Pneumocystis pneumonia
				Chronic Herpes simplex infection
				Esophageal Candidiasis
				Extrapulmonary Tuberculosis
				Disseminated non-TB
				  mycobacterial disease
				Lymphoma
				Progressive Multifocal
				  Leukoencephalopathy
				Isosporiasis
					Cytomegalovirus disease
					Disseminated endemic mycoses
					(Histoplasmosis, Penicilliosis,
					Coccidiomycosis)
					Salmonellosis
					Invasive cervical carcinoma
					Visceral leishmaniasis
					Kaposi sarcoma
					Dementia
					Performance scale 4
					  * Bedridden >50% of the day
					  during the last month

<50/mm³	Disseminated cytomegalovirus (CMV) Disseminated Mycobacterium avium complex	Central nervous system (CNS) lymphoma	NOTE that patients may move from a later stage to an earlier stage if the presenting opportunistic infection is treated.		

* Most complications occur with increasing frequency at lower CD4 cell counts.

TABLE 5A: ADULT ANTIRETROVIRAL THERAPY (ART): WHEN AND WHAT TO START

Overview

- Antiretroviral therapy (ART) in **treatment-naïve adults** *(aidsinfo.nih.gov/guidelines/html/1/adult-and-adolescent-treatment-guidelines/0)*
- Guidelines: www.aidsinfo.nih.gov; iasusa.org; *JAMA 2018; 320:379*

When to Start ART

- **All patients with HIV regardless of CD4 count** *(NEJM 373:795, 2015; NEJM 373:808, 2015)*
- Only exceptions are:
  - Patient is not ready to start (for personal reasons or lack of commitment to take medications)
  - Patient is an "Elite Controller", i.e., HIV RNA undetectable for extended period without ART. Controversy exists about treating such patients, though many experts suggest ART owing to inflammation resulting from ongoing de novo HIV replication.
  - Many clinics are adopting a 'treat now' policy whereby the ARV regimen is started on the first encounter with the clinic. In such instances, resistance tests are obtained and the regimen(s) adjusted as indicated once the resistance test data return.

What Regimen to Start

- Design a regimen consisting of:

Dual nucleoside / nucleotide reverse transcriptase inhibitor **(NRTI component) PLUS** either a	• Non-nucleoside reverse transcriptase inhibitor **(NNRTI) OR** • Protease Inhibitor **(PI) OR** • Integrase strand-transfer inhibitor **(INSTI)**
Note: Prefer combination that includes Tenofovir-AF over original Tenofovir-DF	

NRTI: e.g., Tenofovir (TAF or TDF), Abacavir (ABC), Emtricitabine (FTC), or Lamivudine (3TC)
NNRTI: e.g., Efavirenz (EFV), Rilpivirine (RPV), Doravirine (DOR) or Etravirine (ETV)
PI: e.g., Darunavir (DRV) or Atazanavir (ATV) [both boosted with either Ritonavir (/r) or Cobicistat (Cobi)]
INSTI: e.g., Bictegravir (BIC), Dolutegravir (DTG), Elvitegravir (ETG), or Raltegravir (RAL)

- Selection of components is influenced by many factors, including:
  - HLA-B5701 testing required prior to using Abacavir (ABC)
  - Results of viral resistance testing
  - **Pregnancy:** EFV is now permitted for use in pregnancy; DTG and TAF not recommended yet for pregnant women owing to higher drug levels in fetus and reports of higher than expected neural tube defects in newborn with dolutegravir *(DOI: 10.1056/NEJMc1807653, 2018)*
  - Potential drug interactions or adverse drug effects; special focus on tolerability (even low grade side effects can profoundly affect adherence)
  - Co-morbidities (e.g., lipid effects of PIs, liver or renal disease, cardiovascular disease risk, chemical dependency, psychiatric disease)
  - Convenience of dosing. Co-formulations increase convenience, but sometimes prescribing the two constituents individually is preferred, as when dose-adjustments are needed for renal disease
  - HLA-B5701 testing required prior to using ABC

TABLE 5A (2)

	Frequency & Formulation	Drug/Dose	Components	Comments
Recommended	Once daily, single tablet	**Biktarvy** 1 tablet once daily	Bictegravir (BIC) + FTC + TAF	
		Triumeq 1 tablet once daily	ABC + 3TC + DTV	Only if HLA-B* 5701 neg (See Warnings)
	Once daily, separate tablets	**Descovy** + **Dolutegravir** 1 tablet each once daily	(FTC + TAF) + DTV	
Alternative	Once daily, single tablet combinations	**Atripla** 1 tablet once daily qhs	TDF + FTC + EFV	
		Complera/Eviplera 1 tablet once daily with food	FTC + TDF + RPV	Avoid when VL >100,000 cells/mL
		Delstrigo 1 tablet once daily	Doravirine (DOR) + 3TC + TDF	
		Genvoya 1 tablet once daily	EVG + Cobi + FTC + TAF	
		Stribild 1 tablet once daily	EVG + Cobi + FTC + TDF	
		Symtuza 1 tablet once daily	DRV + Cobi + FTC + TAF	
Alternative	NNRTI-based, multi-tablet	**Efavirenz** (EFV) 1 tablet once daily + (**Descovy** or **Truvada** or **Epzicom/Kivexa**) 1 tablet once daily	Descovy: FTC + TAF; Truvada: FTC + TDF; Epzicom/Kivexa: ABC + 3TC; Evotaz: ATV + Cobi/r (ritonavir boosted); Prezcobix: DRV + Cobi	Epzicom/Kivexa: take qhs. Avoid when VL >100,000 cells/mL. Use only if HLA-B* 5701 neg; see Warnings.
		Rilpivirine (RPV) 1 tablet once daily + (**Descovy** or **Truvada** or **Epzicom/Kivexa**) 1 tablet once daily		
		Doravirine 1 tablet once daily + (**Descovy** or **Truvada** or **Epzicom/Kivexa**) 1 tablet once daily		
	PI-based (boosted), multi-tablet	**Evotaz** 1 tablet once daily + (**Descovy** or **Truvada** or **Epzicom/Kivexa**) 1 tablet once daily		
		Atazanavir/r 1 tablet once daily + (**Descovy** or **Truvada** or **Epzicom/Kivexa**) 1 tablet once daily		
		Prezcobix 1 tablet once daily + (**Descovy** or **Truvada** or **Epzicom/Kivexa**) 1 tablet once daily		
		Darunavir/r 1 tablet once daily + (**Descovy** or **Truvada** or **Epzicom/Kivexa**) 1 tablet once daily		
	INSTI-based, multi-tablet	**Descovy** 1 tablet once daily + **Raltegravir** (RAL) 600 mg 2 tablets once daily		
		Truvada 1 tablet once daily + **RAL** 600 mg 2 tablets once daily		
		Truvada + **Dolutegravir** (DTG) 1 tablet each once daily		
		Epzicom/Kivexa + **DTG** 1 tablet each once daily		
	Dual therapy	**DTG** + (**3TC** or **FTC**) 1 tablet each once daily		
		DTG + **RPV** 1 tablet each once daily		

TABLE 5A (3)

Legend, Warnings and Notes Regarding Regimens

- Legend
  - o **NNRTI** = Non-nucleoside reverse transcriptase inhibitor
  - o **PI** = Protease inhibitor
  - o **INSTI** = Integrase strand-transfer inhibitor
- Warnings
  - o **Epzicom/Kivexa** (ABC/3TC) containing regimens: **Use only in patients who are HLA-B5701 negative.**
  - o Use ABC with caution in those with HIV RNA <100,000 c/mL at baseline (this does not apply when DTG i-s the anchor drug of the regimen).
- Notes
  - o Co-formulations increase convenience, but sometimes prescribing the components individually is preferred, e.g., when dose adjustments are needed for renal impairment.
  - o Rilpivirine (RPV) with 2 nucleosides should be used only in patients with a baseline HIV RNA level < 100,000 c/mL. However, RPV can be used in combination with DTG in those with > 100,000 c/mL.
  - o Higher rates of renal dysfunction occur when TDF is combined with boosted PIs; TAF is the preferred drug in this setting. Conversely, TDF does not have nearly as much renal toxicity when paired with non-boosted PI drugs.
  - o RAL reformulated as 600 mg tablet. Preferred dose is 2 tablets (1200 mg) once daily.

Other drugs that may be used in selected populations (typically not used as initial therapy)

- FDC DTG/RPV can be used to simplify 3-drug regimen to 2-drugs when initial regimen successful (< 50c/ml for > 6 months), no baseline pre-Rx resistance mutations, and no virologic failure.
- ETV and RPV are options for some patients who have NNRTI resistance mutations, e.g., K103N, at baseline. Expert consultation is recommended.
- Boosted PIs can be administered once or twice daily.
- Both Ritonavir and Cobicistat are available as PI-boosting agents.
- Non-boosted PIs are no longer recommended.

Pregnancy Considerations *(See also, Table 8A)*

- Timing of initiation of therapy and drug choice must be individualized.
- Viral resistance testing should be performed.
- Long-term effects of agents are unknown.
- Efavirenz is a permitted alternative in pregnancy.
- DTG, BIC, Cobi, and TAF based regimens should NOT be used in pregnancy until further data are available.
- If recommended drugs are not available, remember that certain drugs are contraindicated, e.g., Didanosine plus Stavudine.

Other Special Populations

- Primary (acute) HIV (INSTI preferred).
- Hepatitis B/C co-infection (See Table 14E & 14F) (Should always use a TDF or TAF-based regimen).
- Opportunistic infection (Treat early in course of Rx of OI; use DTG or BIC if possible owing to fewer drug-drug interactions).

TABLE 5B: FAILURE OF ANTIRETROVIRAL THERAPY (ART)

Definition	**Therapeutic Failure:** Progression of clinical disease, virologic failure, or development of toxicity. **Virologic Failure:** Persistent (confirmed) HIV RNA (VL) >200 copies/mL 6 months after starting ART.
General approach to management	• Evaluate Adherence, tolerability, drug-drug interactions, and psychosocial issues • If tolerability/toxicity issue, identify the most likely offending agent and substitute another agent that is likely to have antiviral activity and not have overlapping toxicities or drug-drug interactions with remaining agents • Obtain/review antiretroviral drug history (including tolerability to prior agents used) • Re-check HIV RNA in 6 - 8 weeks; if still >200 copies/mL check resistance assay and change Rx (Note: Resistance assays may yield results even if HIV RNA <1000 copies/mL). Can use DNA genotype resistance assay when VL is < 200 c/ml (archived virus)
Management of virologic failure	**For documented HIV RNA >200 but less than 500 copies/mL** • Carefully review adherence / barriers to medication access • Improve PK if possible (boosting, drug-drug interactions) **For confirmed HIV RNA >500 – 1000 copies/mL** • Change regimen as soon as possible (prevent emergence of further resistance) • Obtain resistance test while on the failing regimen (genotype preferable in general; phenotype most helpful for complex treatment history) **If no resistance mutations noted:** • Reassess adherence / drug-drug interactions/absorption issues • Check plasma drug levels (optional) **If resistance mutations observed:** • Change regimen based on findings (see below) and antiretroviral history • Expert discussion advised if unfamiliar with mutations or findings
Use of resistance test mutations	**General Rules** • Use at least 2 fully active agents; especially DTG, BIC, or boosted DRV as 'anchor' drugs. Can be active drugs from prior regimen(s). However beware of archived resistant virus • Unclear how to 'count' partially active drugs. 3TC and FTC usually have residual partial activity and are often included in the new regimen (though not considered 'fully active' agents when M184 mutation is present) • Avoid 'double boosted' PIs (i.e., two PI agents + ritonavir) **If many options available** • Choose agent(s) most likely to be (1) better tolerated (2) more convenient/simpler (3) least drug-drug interaction **If only limited active drugs identified** • If 2 fully active drugs not identified / available, generally should defer changing therapy until newer agents are available. If clinical deterioration impending, switch to best alternative. Clinical judgment necessary **Treatment interruption should be avoided** • Even partially active regimens (~ 0.5 - 1.0 log reduction) are better than no therapy
Use of therapeutic drug monitoring (tdm)	**Rationale:** Drug levels can be highly variable (esp. PIs) **Which Drugs:** PIs, NNRTIs, maraviroc **Which Patients:** • Drug-drug interactions suspected • HIV agents with partial activity (desire to get optimal drug levels) • Pregnancy (selected cases) • Concentration-dependent toxicities • Unexplained absence of virologic response (e.g., wild type virus in pt with virologic failure) **Limitations** • Few prospective studies demonstrating benefit • Incomplete knowledge of therapeutic ranges • Considerable inter-individual variation of levels • Little / no role in NRTI medications owing to role of intracellular concentrations • Only a few qualified labs **Target Trough Concentrations for Selected Medications** (levels should be obtained at steady-state) • Atazanavir (150 ng/mL) • Fosamprenavir (400 ng/mL) • Indinavir (100 ng/mL) • Lopinavir (1000 ng/mL) • Nelfinavir (800 ng/mL) • Saquinavir (100-250 ng/mL) • Tipranivir (20,500 ng/mL) • Efavirenz (1000 ng/mL) • Nevirapine (3,000 ng/mL) • Maraviroc (>50 ng/mL)

TABLE 6A: SELECTED CHARACTERISTICS OF ANTIRETROVIRAL (ARV) DRUGS

Selected Characteristics of Antiretroviral Drugs								
Generic/ Trade Name	Pharmaceutical Prep.	Usual Adult Dosage & Food Effect	% Absorbed, po	Serum $T\frac{1}{2}$, hrs	Intracellular $T\frac{1}{2}$, hrs	CPE*	Elimination	Major Adverse Events/Comments (See Table 6B)

1. **Selected Characteristics of Nucleoside or Nucleotide Reverse Transcriptase Inhibitors (NRTIs)**

All NRTIs have Black Box warning: Risk of lactic acidosis/hepatic steatosis. Also, labels note risk of fat redistribution/accumulation with ARV therapy. For combinations, *see warnings for component agents.*

Generic/ Trade Name	Pharmaceutical Prep.	Usual Adult Dosage & Food Effect	% Absorbed, po	Serum $T\frac{1}{2}$, hrs	Intracellular $T\frac{1}{2}$, hrs	CPE*	Elimination	Major Adverse Events/Comments
Abacavir (ABC; Ziagen)	300 mg tabs or 20 mg/mL oral solution	300 mg po bid or 600 mg po q24h. Food OK	83	1.5	20	3	Liver metab., renal excretion of metabolites, 82%	Hypersensitivity reaction: fever, rash, N/V, malaise, diarrhea, abdominal pain, respiratory symptoms (Severe reactions may be ↑ with 600 mg dose). **Do not rechallenge!** Report to 800-270-0425 **Test HLA-B*5701 before use. *See Comment Table 6B.*** Studies raise concerns re ABC/3TC regimens in pts with VL ≥ 100,000 *(www.niaid.nih.gov/news/newsreleases/2008/ actg5202bulletin.htm).* Controversy re increased CV events with use of ABC. Large meta-analysis shows no increased risk *(JAIDS 61, 441, 2012)*
Abacavir (ABC)/ lamivudine (3TC)/ zidovudine (AZT) (Trizivir)	Film-coated tabs: ABC 300 mg + 3TC 150 mg + ZDV 300 mg	1 tab po bid (not recommended for wt <40 kg or CrCl <50 mL/min or impaired hepatic function)			*(See individual components)*			*(See Comments for individual components)* Note: **Black Box warnings** for ABC hypersensitivity reaction & others. Should only be used for regimens intended to include these 3 agents. Black Box warning— limited data for VL >100,000 copies/mL. **Not recommended as initial therapy because of inferior virologic efficacy.**
Didanosine (ddl; Videx or Videx EC)	125, 200, 250, 400 enteric-coated caps; powder for oral solution (final conc 10 mg/mL)	≥60 kg Usually 400 mg enteric-coated po q24h 0.5 hr before or 2 hrs after meal. Do not crush. <60 kg: 250 mg EC po q24h. Food ↓ levels. *See Comment*	30–40	1.6	25–40	2	Renal excretion, 50%	**Pancreatitis,** peripheral neuropathy, lactic acidosis & hepatic steatosis (rare but life-threatening, esp. combined with stavudine in pregnancy). Retinal, optic nerve changes. **The combination ddl + TDF is generally avoided, but if used,** reduce dose of ddl-EC from 400 mg to 250 mg EC q24h (or from 250 mg EC to 200 mg EC for adults <60 kg). **Monitor for ↑ toxicity & possible ↓ in efficacy of this combination; may result in ↓ CD4.** Possibly associated with noncirrhotic portal hypertension.

* **CPE (CNS Penetration Effectiveness) value:** 1= Low Penetration; 2 - 3 = Intermediate Penetration; 4 = Highest Penetration into CNS *(Arch Neurol 2008;65(1):65-70)*

TABLE 6A (2)

								Selected Characteristics of Antiretroviral Drugs
Generic/ Trade Name	Pharmaceutical Prep.	Usual Adult Dosage & Food Effect	% Absorbed, po	Serum T½, hrs	Intracellular T½, hrs	CPE*	Elimination	Major Adverse Events/Comments (See Table 6B)
1. Selected Characteristics of Nucleoside or Nucleotide Reverse Transcriptase Inhibitors (NRTIs) (continued)								
Emtricitabine (FTC, Emtriva)	200 mg caps; 10 mg per mL oral solution. **Note:** caps and sol'n are not interchangeable.	200 mg po q24h. Food OK	93 (caps), 75 (oral sol'n)	Approx. 10	39	3	Renal excretion 86%, minor bio-transforma-tion, 14% excretion in feces	Well tolerated; headache, nausea, vomiting & diarrhea occasionally, skin rash rarely. Skin hyperpigmentation. Differs only slightly in structure from lamivudine (5-fluoro substitution). **Exacerbation of Hep B reported in pts after stopping FTC.** Monitor at least several months after stopping FTC in Hep B pts; some may need anti-HBV therapy.
Emtricitabine/ tenofovir alafenamide fumarate (TAF) (Descovy)	FTC 200 mg + TAF 25 mg	1 tab po q24h ± food			(See individual components)			Before starting: test for Hepatitis B (HBV) infection and obtain estimated CrCl **(not recommended for CrCl <30 mL/min)**, urine glucose and urine protein.
Emtricitabine/ tenofovir disoproxil fumarate (TDF) (Truvada)	1 tab (FTC 200 mg/ TDF 300 mg) po q24h	Tabs (mg FTC/TDF): 100/150, 133/200, 167/250, 200/300 for CrCl ≥50 mL/min. Food OK			(See individual components)			See Comments for individual agents **Black Box warning—Exacerbation of Hep B after stopping FTC;** but preferred therapy for those with Hep B.
Emtricitabine/ tenofovir/efavirenz (Atripla)	Film-coated tabs: FTC 200 mg + TDF 300 mg + efavirenz 600 mg	1 tab po q24h on an empty stomach, preferably at bedtime. Do not use if CrCl <50 mL/min			(See individual components)			Not recommended for pts <18 yrs. (See warnings for individual components). **Exacerbation of Hep B** reported in pts discontinuing component drugs; some may need anti-HBV therapy (preferred anti-Hep B therapy). **Pregnancy category D-** may cause fetal harm. Avoid in pregnancy or in women who may become pregnant.
Emtricitabine/ tenofovir/rilpivirine (Complera/Eviplera)	Film-coated tabs: FTC 200 mg +TDF 300 mg + RPV 25 mg	1 tab po q24h with food			(See individual components)			See individual components. Preferred use in pts with HIV RNA level <100,000 c/mL. Should not be used with PPI agents.
Lamivudine (3TC; Epivir)	150, 300 mg tabs; 10 mg/mL oral solution	150 mg po bid or 300 mg po q24h. Food OK	86	5–7	18	2	Renal excretion, minimal metabolism	**Use HIV dose, not Hep B dose.** Usually well-tolerated. **Risk of exacerbation of Hep B after stopping 3TC.** Monitor at least several months after stopping 3TC in Hep B pts; some may need anti-HBV therapy.

* **CPE (CNS Penetration Effectiveness) value:** 1= Low Penetration; 2 - 3 = Intermediate Penetration; 4 = Highest Penetration into CNS (Arch Neurol. 2008;65(1):65-70).

TABLE 6A (3)

	Selected Characteristics of Antiretroviral Drugs							
Generic/ Trade Name	Pharmaceutical Prep.	Usual Adult Dosage & Food Effect	% Absorbed, po	Serum T½, hrs	Intracellular T½, hrs	CPE*	Elimination	Major Adverse Events/Comments *(See Table 6B)*
1. Selected Characteristics of Nucleoside or Nucleotide Reverse Transcriptase Inhibitors (NRTIs) *(continued)*								
Lamivudine/Abacavir (Epzicom/Kivexa)	Film-coated tabs: 3TC 300 mg + abacavir 600 mg	1 tab po q24h. Food OK Not recommended for CrCl <50 mL/min or impaired hepatic function	*(See individual components)*					*See Comments for individual agents.* **Note abacavir hypersensitivity Black Box warnings** (severe reactions may be somewhat more frequent with 600 mg dose) and 3TC Hep B warnings. Test HLA-B*5701 before use.
Lamivudine/TDF (Cimduo)	Film-coasted tabs: 3TC 300 mg + TDF 300 mg	1 tab po q24h w/wo food. Not recommended for CrCl <50 mL/min	*(See individual components)*					*See Comments for individual agents.* **Black Box warning**—exacerbation of HBV in pts stopping 3TC/TDF
Lamivudine/ Zidovudine (Combivir)	Film-coated tabs: 3TC 150 mg + ZDV 300 mg	1 tab po bid. Not recommended for CrCl <50 mL/min or impaired hepatic function Food OK	*(See individual components)*					*See Comments for individual agents* **Black Box warning**—exacerbation of Hep B in pts stopping 3TC
Stavudine (d4T; Zerit)	15, 20, 30, 40 mg capsules; 1 mg per mL oral solution	≥60 kg: 40 mg po bid <60 kg: 30 mg po bid Food OK	86	1.2–1.6	3.5	2	Renal excretion, 40%	Not recommended by DHHS as initial therapy because of adverse reactions. **Highest incidence of lipoatrophy, hyperlipidemia, & lactic acidosis of all NRTIs.** Pancreatitis. Peripheral neuropathy *(See didanosine comments).*
Tenofovir alafenamide fumarate (TAF)	10 mg po q24h (part of Genvoya, Symtuza) 25 mg po q24h (part of Biktarvy, Descovy, Odefsey)	Food OK with all TAF preps	ND	0.51	ND	ND	ND	
Tenofovir disoproxil fumarate (TDF) (TDF; Viread)— a nucleotide	Tabs: 150, 200, 250, 300 mg Oral powder: 40 mg/scoop	CrCl ≥50 mL/min: 300 mg po q24h Food OK; high-fat meal ↑ absorption	39 (with food) 25 (fasted)	17	>60	1	Renal excretion	Headache, N/V. **Cases of renal dysfunction reported:** check renal function before using (dose reductions necessary if CrCl <50 cc/min); avoid concomitant nephrotoxic agents. Fanconi's syndrome *(See Table 6B, page 38).* Adjust dose of ddI (↓) if used concomitantly but best to avoid this combination *(see ddI Comments).* Atazanavir & lopinavir/ritonavir ↑ tenofovir concentrations: monitor for adverse effects. **Black Box warning— exacerbations of Hep B reported after stopping TDF.** Monitor several months after stopping TDF in Hep B pts; some may need anti-HBV Rx.

* **CPE (CNS Penetration Effectiveness) value:** 1= Low Penetration; 2 - 3 = Intermediate Penetration; 4 = Highest Penetration into CNS (*Arch Neurol.* 2008;65(1):65-70)

TABLE 6A (4)

Selected Characteristics of Antiretroviral Drugs								
Generic/ Trade Name	Pharmaceutical Prep.	Usual Adult Dosage & Food Effect	% Absorbed, po	Serum T½, hrs	Intracellular T½, hrs	CPE*	Elimination	Major Adverse Events/Comments (See Table 6B)
1. Selected Characteristics of Nucleoside or Nucleotide Reverse Transcriptase Inhibitors (NRTIs) *(continued)*								
Zidovudine (ZDV, AZT; Retrovir)	100 mg caps, 300 mg tabs; 10 mg per mL IV solution; 10 mg/mL oral syrup	300 mg po q12h. Food OK	60	0.5-3	11	4	Metabolized to glucuronide & excreted in urine	Bone marrow suppression, GI intolerance, headache, insomnia, malaise, myopathy.
2. Selected Characteristics of Non-Nucleoside Reverse Transcriptase Inhibitors (NNRTIs)								
Delavirdine (Rescriptor, DLV)	100, 200 mg tabs	400 mg po three times daily. Food OK	85	5.8	ND	3	Converted by CYP3A and 2D6 to inactive metabolites; 51% excreted in urine (<5% unchanged), 44% in feces	Rash severe enough to stop drug in 4.3%. ↑ AST/ALT, headaches. **Use of DLV is not recommended.**
Doravirine (DOR, Pifeltro)	100 mg film-coated tabs	100 mg po qd with or without food	64	15	ND	ND	Metabolism; 6% excreted in urine unchanged	Nausea, dizziness, headache, fatigue, diarrhea, abdominal pain, abnormal dreams
Efavirenz (EFV, Sustiva)	50, 200 mg capsules; 600 mg tablet	600 mg po q24h at bedtime, without food. Food may ↑ serum conc., which can lead to ↑ in risk of adverse events.	42	40–55 *See Comment*	ND	3	Metabolized by CYP2B6 and 3A4 to hydroxylated metabolites which are then glucuronidate d and excreted in feces and urine	Rash severe enough to dc use of drug in 1.7%. High frequency of diverse CNS AEs: somnolence, dreams, confusion, agitation. Serious psychiatric symptoms. Certain CYP2B6 polymorphisms may predict exceptionally high plasma levels with standard doses *(CID 45:1230, 2007)*. False-pos. cannabinoid screen. **New Guidelines indicate it is OK to use in pregnant women (WHO Guidelines) or continue EFV in women identified as pregnant (HHS Guidelines).** Very long tissue T½. **If rx to be discontinued, stop efavirenz 1–2 wks before stopping companion drugs.** Otherwise, risk of devel- oping efavirenz resistance, as after 1–2 days only efavirenz in blood &/or tissue. Some authorities bridge this gap by adding a PI to the NRTI backbone if feasible after efavirenz is discontinued. *(CID 42:401, 2006)*

* **CPE (CNS Penetration Effectiveness) value:** 1= Low Penetration; 2 - 3 = Intermediate Penetration; 4 = Highest Penetration into CNS *(Arch Neurol. 2008;65(1):65-70).*

TABLE 6A (5)

			Selected Characteristics of Antiretroviral Drugs					
Generic/ Trade Name	Pharmaceutical Prep.	Usual Adult Dosage & Food Effect	% Absorbed, po	Serum $T\frac{1}{2}$, hrs	Intracellular $T\frac{1}{2}$, hrs	CPE*	Elimination	Major Adverse Events/Comments *(See Table 6B)*
2. Selected Characteristics of Non-Nucleoside Reverse Transcriptase Inhibitors (NNRTIs) *(continued)*								
Efavirenz/TDF/3TC (Symfi, Symfi Lo)	Tabs: EFV 600 mg + 3TC 300 mg + TDF 300 mg (Symfi). Symfi Lo reduces EFV component to 400 mg	1 tab po q24h without food	*(See individual components)*					Symfi is a generic version of Atripla, substituting 3TC for FTC. EFV dose in Symfi Lo is lower than in Symfi, which is associated with lower toxicity, better tolerability, and similar efficacy to the brand name formulation.
Efavirenz/ Tenofovir DF/ Emtricitabine (Atripla)	Tabs: EFV 600 mg + FTC 200 mg + TDF 300 mg	1 tab po q24h without food	*(See individual components)*					Exacerbation of HBV reported in patients discontinuing component drugs (FTC). EFV: potential for fetal harm, neuropsychiatric AEs that dissipate over time, increased plasma lipids, mild rash
Etravirine (ETR, Intelence)	25, 100, 200 mg tablets	200 mg twice daily after a meal. May also be given as 400 mg once daily	Unknown (↓ systemic exposure if taken fasting)	41	ND	2	Hepatic oxidation by CYP450; excreted into feces (>90%), mostly as unchanged drug	For pts with HIV-1 resistant to NNRTIs & others. Active in vitro against most such isolates. Rash common, but rarely can be severe. Potential for multiple drug interactions. Generally, multiple mutations are required for high-level resistance. Because of interactions, do not use with boosted atazanavir, boosted tipranavir, unboosted PIs, or other NNRTIs.
Nevirapine (NVP, Viramune, Viramune XR)	200 mg tabs; 50 mg per 5 mL oral suspension; XR 100, 400 mg tabs	200 mg po q24h x 14 days & then 200 mg po bid *(see comments & **Black Box warning**)* Food OK. **If using Viramune XR, Still need the lead in dosing of 200 mg q24h prior to using 400 mg/d**	>90	25–30	ND	4	Heavily oxidized by CYP450; >80% of dose excreted in urine as glucuronidated metabolites, 10% in feces	**Black Box warning—fatal hepatotoxicity.** Women with CD4 >250 esp. vulnerable, inc. pregnant women. Avoid in this group unless benefits clearly >risks *(www.fda.gov/cderdrug/advisory/nevirapine.htm).* If used, intensive monitoring required. Men with CD4 >400 also at ↑ risk. Rash severe enough to stop drug in 7%, **severe or life-threatening skin reactions** in 2%. Do not restart if any suspicion of such reactions. 2 wk dose escalation period may ↓ skin reactions. As with efavirenz, because of long $T\frac{1}{2}$, consider continuing companion agents for several days if nevirapine is discontinued.

* **CPE (CNS Penetration Effectiveness) value:** 1= Low Penetration; 2 - 3 = Intermediate Penetration; 4 = Highest Penetration into CNS *(Arch Neurol. 2008;65(1):65-70)*

Selected Characteristics of Antiretroviral Drugs

Generic/ Trade Name	Pharmaceutical Prep.	Usual Adult Dosage & Food Effect	% Absorbed, po	Serum $T_{1/2}$, hrs	Intracellular $T_{1/2}$, hrs	CPE*	Elimination	Major Adverse Events/Comments (See Table 6B)
2. Selected Characteristics of Non-Nucleoside Reverse Transcriptase Inhibitors (NNRTIs) (continued)								
Rilpivirine (RPV, Edurant)	25 mg tabs	25 mg daily with food	absolute bioavailabi-lity unknown; 40% lower Cmax in fasted state	45-50	unknown	No data	Oxidized by hepatic CYP3A4; metabolites excreted in feces	QTc prolongation with doses higher than 50 mg per day. Most common side effects are depression, insomnia, headache, and rash. Rilpivirine should not be co-administered with carbamazepine, phenobarbitol, phenytoin, rifabutin, rifampin, rifapentine, proton pump inhibitors, or multiple doses of dexamethasone. A fixed dose combination of rilpivirine + TDF/FTC (Complera/Eviplera) is approved. **Needs stomach acid for absorption. Do not administer with PPI.**
Rilpivirine/ Dolutegravir (Juluca)	Tabs: RPV 25 mg + DTG 50 mg	1 tab po q24h with food	(See individual components)					Complete two-drug substitute regimen for adults who are virologically suppressed on a stable ARV regimen for at least 6 months, with no baseline pre-therapy resistance mutations and no history of virologic failure.
Rilpivirine/ Emtricitabine/ Tenofovir DF (Complera)	Tabs: RPV 25 mg + FTC 200 mg + TDF 300 mg	1 tab po q24h with food	(See individual components)					Less neuropsychiatric AEs, rash, lipid elevation than EFV, not teratogenic. Not recommended if baseline CD4 <200 or viral load >100,000. Avoid acid suppressing drugs (impaired absorption)
Rilpivirine/ Emtricitabine/ Tenofovir AF (Odefsey)	Tabs: RPV 25 mg + FTC 200 mg + TAF 25 mg	1 tab po q24h with food	TAF: ND	TAF: 0.51	TAF: ND	TAF: ND	TAF: >80% metabolized, <1% of dose excreted in urine	Before starting, test for HBV infection and obtain CrCl (not recommended if CrCl <30 mL/min), urine glucose, and urine protein. TAF is a Tenofovir prodrug that has antiretroviral efficacy similar to TDF at less than 1/10th the dose.

* **CPE (CNS Penetration Effectiveness) value:** 1= Low Penetration; 2 - 3 = Intermediate Penetration; 4 = Highest Penetration into CNS (Arch Neurol. 2008;65(1):65-70).

TABLE 6A (7)

			Selected Characteristics of Antiretroviral Drugs				
Generic/Trade Name	Pharmaceutical Prep.	Usual Adult Dosage & Food Effect	% Absorbed, po	Serum T T½, hrs	CPE*	Elimination	Major Adverse Events/Comments (See Table 6B)
3. Selected Characteristics of Protease Inhibitors (PIs)							
Atazanavir (ATV, Reyataz)	150, 200, 300 mg capsules 50 mg oral powder	400 mg po q24h with food. RTV-boosted dose (ATV 300 mg + RTV 100 mg po q24h, with food) is recommended for ART-experienced patients. The boosted dose is also used when combined with either efavirenz 600 mg po q24h or TDF 300 mg po q24h. If used with buffered ddl, take with food 2 hrs pre or 1 hr post ddl.	Absorption decreased by antacids, H2-blockers, and proton pump inhibitors. Administer ATV 2 hr before or 1 hr after antacids. Avoid unboosted ATV with PPIs/H2-blockers. ATV/r can be used with or >10 hr after H2-blockers or >12 hr after a PPI, as long as limited doses of the acid-lowering agents are used (see drug label for a complete summary).	Approx. 7	2	Extensively metabolized; 20% and 7% of a dose eliminated as unchanged drug in the feces and urine, respectively.	Lower potential for ↑ lipids. Asymptomatic unconjugated hyperbilirubinemia common; jaundice especially likely in Gilbert's syndrome (JID 192:1381, 2005). Headache, rash, GI symptoms. Prolongation of PR interval (1st degree AV block) reported. Caution in pre-existing conduction system disease. Efavirenz & tenofovir ↓ atazanavir exposure: use atazanavir/ritonavir regimen; also, atazanavir ↑ tenofovir concentrations—watch for adverse events. In rx-experienced pts taking TDF and needing H2 blockers, atazanavir 400 mg with ritonavir 100 mg can be given; do not use PPIs. Rare reports of renal stones.
Atazanavir/ Cobicistat (ATV/c, Evotaz)	Tabs: ATV 300 mg + Cobi 150 mg	1 tab po q24h with food	(See individual components)				Not recommended for use with regimens containing RTV, other PIs, or EVG. Contraindicated if previous hypersensitivity reaction to either component.
Darunavir (DRV, Prezista)	75, 150, 600, 800 mg tabs; 100 mg/mL oral susp	[600 mg darunavir + 100 mg ritonavir] po bid, with food or **[800 mg darunavir (two 400 mg tabs or one 800 mg tab) + 150 mg cobicistat] po once daily with food (Preferred regimen in ART naïve pts)**	82% absorbed (taken with ritonavir). Food ↑ absorption.	Approx 15 hr (with ritonavir)	3	Extensively metabolized mainly by CYP3A, eliminated in feces	Once daily dosing regimen mostly in 1st line therapy. Contains sulfa moiety. Rash, nausea, headaches seen. Co-admin of certain drugs cleared by CYP3A is contraindicated (see label). Use with caution in pts with hepatic dysfunction. (Recent FDA warning about occasional hepatic dysfunction early in the course of treatment). Monitor carefully, esp. first several months and with pre-existing liver disease. May cause hormonal contraception failure.
Darunavir/ Cobicistat (DRV/c, Prezcobix)	DRV 800/Cobi 150 mg tabs						
Darunavir/ Cobicistat/FTC/TAF (Symtuza)	Tabs: DRV 800 mg + Cobi 150 mg + FTC 200 mg + TAF 10 mg	1 tab q24h with food	(See individual components)				4-drug combo formulation for treatment of adults who are treatment naive or are virologically suppressed on another ARV regimen for at least 6 months (and no resistance to DRV or TAF). Test for HBV co-infection before starting. Not recommended for use in pregnancy or during lactation (substantially reduced exposures of DRV and cobicistat).

* **CPE (CNS Penetration Effectiveness) value:** 1= Low Penetration; 2 - 3 = Intermediate Penetration; 4 = Highest Penetration into CNS (Arch Neurol. 2008;65(1):65-70)

TABLE 6A (8)

Selected Characteristics of Antiretroviral Drugs

Generic/Trade Name	Pharmaceutical Prep.	Usual Adult Dosage & Food Effect	% Absorbed, po	Serum T T½, hrs	CPE*	Elimination	Major Adverse Events/Comments (See Table 6B)
3. Selected Characteristics of Protease Inhibitors (PIs) *(continued)*							
Fosamprenavir (FPV, Lexiva)	700 mg tablet, 50 mg/mL oral suspension	1400 mg (two 700 mg tabs) po bid **OR** with ritonavir: [1400 mg fosamprenavir (2 tabs) + ritonavir 200 mg] po q24h **OR** [1400 mg fosamprenavir (2 tabs) + ritonavir 100 mg] po q24h **OR** [700 mg fosamprenavir (1 tab) + ritonavir 100 mg] po bid	Bioavailability not established. Food OK	7.7 Amprenavir	3	Hydrolyzed to amprenavir, then metabolized by CYP3A4. The two major metabolites are excreted mainly in feces.	Amprenavir prodrug. Contains sulfa moiety. Potential for serious drug interactions (*see label*). Rash, including Stevens-Johnson syndrome. Once daily regimens: (1) not recommended for PI-experienced pts, (2) additional ritonavir needed if given with efavirenz (*see label*). Boosted twice daily regimen is recommended for PI-experienced pts. Potential for PI cross-resistance with darunavir.
Indinavir (IDV, Crixivan)	100, 200, 400 mg capsules Store in original container with desiccant	Two 400 mg caps (800 mg) po q8h, without food or with light meal. Can take with enteric-coated Videx. *[If taken with ritonavir (e.g., 800 mg indinavir + 100 mg ritonavir po q12h), no food restrictions]*	65	1.2–2	4	Oxidized by CYP3A4 to multiple metabolites that are mainly excreted in feces	**Maintain hydration. Nephrolithiasis,** nausea, inconsequential ↑ of indirect bilirubin (jaundice in Gilbert syndrome), ↑ AST/ALT, headache, asthenia, blurred vision, metallic taste, hemolysis. ↑ urine WBC (>100/hpf) has been assoc. with nephritis/ medullary calcification, cortical atrophy.
Lopinavir + ritonavir (LPV/r, Kaletra)	(200 mg lopinavir + 50 mg ritonavir), and (100 mg lopinavir + 25 mg ritonavir) tablets. Tabs do not need refrigeration. Oral solution: (80 mg lopinavir + 20 mg ritonavir) per mL. Refrigerate, but can be kept at room temp. (≤77 °F) x 2 mos.	(LPV 200/RTV 50 mg) tabs: 2 tabs po bid. Higher dose may be needed in non-Rx-naive pts when used with efavirenz, nevirapine, or unboosted fosamprenavir. [Dose adjustment in concomitant drugs may be necessary]	No food effect with tablets; take oral solution with food.	5-6 (lopinavir)	3	Substrate of CYP3A4; inhibits 3A4	Nausea/vomiting/diarrhea (worse when administered with zidovudine), ↑ AST/ ALT, pancreatitis. Oral solution 42% alcohol. Lopinavir + ritonavir can be taken as a single daily dose of 4 tabs (total 800 mg lopinavir + 200 mg ritonavir), except in treatment-experienced pts or those taking concomitant efavirenz, nevirapine, amprenavir, or nelfinavir. Possible PR and QT prolongation. Use with caution in those with cardiac conduction abnormalities or when used with drugs with similar effects.

∗ **CPE (CNS Penetration Effectiveness) value:** 1= Low Penetration; 2 - 3 = Intermediate Penetration; 4 = Highest Penetration into CNS (*Arch Neurol. 2008;65(1):65-70*).

TABLE 6A (9)

	Selected Characteristics of Antiretroviral Drugs						
Generic/Trade Name	Pharmaceutical Prep.	Usual Adult Dosage & Food Effect	% Absorbed, po	Serum T T½, hrs	CPE*	Elimination	Major Adverse Events/Comments (See Table 6B)
3. Selected Characteristics of Protease Inhibitors (PIs). (continued)							
Nelfinavir (NFV, Viracept)	625, 250 mg tabs; 50 mg/gm oral powder (1 level scoopful = 1 gm oral powder)	Two 625 mg tabs (1250 mg) po bid, with food	20–80 Food ↑ exposure & ↓ variability	3.5–5	1	Eliminated primarily in the feces, mainly as numerous oxidative metabolites	Diarrhea. Coadministration of drugs with life-threatening toxicities & which are cleared by CYP34A is contraindicated. Not recommended in initial regimens because of inferior efficacy; **prior concerns about EMS now resolved. Acceptable choice in pregnant women although it has inferior virologic efficacy than most other ARV anchor drugs.**
Ritonavir (RTV, Norvir)	100 mg tabs, 80 mg/mL oral solution, 100 mg oral powder packets	Full dose not recommended (see comments). **With rare exceptions, used exclusively to enhance pharmacokinetics of other PIs, using lower ritonavir doses.**	Food ↑ absorption	3–5	1	Metabolized mainly by CYP3A4, metabo ites eliminated in feces.	Nausea/vomiting/diarrhea, extremity & circumoral paresthesias, hepatitis, pancreatitis, taste perversion, ↑ CPK & uric acid. **Black Box warning—**potentially fatal drug interactions. Many drug interactions.
Saquinavir (SQV, Invirase) Must be used with **Ritonavir**	Saquinavir 200 mg caps, 500 mg film-coated tabs	[2 tabs saquinavir (1000 mg) + 1 cap ritonavir (100 mg)] po bid with food	Erratic, 4 (saquinavir alone). Much more reliably absorbed when boosted with ritonavir.	1–2	1	Metabolized by CYP450 (mainly 3A4) to multiple inactive compounds excreted mainly in feces	Nausea, diarrhea, headache, ↑ AST/ALT. Avoid rifampin with saquinavir + ritonavir: ↑ hepatitis risk. **Black Box warning—**Invirase to be used only with ritonavir. Possible QT prolongation. Use with caution in those with cardiac conduction abnormalities or when used with drugs with similar effects.
Tipranavir (TPV, Aptivus)	250 mg caps (refrigerate unopened bottles), 100 mg/mL oral solution (store at room temp). Use opened bottles of caps and soln within 60 days.	[500 mg (two 250 mg caps) + ritonavir 200 mg] po bid with food.	Absorption low, ↑ with high fat meal, ↓ with Al+++ & Mg++ antacids.	5.5-6	1	Metabolism in the presence of RTV is minimal; eliminated in feces mcstly as unchanged drug.	Contains sulfa moiety. **Black Box warning—reports of fatal/nonfatal intracranial hemorrhage, hepatitis, fatal hepatic failure.** Use cautiously in liver disease, esp. Hep B, Hep C; contraindicated in Child-Pugh class B-C. Monitor LFTs. Coadministration of certain drugs contraindicated (see label). **For highly ART-experienced pts or for multiple-PI resistant virus.** Do not use tipranavir and etravirine together owing to 76% reduction in etravirine levels.

* **CPE (CNS Penetration Effectiveness) value:** 1= Low Penetration; 2 - 3 = Intermediate Penetration; 4 = Highest Penetration into CNS (*Arch Neurol* 2008;65(1):65-70)

TABLE 6A (10)

Selected Characteristics of Antiretroviral Drugs

Generic/ Trade Name	Pharmaceutical Prep.	Usual Adult Dosage	% Absorbed	Serum T½, hrs	CPE*	Elimination	Major Adverse Events/Comments (See Table 6B)
4. Selected Characteristics of Fusion Inhibitors							
Enfuvirtide (T20, Fuzeon)	Single-use vials of 90 mg/mL when reconstituted. Vials should be stored at room temperature. Reconstituted vials can be refrigerated for 24 hrs only.	90 mg (1 mL) subcut. bid. Rotate injection sites, avoiding those currently inflamed.	84	3.8	1	Catabolism to its constituent amino acids with subsequent recycling of the amino acids in the body pool. Elimination pathway studies have not been performed in humans.	Local reaction site reactions 98%, 4% discontinue; erythema/induration ~80–90%, nodules/cysts ~80%. **Hypersensitivity reactions reported** (fever, rash, chills, N/V, ↓ BP, &/or ↑ AST/ALT)—do not restart if occur. Including background regimens, peripheral neuropathy 8.9%, insomnia 11.3%, ↓ appetite 6.3%, myalgia 5%, lymphadenopathy 2.3%, eosinophilia ~10%. ↑ incidence of bacterial pneumonias: Alone offers little benefit to a failing regimen (NEJM 348:2249, 2003).
5. Selected Characteristics of CCR-5 Co-receptor Antagonists							
Maraviroc (MVC, Selzentry)	25 mg, 75 mg, 150 mg, 300 mg tablets; 20 mg/mL oral solution	Without regard to food: • 150 mg bid if concomitant meds include CYP3A inhibitors including PIs (except tipranavir/ritonavir) and delavirdine (with/without CYP3A inducers) • 300 mg bid without significantly interacting meds including NRTIs, tipranavir/ritonavir, nevirapine • 600 mg bid if concomitant meds include CYP3A inducers, including efavirenz (without strong CYP3A inhibitors)	Est. 33% with 300 mg dosage	14-18	3	Metabolites (via CYP3A) excreted feces > urine	**Black Box Warning-Hepatotoxicity,** may be preceded by rash, ↑ eos or IgE. NB: no hepatoxicity was noted in MVC trials. Black box inserted owing to concern about potential CCR5 class effect. Data lacking in hepatic/renal insufficiency; ↑ concern with either could ↑ risk of ↓ BP. Currently for treatment-experienced patients with multi-resistant strains. **Document CCR-5-tropic virus before use, as treatment failures assoc. with appearance of CXCR-4 or mixed-tropic virus.**
6. Selected Characteristics of Integrase Strand Transfer Inhibitors							
Bictegravir/ FTC/TAF (Biktarvy)	BIC 50 mg + FTC 200 mg + TAF 25 mg	1 tab po q24h with food			(See individual components)		**Black Box Warning** for HBV exacerbation in co-infected patients who discontinue Biktarvy. Expect Scr to increase slightly (0.1-0.15 mg/dL) when initiating Biktarvy due to inhibition of proximal tubular secretion of creatinine (NOTE: not a reflection of a true change in GFR).

* **CPE (CNS Penetration Effectiveness) value:** 1= Low Penetration; 2 - 3 = Intermediate Penetration; 4 = Highest Penetration into CNS (Arch Neurol. 2008;65(1):65-70).

TABLE 6A (11)

				Selected Characteristics of Antiretroviral Drugs			
Generic/ Trade Name	Pharmaceutical Prep.	Usual Adult Dosage	% Absorbed	Serum $T_{1/2}$, hrs	CPE*	Elimination	Major Adverse Events/Comments (See Table 6B)
6. Selected Characteristics of Integrase Strand Transfer Inhibitors (continued)							
Raltegravir (RAL, Isentress)	400 mg film-coated tabs 25, 100 mg chewable tabs 100 mg/5 ml oral susp (single use packets) 600 mg tablets	400 mg po bid, without regard to food OR 1200 mg (two 600 mg tabs) once daily	Unknown	~ 9	3	Glucuronidation via UGT1A1, with excretion into feces and urine. (Therefore does NOT require ritonavir boosting)	For naïve patients and treatment experienced pts with multiply-resistant virus. Well-tolerated. Nausea, diarrhea, headache, fever similar to placebo. CK↑ & rhabdomyolysis reported: unclear relationship. Increased depression in those with a history of depression. Low genetic barrier to resistance. Increase in CPK, myositis, rhabdomyolysis have been reported. Rare Stevens Johnson Syndrome. Better oral absorption if chewed (CID 57:480, 2013).
Elvitegravir/ Cobicistat/ Emtricitabine/ Tenofovir DF (Stribild) Ref: CID 58:93, 2014	EVG 150 mg + Cobi 150 mg + FTC 200 mg + TDF 300 mg	1 tab po q24h Food OK			See individual components		For both treatment naïve patients and treatment experienced pts with multiply-resistant virus. Generally well-tolerated. Use of cobicistat increases serum creatinine by ~ 0.1 mg/dl via inhibition of proximal tubular enzyme; this does not result in reduction in true GFR but will result in erroneous apparent reduction in eGFR by MDRD or Cockcroft Gault calculations. Usual AEs are similar to those observed with ritonavir (cobi) and tenofovir/FTC.
Dolutegravir (DTG, Tivicay) Ref: CID 59:265, 2014	25 mg, 75 mg, 150 mg, 300 mg tablets; 20 mg/mL oral solution	50 mg po once daily 50 mg po BID (if STII resistance present or if co-admin with EFV, FOS-RTV, TIP-RTV, or Rifampin	Unknown	14	4	Primarily metabolized and eliminated by the liver	Hypersensitivity (rare); Most common: insomnia (3%) headache (2%), N/V (1%), rash (<1%). Watch for IRIS; Watch for elevated LFTs in those with HCV
Dolutegravir/ Abacavir/ Lamivudine (Triumeq)	Tabs: DTG 50 mg + ABC 600 mg + 3TC 300 mg	1 tab po q24h (Food OK)			(See individual components)		DTG-based regimens superior to EFV-based regimens in treatment-naïve patients. DTG blunts tubular secretion of creatinine; SCr increases <0.6 mg/dL, no change in GFR. Test for HLA-B*5701 before use (ABC). Avoid antacids (decreased DTG absorption)
Elvitegravir/ Cobicistat/ Emtricitabine/ Tenofovir AF (Genvoya)	Tabs: EVG 150 + Cobi 150 mg + FTC 200 mg + TAF 10 mg	1 tab po q24h with food	TAF: ND	TAF: 0.51	TAF: ND	TAF: >80% metabolized, <1% of dose excreted in urine	TAF is a Tenofovir prodrug that has antiretroviral efficacy similar to TDF at less than 1/10th the dose.

* **CPE (CNS Penetration Effectiveness) value:** 1= Low Penetration; 2 - 3 = Intermediate Penetration; 4 = Highest Penetration into CNS (Arch Neurol. 2008;65(1):65-70).

Selected Characteristics of Antiretroviral Drugs

Other Considerations in Selection of Therapy

Caution: Initiation of ART may result in immune reconstitution syndrome with significant clinical consequences. *See Table 11B, page 112 (AIDS Reader 16:199, 2006).*

1. **Resistance testing:** Given current rates of **resistance, resistance testing is recommended in all patients prior to initiation of therapy,** including those with acute infection syndrome (may initiate therapy while waiting for test results and adjusting Rx once results return), at time of change of therapy owing to antiretroviral failure, when suboptimal virologic response is observed, and in pregnant women. **Resistance testing NOT recommended if pt is off ART for >4 weeks or if HIV RNA is <1000 c/mL.** *See Table 6F, page 49.*
2. Drug-induced disturbances of glucose & lipid metabolism *(see Table 6C)*
3. Drug-induced lactic acidosis & other FDA "box warnings" *(see Table 6C)*
4. Drug-drug interactions *(see https://www.hiv-druginteractions.org/checker)*
5. Risk in pregnancy *(see Table 17)*
6. Use in women & children *(see Table 8A)*
7. Dosing in patients with renal or hepatic dysfunction *(see Table 15A & Table 15C)*

✲ **CPE (CNS Penetration Effectiveness) value:** 1= Low Penetration; 2 - 3 = Intermediate Penetration; 4 = Highest Penetration into CNS *(Arch Neurol. 2008;65(1):65-70).*

TABLE 6B: ANTIRETROVIRAL DRUGS & ADVERSE EFFECTS

(See also www.aidsinfo.nih.gov; for combinations, see individual components)

DRUG NAME(S): GENERIC (TRADE)	MOST COMMON ADVERSE EFFECTS	MOST SIGNIFICANT ADVERSE EFFECTS
Nucleoside Reverse Transcriptase Inhibitors (NRTI) Black Box warning for all nucleoside/nucleotide RTIs: lactic acidosis/hepatic steatosis, potentially fatal. Also carry Warnings that fat redistribution and immune reconstitution syndromes (including autoimmune syndromes with delayed onset) have been observed		
Abacavir (Ziagen)	Headache 7–13%, nausea 7–19%, diarrhea 7%, malaise 7-12%	**Black Box warning-Hypersensitivity reaction (HR)** in 8% with malaise, fever, GI upset, rash, lethargy & respiratory symptoms most commonly reported; myalgia, arthralgia, edema, paresthesia less common. **Discontinue immediately if HR suspected. Rechallenge contraindicated; may be life-threatening.** Severe HR may be more common with once-daily dosing. **HLA-B*5701 allele** predicts ↑ risk of HR in Caucasian pop.; excluding pts with B*5701 markedly ↓'d HR incidence *(NEJM 358:568, 2008; CID 46:1111-1118, 2008)*. Use abacavir-containing regimens only if HLA-B*5701 negative; Vigilance essential in all groups. Possible increased risk of MI with use of abacavir had been suggested *(JID 201:318, 2010)*. Other studies found no increased risk of MI *(CID 52: 929, 2011)*. A meta-analysis of randomized trials by FDA also did not show increased risk of MI *(www.fda.gov/drugs/drugsafety/ucm245164.htm)*. VA study found current use of abacavir associated with increased risk of cardio-vascular events *(CID 61: 445, 2015)*. Care is advised to optimize potentially modifiable risk factors when abacavir is used.
Didanosine (ddI) (Videx)	Diarrhea 28%, nausea 6%, rash 9%, headache 7%, fever 12%, hyperuricemia 2%	**Pancreatitis 1–9%. Black Box warning—Cases of fatal & nonfatal pancreatitis** have occurred in pts receiving ddI, especially when used in combination with d4T or d4T + hydroxyurea. Fatal lactic acidosis in pregnancy with ddI + d4T. Peripheral neuropathy in 20%, 12% required dose reduction. ↑ toxicity if used with ribavirin. Use with TDF generally avoided (but would require dose reduction of ddI) because of ↑ toxicity and possible ↓ efficacy; may result in ↓ CD4. Rarely, retinal changes or optic neuropathy. Diabetes mellitus and rhabdomyolysis reported in post-marketing surveillance. Possible increased risk of MI under study *(www.fda.gov/CDER; JID 201:318, 2010)*. Non-cirrhotic portal hypertension with ascites, varices, splenomegaly reported in post-marketing surveillance. *See also Clin Infect Dis 49:626, 2009; Amer J Gastroenterol 104:1707, 2009*. This entity has been associated with SNPs in 5'-nucleotidase and xanthine oxidase genes *(CID 56:1117, 2013)*.
Emtricitabine (FTC) (Emtriva)	Well tolerated. Headache, diarrhea, nausea, rash, skin hyperpigmentation	Potential for lactic acidosis (as with other NRTIs). Also **in Black Box—severe exacerbation of hepatitis B on stopping drug reported—monitor clinical/labs for several months after stopping in pts with Hep B.** Anti-HBV rx may be warranted if FTC stopped.
Lamivudine (3TC) (Epivir)	Well tolerated. Headache 35%, nausea 33%, diarrhea 18%, abdominal pain 9%, insomnia 11% (all in combination with ZDV). Pancreatitis more common in pediatrics.	**Black Box warning.** Make sure to use HIV dosage, not Hep B dosage. **Exacerbation of hepatitis B on stopping drug. Patients with Hep B who stop lamivudine require close clinical/lab monitoring for several months.** Anti-HBV rx may be warranted if 3TC stopped.
Stavudine (d4T) (Zerit)	Diarrhea, nausea, vomiting, headache	**Peripheral neuropathy** 15–20%. Pancreatitis 1%. Appears to produce lactic acidosis, hepatic steatosis and lipoatrophy/lipodystrophy more commonly than other NRTIs. **Black Box warning—Fatal & nonfatal pancreatitis with d4T + ddI.** Use with TDF generally avoided (but would require dose reduction of ddI) because of ↑ toxicity and possible ↓ efficacy; may result in ↓ CD4. Rarely, retinal changes or optic neuropathy. Diabetes mellitus and rhabdomyolysis reported in post-marketing surveillance. **Fatal lactic acidosis/steatosis in pregnant women receiving d4T + ddI.** Fatal and non-fatal lactic acidosis and severe hepatic steatosis can occur in others receiving d4T. Use with particular caution in patients with risk factors for liver disease, but lactic acidosis can occur even in those without known risk factors. Possible ↑ toxicity if used with ribavirin. Motor weakness in the setting of lactic acidosis mimicking the clinical presentation of Guillain-Barré syndrome (including respiratory failure) (rare).

TABLE 6B (2)

DRUG NAME(S): GENERIC (TRADE)	MOST COMMON ADVERSE EFFECTS	MOST SIGNIFICANT ADVERSE EFFECTS
Nucleotide Reverse Transcriptase Inhibitor (NtRTI) Black Box warning for all nucleoside/nucleotide RTIs: lactic acidosis/hepatic steatosis, potentially fatal. Also carry Warnings that fat redistribution and immune reconstitution syndromes (including autoimmune syndromes with delayed onset) have been observed *(continued)*		
Zidovudine (ZDV, AZT) (Retrovir)	Nausea 50%, anorexia 20%, vomiting 17%, **headache 62%.** Also reported: asthenia, insomnia, myalgias, nail pigmentation. Macrocytosis expected with all dosage regimens.	**Black Box warning—hematologic toxicity, myopathy. Anemia** (<8 gm, 1%), granulocytopenia (<750, 1.8%). Anemia may respond to epoetin alfa if endogenous serum erythropoietin levels are ≤500 milliUnits/mL. Possible ↑ toxicity if used with ribavirin. Co-administration with Ribavirin not advised. Hepatic decompensation may occur in HIV/HCV co-infected patients receiving zidovudine with interferon alfa ± ribavirin.
Tenofovir alafenamide fumarate (TAF) Currently as Descovy (with emtricitabine) or Genvoya (with emtricitabine, elvitegravir, cobicistat)	In studies with Genvoya: nausea (10%), diarrhea (7%), headache (6%), fatigue (5%). Increase in serum lipids.	**Black Box Warning**—Lactic acidosis and hepatic steatosis; potential for post-therapy exacerbation of chronic hepatitis B infection. Not approved for treatment of hepatitis B. Renal—serious renal effects in <1% of those with initial CrCl >50. Discontinue with evidence of decreasing renal function or Fanconi syndrome. Bone mineral density—potential for decreased bone mineral density. Reduced potential for renal dysfunction and bone mineral abnormalities with TAF compared with TDF *(JAIDS 72:58, 2016; Lancet HIV 3: e158, 2016).*
Tenofovir disoproxil fumarate (TDF) (Viread)	Diarrhea 11%, nausea 8%, vomiting 5%, flatulence 4% (generally well tolerated)	• **Nephrotoxicity:** Several studies associate TDF therapy with renal injury *(CID 51:296, 2010; AIDS 26:567, 2012).* In VA study of >10,000 HIV pts, more proteinuria and renal function decline with TDF. Further, even if TDF therapy stopped, 1/3 of pts do not recover renal function *(JID 210:363, 2014).* • **Fanconi's syndrome:** Proximal tubular injury can cause renal Fanconi's syndrome manifest by: hypophosphatemia and hypokalemia due to excessive urine loss. Result is non-anion gap acidosis. Concomitant glycosuria, proteinuria, low serum uric acid and elevated serum creatinine. • **Osteomalacia:** Phosphate loss can cause osteomalacia, increased alk. Phosphaturia and reduced bone density *(NEJM 370:959, 2014).* **Black Box warning**—before using TDF-FTC as pre-exposure prophylaxis (PrEP), confirm HIV-1 negative status immediately before start and at least Q3Months; do not start PrEP in presence of any symptoms suggesting acute HIV infection until this is excluded. Caution when used with sofosbuvir/ledipasvir as TDF levels can increase, with potential for greater toxicity.
Non-Nucleoside Reverse Transcriptase Inhibitors (NNRTI). Labels caution that fat redistribution and immune reconstitution can occur with ART.		
Delavirdine (Rescriptor)	Nausea, diarrhea, vomiting, headache	**Skin rash** has occurred in 18%; can continue or restart drug in most cases. Stevens-Johnson syndrome & erythema multiforme have been reported rarely. ↑ in liver enzymes in <5% of patients.
Efavirenz (Sustiva)	**CNS side effects 52%;** symptoms include dizziness, insomnia, somnolence, impaired concentration, psychiatric sx, & abnormal dreams; symptoms are worse after 1st or 2nd dose & improve over 2–4 weeks; discontinuation rate 2.6%. Rash 26% (vs. 17% in comparators); often improves with oral antihistamines; discontinuation rate 1.7%. Can cause false-positive urine test results for cannabinoid with CEDIA DAU multi-level THC assay. Metabolite can cause false-positive urine screening test for benzodiazepines *(CID 48:1787, 2009).*	**Caution:** CNS effects may impair driving and other hazardous activities. Serious neuropsychiatric symptoms reported, including severe depression (2.4%) & suicidal ideation (0.7%). In treatment-naïve pts, 2-fold increase in suicide thoughts, attempts or success if regimen included Efavirenz *(AnIM 161:1, 2014).* Elevation in liver enzymes. Fulminant hepatic failure has been reported *(see FDA label).* **New Guidelines indicate it is OK to use in pregnant women** *(WHO Guidelines)* **or continue EFV in women identified as pregnant** *(DHHS Guidelines) (see Table 8A).* NOTE: No single method of contraception is 100% reliable. Barrier + 2nd method of contraception advised, continued 12 weeks after stopping efavirenz. Contraindicated with certain drugs metabolized by CYP3A4. Slow metabolism in those homozygous for the CYP-2B6 G516T allele can result in exaggerated toxicity and intolerance. This allele much more common in blacks and women *(CID 42:408, 2006).* Stevens-Jonson syndrome and erythema multiforme reported in post-marketing surveillance.

TABLE 6B (3)

DRUG NAME(S): GENERIC (TRADE)	MOST COMMON ADVERSE EFFECTS	MOST SIGNIFICANT ADVERSE EFFECTS
Non-Nucleoside Reverse Transcriptase Inhibitors (NNRTI) *(continued)*		
Etravirine (Intelence)	Rash 9%, generally mild to moderate and spontaneously resolving; 2% dc clinical trials for rash. More common in women. Nausea 5%.	Severe rash (erythema multiforme, toxic epidermal necrolysis, Stevens-Johnson syndrome) has been reported. Hypersensitivity reactions can occur with rash, constitutional symptoms and organ dysfunction, including hepatic failure *(see FDA label)*. Potential for CYP450-mediated drug interactions. Rhabdomyolysis has been reported in post-marketing surveillance.
Nevirapine (Viramune)	**Rash 37%:** usually occurs during 1st 6 wks of therapy. Follow recommendations for 14-day lead-in period to ↓ risk of rash *(see Table 6A)*. Women experience 7-fold ↑ in risk of severe rash *(CID 32:124, 2001)*. 50% resolve within 2 wks of dc drug & 80% by 1 month. 6.7% discontinuation rate. In a Malawi cohort, HLA-C*04:01 was a risk factor for nevirapine-related Stevens-Johnson syndrome or TEN *(CID 56:1330, 2013)*.	**Black Box warning—Severe life-threatening skin reactions reported:** Stevens-Johnson syndrome, toxic epidermal necrolysis, & hypersensitivity reaction or drug rash with eosinophilia & systemic symptoms (DRESS) *(ArIM 161:2501, 2001)*. For severe rashes, dc drug immediately & do not restart. In a clinical trial, the use of prednisone ↑ the risk of rash. **Black Box warning—Life-threatening hepatotoxicity reported**, 2/3 during the first 12 wks of rx. Overall 1% develops hepatitis. Pts with pre-existing ↑ in ALT or AST &/or history of chronic Hep B or C ↑ susceptible *(Hepatol 35:182, 2002)*. Women with CD4 >250, including pregnant women, at ↑ risk. Avoid in this group unless no other option. Men with CD4 >400 also at ↑ risk. Monitor pts intensively (clinical & LFTs), esp. during the first 12 wks of rx. If clinical hepatotoxicity, severe skin or hypersensitivity reactions occur, dc drug & never rechallenge.
Rilpivirine (Edurant)	Headache (3%), rash (3%; led to discontinuation in 0.1%), insomnia (3%), depressive disorders (8%). Psychiatric disorders led to discontinuation in 1%. Increased liver enzymes observed.	Drugs that induce CYP3A or increase gastric pH may decrease plasma concentration of rilpivirine and co-administration with rilpivirine should be avoided. Among these are certain anticonvulsants, rifamycins, PPIs, dexamethasone and St. John's wort. At supra-therapeutic doses, rilpivirine can increase QTc interval; use with caution with other drugs known to increase QTc. May cause depressive disorder, including suicide attempts or suicidal ideation. Overall, appears to cause fewer neuropsychiatric side effects than efavirenz *(JAIDS 60:33, 2012)*. Hepatitis especially with pre-existing liver disease, including HBV and HCV; monitor LFTs. Nephrolithiasis and nephrotic syndrome reported. Potential for weight gain, skin hypersensitivity reactions and DRESS (Complera).

Protease inhibitors (PI)

Abnormalities in glucose metabolism, dyslipidemias, fat redistribution syndromes are potential problems. Pts taking PI may be at increased risk for developing osteopenia/osteoporosis. *(See Table 6C, page 46)*. Spontaneous bleeding episodes have been reported in HIV+ pts with hemophilia being treated with PI. Rheumatoid complications have been reported with use of PIs *(Ann Rheum Dis 61:82, 2002)*. Potential of some PIs for QTc prolongation has been suggested *(Lancet 365:682, 2005)*. **Caution for all PIs**—Coadministration with certain drugs dependent on CYP3A or other enzymes for elimination & for which ↑ levels can cause serious toxicity may be contraindicated. As with other classes, rx may result in immune reconstitution syndromes, which may include early or late presentations of autoimmune syndromes. Taking into account both spontaneous and induced deliveries, a French cohort study demonstrated increased premature births among women receiving ritonavir-boosted PIs as compared with those receiving other antiretroviral therapy, even after accounting for other potential risk factors *(CID 54: 1348, 2012)*.

DRUG NAME(S): GENERIC (TRADE)	MOST COMMON ADVERSE EFFECTS	MOST SIGNIFICANT ADVERSE EFFECTS
Atazanavir (Reyataz)	Asymptomatic unconjugated hyperbilirubinemia in up to 60% of pts; jaundice in 7–9% [especially with Gilbert syndrome *(JID 192: 1381, 2005)*]. Moderate to severe events: Diarrhea 1–3%, nausea 6–14%, abdominal pain 4%, headache 6%, rash 20%.	Prolongation of PR interval (1st degree AV block in 5-6%) reported; rarely 2° AV block. QTc increase and torsades reported *(CID 44:e67, 2007)*. Acute interstitial nephritis *(Am J Kid Dis 44:E81, 2004)* and urolithiasis (atazanavir stones) reported *(AIDS 20:2131, 2006; NEJM 355:2158, 2006)*. 10-fold increased risk of renal stones compared with pts receiving other PIs *(CID 55: 1262, 2012)*. D:A:D study found Atazanavir/ritonavir to be an independent risk factor for eGFR ≤70 in those with normal baseline renal function *(JID 207:1359, 2013)*. However, another study no deterioration of renal function in patients switched to atazanavir from other PIs *(AIDS 29: 392, 2015)*. Potential ↑ transanimases in pts co-infected with HBV or HCV. Severe skin eruptions (Stevens-Johnson syndrome, erythema multiforme, and toxic eruptions, or DRESS syndrome) have been reported.
Darunavir (Prezista)	With background regimens, headache 15%, nausea 18%, diarrhea 20%, ↑ amylase 17%. Rash in 10% of treated; 0.5% discontinuation.	Hepatitis in 0.5%, some with fatal outcome. Use caution in pts with HBV or HCV co-infections or other hepatic dysfunction. Monitor for clinical symptoms and LFTs. Stevens-Johnson syndrome, toxic epidermal necrolysis, erythema multiforme. Contains sulfa moiety. Potential for major drug interactions. May cause failure of hormonal contraceptives.

TABLE 6B (4)

DRUG NAME(S): GENERIC (TRADE)	MOST COMMON ADVERSE EFFECTS	MOST SIGNIFICANT ADVERSE EFFECTS
Protease inhibitors (PI) (continued)		
Fosamprenavir (Lexiva)	Skin rash ~ 20% (moderate or worse in 3–8%), nausea, headache, diarrhea.	Rarely Stevens-Johnson syndrome, hemolytic anemia. Pro-drug of amprenavir. Contains sulfa moiety. Angioedema and nephrolithiasis reported in post-marketing experience. Angioedema, oral paresthesias, myocardial infarction and nephrolithiasis reported in post-marketing experience. Elevated LFTs seen with higher than recommended doses; increased risk in those with pre-existing liver abnormalities. Acute hemolytic anemia reported with amprenavir.
Indinavir (Crixivan)	↑ in indirect bilirubin 10–15% (≥2.5 mg/dl), with overt jaundice especially likely in those with Gilbert syndrome (*JID 192: 1381, 2005*). Nausea 12%, vomiting 4%, diarrhea 5%. Metallic taste. Paronychia and ingrown toenails reported (*CID 32:140, 2001*).	**Kidney stones.** Due to indinavir crystals in collecting system. Nephrolithiasis in 12% of adults, higher in pediatrics. Minimize risk with good hydration (at least 48 oz. water/day) (*AAC 42:332, 1998*). Tubulointerstitial nephritis/renal cortical atrophy reported in association with asymptomatic ↑ urine WBC. Severe hepatitis reported in 3 cases (*Ln 349:924, 1997*). Hemolytic anemia reported.
Lopinavir/Ritonavir (Kaletra)	GI: **diarrhea** 14–24%, nausea 2–16%. More diarrhea with q24h dosing.	Lipid abnormalities in up to 20–40%. Possible increased risk of MI with cumulative exposure (*JID 201:318, 2010*). ↑ PR interval, 2º or 3º heart block described. Post-marketing reports of ↑ QTc and torsades: avoid use in congenital QTc prolongation or in other circumstances that prolong QTc or increase susceptibility to torsades. Hepatitis, with hepatic decompensation; caution especially in those with pre-existing liver disease. Pancreatitis. Inflammatory edema of legs (*AIDS 16:673, 2002*). Stevens-Johnson syndrome & erythema multiforme reported. Note high drug concentration in oral solution. Toxic potential of oral solution (contains ethanol and propylene glycol) in neonates. *ARV Pregnancy Register 1-800-258-4263.*
Nelfinavir (Viracept)	Mild to moderate **diarrhea** 20%. Oat bran tabs, calcium, or oral anti-diarrheal agents (e.g., loperamide, diphenoxylate/atropine sulfate) can be used to manage diarrhea.	Potential for drug interactions. Powder contains phenylalanine.
Ritonavir (Norvir) (Primary use is to boost levels of other anti-retrovirals, because of ↑ toxicity/ interactions with full-dose ritonavir)	GI: bitter aftertaste ↓ by taking with chocolate milk, Ensure, or Advera; nausea 23%, ↓ by initial dose esc (titration) regimen; vomiting 13%; diarrhea 15%. Circumoral paresthesias 5–6%. Dose >100 mg bid assoc. with ↑ GI side effects & ↑ in lipid abnormalities.	**Black Box** warning relates to many important drug-drug interactions—inhibits P450 CYP3A & CYP2 D6 system—may be life-threatening. Several cases of iatrogenic Cushing's syndrome reported with concomitant use of ritonavir and corticosteroids, including dosing of the latter by inhalation, epidural injection or a single IM injection. Rarely Stevens-Johnson syndrome, toxic epidermal necrolysis anaphylaxis. Primary A-V block (and higher) and pancreatitis have been reported. Hepatic reactions, including fatalities. Monitor LFTs carefully during therapy, especially in those with pre-existing liver disease, including HBV and HCV. Small % pts with ritonavir-induced diarrhea may benefit from crofelemer 125 mg po bid (*Med Lett 55:59, 2013*).
Saquinavir (Invirase: hard cap, tablet)	**Diarrhea,** abdominal discomfort, nausea, headache	**Warning—Use Invirase only with ritonavir.** Avoid garlic capsules (may reduce SQV levels) and use cautiously with proton-pump inhibitors (increased SQV levels significant. Use of saquinavir/ritonavir can prolong QTc interval or may rarely cause 2º or 3º heart block; torsades reported. Contraindicated in patients with prolonged QTc or those taking drugs or who have other conditions (e.g., low K+ or Mg++) that pose a risk with prolonged QTc (*http://www.fda.gov/drugs/DrugSafety/ucm230096.htm, accessed May 25, 2011*). Contraindicated in patients with complete AV block, or those at risk, who do not have pacemaker. Hepatic toxicity encountered in patients with pre-existing liver disease or in individuals receiving concomitant rifampin. Rarely, Stevens Johnson syndrome. Not recommended for use with cobicistat.

TABLE 6B (5)

DRUG NAME(S): GENERIC (TRADE)	MOST COMMON ADVERSE EFFECTS	MOST SIGNIFICANT ADVERSE EFFECTS
Protease inhibitors (PI) *(continued)*		
Tipranavir (Aptivus)	Nausea & vomiting, diarrhea, abdominal pain. Rash in 8-14%, more common in women, & 33% in women taking ethinyl estradiol. Major lipid effects.	**Black Box Warning—associated with hepatitis & fatal hepatic failure.** Risk of hepatotoxicity increased in HBV or HCV co-infection. Possible photosensitivity skin reactions. Contraindicated in Child-Pugh Class B or C hepatic impairment. **Associated with fatal/nonfatal intracranial hemorrhage (can inhibit platelet aggregation).** Caution in those with bleeding risks. Potential for major drug interactions. Contains sulfa moiety and vitamin E.
Fusion Inhibitor		
Enfuvirtide (T20, Fuzeon)	Local injection site reactions (98% at least 1 local ISR, 4% dc because of ISR) (pain & discomfort, induration, erythema, nodules & cysts, pruritus, & ecchymosis). Diarrhea 32%, nausea 23%, fatigue 20%.	↑ Rate of bacterial pneumonia (3.2 pneumonia events/100 pt yrs), **hypersensitivity reactions** ≤1% (rash, fever, nausea & vomiting, chills, rigors, hypotension, & ↑ serum liver transaminases); can occur with reexposure. Cutaneous amyloid deposits containing enfuvirtide peptide reported in skin plaques persisting after discontinuation of drug *(J Cutan Pathol 39:220, 2012).*
CCR5 Co-receptor Antagonists		
Maraviroc (Selzentry)	With ARV background: cough 13%, fever 12%, rash 10%, abdominal pain 8%. Also, dizziness, myalgia, arthralgias. ↑ Risk of URI, HSV infection.	**Black box warning-Hepatotoxicity.** May be preceded by allergic features (rash, ↑ eosinophils or ↑ IgE levels). Use with caution in pt with Hep B or Hep C. Cardiac ischemia/infarction in 1.3%. May cause ↓BP, orthostatic syncope, especially in patients with renal dysfunction. Significant interactions with CYP3A inducers/inhibitors. Long-term risk of malignancy unknown. Stevens-Johnson syndrome reported post-marketing. Generally favorable safety profile during trial of ART-naïve individuals *(JID 201: 803, 2010).* Immune reconstitution syndrome, including autoimmune manifestations, may occur in those receiving ART, including maraviroc.
Integrase Strand Transfer Inhibitors (INSTI)		
Raltegravir (Isentress)	Diarrhea, headache, insomnia, nausea. LFT ↑ may be more common in pts co-infected with HBV or HCV.	Hypersensitivity reactions can occur. Rash, Stevens-Johnson syndrome, toxic epidermal necrolysis reported. Hepatic failure reported. ↑ CK, myopathy and rhabdomyolysis reported *(AIDS 22:1382, 2008).* ↑ of preexisting depression reported in 4 pts; all could continue raltegravir after adjustment of psych. meds *(AIDS 22:1890, 2008).* Chewable tablets contain phenylalanine. Immune reconstitution syndrome, including autoimmune manifestations, may occur in those receiving ART, including raltegravir.
Elvitegravir (Vitekta) (Used in combinations only)	Diarrhea (7%), nausea (4%) and headache (3%) are most common. *See adverse effects* from co-administered protease inhibitor and ritonavir, Tybost or cobicistat.	<2% Rash, abdominal pain, dyspepsia. Depression, insomnia, suicide ideation/attempt in <1%.
Dolutegravir (Tivicay)	Insomnia, headache. Diarrhea uncommon. Small increase in serum creatinine due to inhibition of tubular secretion of creatinine; no change in GFR *(CID 59:265, 2014).* Increases in ALT/AST, cholesterol, glucose.	Hypersensitivity reactions, which may include fever, rash, fatigue/malaise, myalgia/arthralgia, angioedema, hepatitis, eosinophilia: stop immediately and do not rechallenge. Elevation of transaminases in HBV, HCV. Neutropenia (1%). Fat redistribution and immune reconstitution syndrome, including autoimmune manifestations, may occur. Pancreatitis reported after starting dolutegravir with abacavir and lamivudine, with rapid resolution after discontinuation *(AIDS 29: 390, 2015).*
Other		
Cobicistat (Tybost) Boosts serum levels of ARVs by blocking CYP3A, no HIV activity.	Nausea, rash, jaundice (with atazanavir + Truvada) all ≤5%. Competes with creatinine for tubular secretion; can increase serum creatinine ≤0.4 mg/dL without change in GFR. Compared to ritonavir, less impact on function of fat cells & better solubility.	See package insert for list of drugs metabolized by CYP3A that are contraindicated for concomitant use. Nephrolithiasis with boosted atazanavir. Fanconi syndrome and/or acute renal failure reported when used with TDF. Abdominal pain, depression, insomnia, rhabdomyolysis all <2%.

TABLE 6C: DRUG ADVERSE EFFECTS BY CLINICAL PRESENTATION[1]

Clinical Presentation	Implicated Drug Class or Drug(s)	Onset; Clinical Signs & Symptoms (S&S)	Estimated Frequency	Risk Factors	Prevention/ Monitoring	Clinical Management
LIFE THREATENING ADVERSE EFFECTS (in alphabetical order)						
Drug-induced hepatitis: Nevirapine	**Nevirapine (Viramune) hypersensitivity reaction most important**	Onset: 1st 6-18 weeks of rx. S&S: nausea/vomiting/icterus. Skin rash in 50%. Stomatitis, conjunctivitis, eosinophilia	2.5–11% in clinical trials	Females with CD4 >250; men with CD4 >400.	Gradual increase over 2 wks. Monitor ALT/AST q2 wks x 1 mo., then every month x 3, then q3 mos.	DC all antiretrovirals + other potential hepatotoxic drugs. **Never use nevirapine for PEP in pts with hepatic insufficiency**
Lactic acidosis/ hepatic steatosis ± pancreatitis (Mitochondrial toxicity: *JAC 61:8, 2008*)	Nucleoside reverse transcriptase inhibitors: **stavudine (Zerit), didanosine (Videx), zidovudine (Retrovir)**	Onset: Months after starting therapy. S&S: Nausea, vomiting, fatigue, dyspnea, icterus. Lab: Metabolic acidosis with anion gap & elevated lactate	Rare: 0.85 cases/ 1000 pt yrs, mortality up to 50% if lactate >10 mmol/L	Didanosine + stavudine. Female gender, pregnancy, obesity.	Lactic acid levels if suggestive symptoms and low serum HCO_3 and/or high anion gap. Routine lactate levels **not** recommended	DC all antiretrovirals. IV thiamine &/or riboflavin reported helpful. If needed, use NRTIs[2] with low potential for mitochondrial toxicity: i.e., abacavir, tenofovir, lamivudine, emtricitabine.
Lactic acidosis/rapid progressive ascending neuromuscular weakness	**Stavudine (Zerit) & other nucleoside analogues, esp. ddI , ZDV,** d4T	Onset: After months, insidious S&S: Rapid progressive ascending polyneuropathy that mimics Guillain-Barré. Lab: Metabolic acidosis with anion gap & elevated lactate + high CPK	Rare	Prolonged stavudine use; female gender; obesity.	Early recognition	DC all antiretrovirals, mechanical ventilation. Unclear benefit from plasmapheresis, IVIG, corticosteroids. **Do not rechallenge with stavudine.**
Stevens-Johnson syndrome/toxic epidermal necrosis (*see drug-induced hepatitis above*)	ddI, ZDV Rare case reports with other classes of ARVs. TMP-SMX	Onset: 1st few days to weeks S&S: Skin eruption with mucosal ulcers ± epidermal detachment	Nevirapine (Viramune) 0.3–1% Efavirenz (Sustiva) & delavirdine (Rescriptor) 0.1%	Nevirapine— female, black, Asian, Hispanic.	Educate pts for early recognition	DC all antiretrovirals + other possible drug etiology, e.g., TMP/SMX. Usually requires ICU care.
Systemic hyper- sensitivity reaction (HSR)	**Abacavir (Ziagen) DO NOT rechallenge with abacavir. Etravirine (Intelence)**	Onset: Median 9 days; 90% within 1st 6 wks. S&S: Fever, diffuse rash, nausea/vomiting/diarrhea/ arthralgia, dypsnea, cough, or pharyngitis	8% in clinical trials (range 2–9%)	**HLA-DR7 or HLA-B*5701 positive.**	**Screen for HLA-B*5701**	DC all antiretrovirals; Resolution within 48 hrs; do not rechallenge.
	Nevirapine (Viramune)	Severe skin reactions	2%		Do not restart	*See drug-induced Hepatitis.*
	Raltegravir	Fever, rash	Rare	Combination with other drugs that cause HSR		Stop ART

[1] Adapted from *aidsinfo.nih.gov/guidelines/html/1/adult-and-adolescent-treatment-guidelines/0*
[2] **NRTI** = nucleoside reverse transcr ptase inhibitor

TABLE 6C (2)

Clinical Presentation	Implicated Drug Class or Drug(s)	Onset; Clinical Signs & Symptoms (S&S)	Estimated Frequency	Risk Factors	Prevention/ Monitoring	Clinical Management
SERIOUS ADVERSE EFFECTS (in alphabetical order)						
Bleeding events:						
CD8 Encephalitis	ART	Cognitive impairment, confusion, seizure, CD8 lymphocyte pleocytosis	Rare	CNS IRIS, ART interruption	Gadolinium enhanced MRI for Dx	Glucocorticoids *(CID 57:101, 2013)*
Hemophiliac patients	Protease inhibitors	Spontaneous bleeding: hematuria	Unknown	Protease inhibitor use	Try to avoid PIs	Increased use of Factor VIII.
Intracranial hemorrhage	Ritonavir boosted tipranavir (TPV/r)	Median time to hemorrhage: 525 days of TPV/r therapy	24 cases with TPV/r; 2 deaths	CNS disease, injury or surgery, anti-coagulants, Vitamin E	Avoid vitamin E supplements.	Discontinue TPV/r.
Bone marrow suppression	Zidovudine (Retrovir)	Onset: Weeks to months S&S: Fatigue Lab: Anemia &/or neutropenia	Severe anemia 1.1–4% Severe neutropenia 1.8–8%	AIDS; high dose concomitant marrow-suppressive drug(s)	Avoid marrow suppressive drugs. CBC & differential at least q3 mos.	If severe, could use G-CSF &/or erythropoietin.
Hepatitis	**TAF, TDF, 3TC, FTC**	Flare of HBV if/when NRTI discontinued				All PIs can cause drug-induced hepatitis. Greatest risk with TPV
Hepatotoxicity: steatosis to NASH *(see drug-induced hepatitis, page 43)*	**All NNRTIs, all PIs, most NRTIs, maraviroc.** **Steatosis:** most common with ZDV, d4T, ddI, nevirapine.	PIs: clinical hepatitis reported with TPV/r Onset: variable NRTI: Asym ↑ ed AST/ALT + lactic acidosis (ZDV, ddI, d4T)	Variable with different drugs	Co-infection: Hep B, Hep C, alcoholism, other hepatotoxic drugs	Nevirapine: monitor LFTs frequently; especially females. TPV/r: avoid in pts with hepatic insufficiency.	Test for Hep B&C. If symptomatic, discontinue all retroviral drugs. HBV may "flare" if stop TDF, 3TC or FTC.
Nephrolithiasis/ urolithiasis/ crystalluria	**Indinavir (Crixivan) most often, rarely atazanavir**	Onset: Any time S&S: Flank pain & dysuria Lab: Hematuria, crystalluria, pyuria	Range in clinical trials: 4.7–34.4%	Dehydration; history of nephrolithiasis	Intake of 1.5–2 liters water/day.	Hydration
Nephrotoxicity — TDF *(Topics in Antiviral Med 22:655, 2014; JID 210:363, 2014)*	**TDF:** toxic to proximal tubular cells Inhibition of creatinine secretion with no increase in GFR: Cobi, DTV, RPV, RTV, trimethoprim. **TAF:** less toxic potential compared to TDF.	Gradual onset due to TDF proximal tube wasting of phosphorous, glucose, amino acids, uric acid, bicarbonate. Can present early as Fanconi's syndrome: non gap acidosis, hypokalemia, hypophosphatemia. Phosphate loss can cause osteomalacia *(NEJM 370:959, 2014)*.	Estimates vary: 2.2% in expanded access. Subtle abnormalities more often.	Other nephrotoxins	Monitor for evidence of tubular wasting. Lower TDF dose if CrCl <50 mL/min	Early injury is reversible. Discontinue TDF if possible. Avoid drug-drug interactions. **Use TAF when possible.**

Clinical Presentation	Implicated Drug Class or Drug(s)	Onset; Clinical Signs & Symptoms (S&S)	Estimated Frequency	Risk Factors	Prevention/ Monitoring	Clinical Management
SERIOUS ADVERSE EFFECTS (in alphabetical order) *(continued)*						
Pancreatitis	**Didanosine (Videx); didanosine + stavudine (Zerit);** ddI + ribavirin or tenofovir.	Onset: Weeks to months S&S: Abd./back pain, nausea/ vomiting Lab: ↑ amylase/lipase	Didanosine alone 1–7%. Increased frequency if ddI with d4T, TDF or ribavirin.	High serum/cell didanosine levels; alcoholism; hypertriglycerid-emia. Failure to ↓ dose of didanosine if given with tenofovir	No didanosine if history of pancreatitis. Adjust dose of didanosine if tenofovir used. Avoid use of ddI with d4T, TDF or ribavirin.	Discontinue antiretrovirals.
Polyneuropathy	**D4T (Stavudine) >ddI and ddC**	d4T-induced: Rapidly progressive ascending polyneuropathy mimics Guillain-Barré syndrome.	Rare	Prolonged use of d4T	Early recognition	DC all ARVs. Variable success with plasmapheresis, steroids, IVIG, carnitine.
Psychiatric	**EFV, INSTIs**	EFV: somnolence; INSTIs: insomnia				Rare suicidal ideation
ADVERSE EFFECTS WITH LONG-TERM COMPLICATIONS (in alphabetical order) Ref: *HIV & Aging: JAIDS 60 (Suppl 1):S1, 2012.*						
Atherosclerotic MIs & CVAs. Suggested pathogenesis: low grade viral replication → microbial GI translocations → T-cell monocyte mediated inflammation → non-calcified plaques. *Ref: AnIM 160:458 & 509, 2014*	Traditional risk factors and uncontrolled HIV infection most important. Selected HIV drugs suspected but unproven risk factors. Abacavir considered then rejected as risk factor *(CID 52:929, 2011; CID 53:84 & 92, 2011).*	Onset: Months to years S&S: Premature or accelerated atherosclerotic vascular disease (e.g., MI, stroke)	50% increase in relative risk of MI.	Tobacco use, age, hyperlipidemia, hypertension, diabetes, obesity, HIV infection + lower CD4 count & longer duration of ART *(AnIM 160:458 & 509, 2014).*	Address risk factors; suppress HIV viremia.	Manage risk factors; control HIV viremia. Stop tobacco use. Start statin. *See Topics in Antiviral Med 23:169, 2015.*
Cholelithiasis	Atazanavir	May have concomitant gallstones & nephrolithiasis		Median onset 42 mos		
Hyperlipidemia *(JID 205 (Suppl 3): S383, 2012; CID 52:387, 2011)*	**All protease inhibitors (PIs) except atazanavir; stavudine; efavirenz.** Ritonavir boosting elevates triglyceride levels.	Associated elevation of TG, LDL, HDL: • Stavudine > ZDV > ABC • Efavirenz • All RTV-boosted PIs (LPV/r > DRV/r > ATV/r)	1.7-2.3 fold increase with PIs other than atazanavir	PIs: ritonavir boosted lopinavir NNRTI: Efavirenz NRTI: Stavudine	ART causes modest increase in serum lipids; manage with statins. Check fasting lipid panel at base-line at 3-6 months, then annually.	Check for drug-drug interactions: statins and PIs. In general, prefer treatment with atorvastatin or rosuvastatin *(AIDS 24:77, 2010; CID 52:387, 2011).*
Insulin resistance/ diabetes mellitus *(JID 205 (Suppl 3): S383, 2012)*	**ZDV, Stavudine, ddI. Relation to PIs unclear.**	Onset: Weeks to months S&S: Polydipsia, polyuria, polyphagia	Diabetes in 3-5%	Obesity, genetics, dyslipidemia.	Avoid ZDV & Stavudine	Diet & exercise, metformin, "glitazones," sulfonylureas, insulin.

TABLE 6C (4)

Clinical Presentation	Implicated Drug Class or Drug(s)	Onset; Clinical Signs & Symptoms (S&S)	Estimated Frequency	Risk Factors	Prevention/ Monitoring	Clinical Management
ADVERSE EFFECTS WITH LONG-TERM COMPLICATIONS (in alphabetical order) Ref: *HIV & Aging: JAIDS 60 (Suppl 1):S1, 2012. (continued)*						
Osteonecrosis (Avascular necrosis) *CID 51:937, 2010*	**HIV itself, tenofovir** *(CID 51:963, 2010),* **boosted atazanavir & efavirenz suspect.**	Onset: Can be abrupt S&S: 85% involve one or both femoral heads, humeral heads, proximal tibia	4.8/100 person yrs. Asymptomatic by MRI 4%	Diabetes; prior steroid use; alcohol use; Vitamin D deficiency low CD4 count.	No steroids. Periodic MRIs to assess disease progression. Check Vitamin D levels.	Remove risk factors; less weight-bearing; some require total joint arthroplasty. Vitamin D supplement if levels low.
ADVERSE EFFECTS THAT INFLUENCE QUALITY OF LIFE						
Fat Maldistribution: Association with elevated intracellular concentration of stavudine *(CID 50:1033, 2010)*						
Lipoatrophy *(JID 205 (Suppl 3): S383, 2012)*	**NRTIs, especially Stavudine > zidovudine. > TDF, ABC, 3TC, FTC, esp. when combined with EFV** *(CID 51:591, 2010).*	Loss of subcutaneous fat on face, buttocks & extremities. Note: HLA-B*4001 presence risk factor for stavudine-associated lipodystrophy *(CID 50:597, 2010).*	Precise frequency unknown	Low nadir CD4 count, older age. Low baseline body mass index (BMI).	If possible, avoid stavudine and zidovudine.	• Change NRTI to ABC or TDF/TAF • FDA-approved fillers: Poly-L-lactic acid (Sculptra); Ca hydroxyapatite (Radiesse) • If insulin resistant: Pioglitazone *(JID 195:1731, 2007).*
Fat Accumulation: Lipodistrophy (Lipohyper-trophy)	PI or NNRTI combined with d4T or ZDV.	Excess adipose tissue in abdominal viscera, breast size, dorsocervical fat pad. Management: Tesamorelin responders had ↓ in triglycerides & adiponectin levels *(CID 54:1642, 2012).*	Precise frequency unknown	Obesity prior to HIV infection; low CD4 count prior to therapy; older age; low baseline BMI.	Avoid combination of PI or NNRTI with d4T or AZT. Switching from LPV/r to ATV/r ↓ visceral fat *(AIDS 23:1349, 2009).*	**What helps?** Growth hormone releasing factor (tesamorelin -EGRIFTA) ↓ visceral fat by 18% *(JAIDS 53:311, 2010, Med Lett 53:33, 2011).* If type 2 DM: metformin. Limited role for surgery.
Gastrointestinal— Diarrhea	**All protease inhibitors (PIs), didanosine (Videx)**	Onset: 1st dose Symptoms: Perhaps worst with lopinavir/ritonavir, nelfinavir, & buffered didanosine	Varies	All patients	Antidiarrheals	Loperamide, diphenoxylate/atropine, calcium tabs, psyllium products, pancreatic enzymes, L-glutamate.
Osteopenia & Osteoporosis *(see Osteonecrosis, page 46)*	Bone loss, 2° HIV, TDF, boosted atazanavir, EFV *(JID 205 (Suppl 3): S391, 2012)*	Months to years; increased risk of fractures	Unclear but higher than general population	Low vitamin D levels *(CID 52:396, 2011)*	Vitamin D supplements	Perhaps increased risk with stavudine & TDF; consider bisphosphonates
Peripheral neuropathy	**Didanosine (Videx), stavudine (Zerit) > ddI & ddC**	Onset: Weeks to months S&S: Usually legs. Numbness & paresthesias. Often irreversible even if drug(s) stopped.	Didanosine 12–34% Stavudine 52%.	Pre-existing neuropathy; advanced HIV; concomitant drugs that ↑ intracellular didanosine, e.g., ribavirin, tenofovir.	Avoid use, esp. in combination	If painful can try gabapentin or tricyclic antidepressants; lamotrigine, carbamazepine (watch for drug interactions), topiramate, tramadol, narcotics, topical capsacin.

TABLE 6D: OVERLAPPING TOXICITIES BETWEEN ANTIRETROVIRALS AND OTHER DRUGS COMMONLY USED IN HIV PATIENTS (Anti-HIV Drugs are BOLD)

Bone Marrow Suppression	Periperal Neuropathy	Pancreatitis	Nephrotoxicity	Hepatotoxicity	Rash	Diarrhea	Ocular Effects
Amphotericin B	**Didanosine**	Cotrimoxazole	Acyclovir (IV, HD)	Azithromycin	**Abacavir**	Atovaquone	Cidofovir
Cidofovir	Isoniazid	**Didanosine**	Adefovir	Clarithromycin	**Atazanavir**	Clindamycin	**Didanosine**
Cotrimoxazole	Linezolid	**Lamivudine** (child)	Aminoglycosides	**Darunavir**	Atovaquone	**Darunavir**	Ethambutol
Cytotoxic chemotherapy	**Stavucine**	Pentamidine	Amphotericin B	**Delavirdine**	Cotrimoxazole	**Fosemprenavir**	Linezolid
Dapsone		**Ritonavir**	Atazanavir (stones)	Didanosine (portal hypertension)	Dapsone	**Lopinavir/ritonavir**	Rifabutin
Flucytosine		**Stavudine**	Bictegravir*	Dolutegravir	**Darunavir**	**Nelfinavir**	
Ganciclovir			Cidofovir	**Efavirenz**	**Delavirdine**	**Ritonavir**	
Hydroxyurea			**Cobicistat***	Fluconazole	**Efavirenz**	**Tipranavir**	
Interferon-alpha			Dolutegravir*	Isoniazid	**Fosamprenavir**		
Linezolid			Foscarnet	Itraconazole	**Maraviroc**		
Peg-interferon alpha			**Indinavir** (stones)	Ketoconazole	**Nevirapine**		
Primaquine			Pentamidine	**Maraviroc**	Raltegravir		
Pyrimethamine			Ritonavir*	**Nevirapine**	Sulfadiazine		
Ribavirin			**Tenofovir-DF**	**Didanosine** (hepatic steatosis)	**Tipranavir**		
Rifabutin			(↓ with TAF)	**PIs** (esp. tipranavir)	Trimethoprim/		
Sulfadiazine			* ↑ creatinine,	Rifabutin	sulfamethoxazole		
Trimetrexate			no effect on GFR	Rifampin			
Valganciclovir				Voriconazole			
Zidovudine							

Ref: *Guidelines for use of antiretroviral agents in HIV-1 infected adults and adolescents, DHHS, http://aidsinfo.nih.gov*

TABLE 6E: SELECTED ANTIRETROVIRAL DRUGS IN DEVELOPMENT
(Late 2018)

Drug Name(s), Number, (Manufacturer)	Drug Class (Site of Anti-HIV Activity)	Dose	Comments
Apricitabine (ATC)	NRTI	600 mg twice daily Dose being finalized in current studies	3TC-like agent with activity against virus harboring an M184V mutation. Antagonistic against 3TC and FTC. **Drug back in development.**
BMS-995176	Maturation Inhibitor	Dose finding underway (120 mg po daily)	2nd generation maturation inhibitor. Broader coverage against the gag region of the virus. Binds tightly and reversibly to most gag proteins. Active against multiple PI-resistant viruses. Total bilirubin increases in majority of recipients.
Cabotegravir	INSTI	600 mg IM q 8 weeks OR 800 IM q12 w	Nanotechnology formulation of Dolutegravir, permitting long-exposure, less frequent (e.g., every 2 - 3 month) dosing. Antiviral activity the same as dolutegravir. Needs to be co-administered with other long-acting agents, such as long-acting formulation of rilpivirine; In the future might be paired with EFdA (above). Promising as an approach to PrEP.
Cenicriviroc (TBR-652)	CCR5 - CCR2 Inhibitor	100 mg or 200 mg daily Dose still being determined	Phase III trials about to begin. CCR2 inhibition may produce anti-inflammatory effect.
Fostemsavir (BMS 663068)	Attachment Inhibitor	1200 mg oral once daily dose	Blocks entry of virus by binding to viral gp120 and preventing attachment of virus to CD4 receptor. Inherent 'resistance' in 12% of patients who harbor a virus that has a polymorphism in gp120 that results in decreased binding affinity of the drug.
MK-8591 (EFdA)	NRTTI (Nucleoside reverse transcriptase translocation inhibitor)	10 mg oral daily or parenteral extended release (once q 3 monthly)	Inhibits NT by preventing translocation. Active against HIV 1, HIV2 and MDR strains. Long-acting (>180 days in rat model); potential to be administered once a year.
Pro-140	CCR5 Antagonist	324 mg SQ once weekly or biweekly	Studies underway to determine dose, safety, activity.

TABLE 6F: LIQUID FORMULATIONS OF ART DRUGS

See http://www.hivclinic.ca/main/drugs_extra_files/Crushing%20and%20Liquid%20ARV%20Formulations.pdf

Drug	Dosage Forms Available	Liquid Formulation	Special Instructions for Liquid Formulations	Crush Tablet or Open Capsule	Stability of Tablet/Capsule or Liquid when Mixed
Nucleos(t)ide Reverse Transcriptase Inhibitors (NRTIs)					
Abacavir (Ziagen)[1]	Tablet: 300 mg **Scored tablet** (available in '09-'10): 300 mg[2] Oral Solution	Oral Solution: 20 mg/mL	No reconstitution necessary	Tablets may be crushed and contents mixed with a small amount of water or food and immediately ingested.	
Didanosine (Videx)[1,2]	EC Capsules: 125 mg, 200 mg, 250 mg, 400 mg Generic EC capsules: 200 mg, 250 mg, 400 mg Pediatric Powder for Oral Solution	Powder for oral soln: 2 gm or 4 gm btl (final conc 10 mg/mL)	Reconstitute powder to 20 mg/mL by adding 100 or 200 mL Purified Water to the 2 gm or 4 gm pwd btl. Then mix one part of the 20 mg/mL initial soln with one part Max Strength Mylanta for a final conc of 10 mg/mL. **Shake well and take on empty stomach.** Preferred dosing of liquid is twice daily dosing although once daily may be used to increase compliance—**more PK data with solution to support BID dosing[2].**	Beads in capsules are enteric coated. Capsules may be opened and sprinkled on a small amount of food.	The Videx powder final admixture may be stored up to 30 days in **refrigerator[1,2].**
Emtricitabine (Emtriva)[1,2]	Capsule: 200 mg Oral Solution	Oral Solution: 10 mg/mL	No reconstitution necessary. The solution bioavailability is 80% that of the capsule, therefore dose is 240 mg of solution vs 200 mg for capsule. Store in refrigerator.	No data	Oral solution should be stored in refrigerator[2]. Stable at room temperature for 3 months[2].
Lamivudine (Epivir)[1,2]	Tablets: 100 mg, 150 mg, 300 mg **Scored tablet:** 150 mg[2] Oral Solution	Oral Solution: 10 mg/mL	No reconstitution necessary	Tablets can be crushed and contents mixed with small amount of water or food and immediately taken.	Store oral solution at room temperature[2]
Stavudine (Zerit)[1,2]	Capsules 15 mg, 20 mg, 30 mg, 40 mg (available as Brand and generic) Oral Solution	Powder for Oral Soln: 1 mg/mL (200 mL btl)	Add 202 mL purified water to powder container. Shake container vigorously until powder dissolves completely. This produces 200 mL of 1 mg/mL stavudine solution.	Capsules can be opened and contents mixed with small amounts of food or water (stable in solution for 24 hrs if kept refrigerated).	Prepared solution may be stored up to 30 days in **refrigerator[1,2].** Shake well prior to use. Capsule contents mixed with food or water and in solution are stable for 24 hours if kept refrigerated.

TABLE 6F (2)

Drug	Dosage Forms Available	Liquid Formulation	Special Instructions for Liquid Formulations	Crush Tablet or Open Capsule	Stability of Tablet/Capsule or Liquid when Mixed
Nucleos(t)ide Reverse Transcriptase Inhibitors (NRTIs) *(continued)*					
Tenofovir-DF (Viread)[1]	Tablet: 150 mg, 200 mg, 250 mg, 300 mg	40 mg TDF per 1 gm oral powder	Mix oral powder in 2 - 4 oz of soft food. Tablets dissolve in water, orange juice or grape juice	Consume quickly to avoid taste. DO NOT MIX WITH LIQUIDS. Use soft food only. Tenofovir-AF powder formulation not available (yet)	
Zidovudine (Retrovir)[1,2] All products available as generic	Tablet: 300 mg Capsule: 100 mg Oral Solution Intravenous Solution	Oral Solution: 10 mg/mL Intravenous soln: 10 mg/mL	No reconstitution necessary	Capsules may be opened and dispersed in water or onto a small amount of food and ingested immediately. Tablets may be crushed and combined with a small amount of food or water and ingested immediately.	Capsules and/or tablets opened or crushed and mixed with food or water must be taken immediately.
Non-Nucleoside Reverse Transcriptase Inhibitors (NNRTIs)					
Delavirdine (Rescriptor)[1]	Tablet: 100 mg, 200 mg	None		100 mg tablets may be dispersed in water; place 4 tablets in at least 90 mL, let stand then stir for uniform dispersion, consume promptly, rinse glass and swallow rinse to ensure entire dose[1] 200 mg tablets do **not** disperse in water.	Unknown – take **immediately** upon dispersion of 100 mg tablets in water[1].
Efavirenz (Sustiva)[1,2]	Capsules: 50 mg, 200 mg Tablet: 600 mg	None *Liquid formulation is undergoing current studies[2].*	Capsules may be opened and added to 1-2 tsp of liquids or foods (e.g. applesauce, grape jelly, yogurt, reconstituted infant formula at room temperature) but may result in peppery taste. Grape jelly may mask taste. Specific instructions: *(AJHP 2010;67(3):217-22; DHHS 2017).*	Capsules may be opened and added to liquids or small amounts of food[2]. Capsules may have very peppery taste so may be better to mix with something sweet to disguise taste.	
Etravirine (Intelence)[1]	Tablet: 25 mg, 100 mg, 200 mg	None (but tablets can be dissolved to form liquid slurry)	Place one 200 mg tablets in a glass of water. Stir well until the water looks milky and drink it immediately. Rinse glass several times with water and swallow rinse each time[1,2].	Yes – Tablets may be dissolved.	Unknown, should be used immediately[2].
Nevirapine (Viramune)[1]	**Scored tablet:** 200 mg Oral Suspension.	Oral Suspension: 10 mg/mL.	No reconstitution necessary. Shake well before use. Store at room temperature[2].	Tablets can be crushed and combined with a small amount of food or water and administered immediately.	Crushed tablets mixed with food or water should be administered immediately.
Rilpivirine	25 mg	None		No data	

TABLE 6f (3)

Drug	Dosage Forms Available	Liquid Formulation	Special Instructions for Liquid Formulations	Crush Tablet or Open Capsule	Stability of Tablet/Capsule or Liquid when Mixed
Protease Inhibitors (PIs)					
Atazanavir (Reyataz)[2]	Capsules: 50 mg, 200 mg, 300 mg	50 mg packet		Mix atazanavir oral powder with at least 1 tablespoon of food such as applesauce or yogurt. Oral powder mixed with a beverage (at least 30 mL of milk or water) may be used for adults or older infants who can drink from a cup. For young infants (<6 months) who cannot eat solid food or drink from a cup, oral powder should be mixed with at least 10 mL of infant formula and given using an oral dosing syringe.	
Darunavir (Prezista)[2]	Tablets: 75 mg, 150 mg, 400 mg, 600 mg (75 mg tab available in '09-'10)[2].	100 mg/mL oral suspension		Must be given with 100 mg of ritonavir, either liquid or capsule formulation. Administer darunavir with food.	Store oral suspension in the original container at room temperature (25° C / 77° F) and shake well before dosing.
Fosamprenavir (Lexiva)[2]	Tablets: 700 mg Oral Suspension	Oral Suspension: 50 mg/mL	Adults should take suspension **without** food. Pediatric pts should take suspension **with** food[2]. Shake well prior to use. Store at room temperature[2].	No data	
Indinavir (Crixivan)[2]	Capsules 100 mg, 200 mg, 333 mg, 400 mg	None		No data	
Lopinavir/ritonavir (Kaletra)[2]	Tablets: 100/25 mg, 200/50 mg Pediatric tablets: 100/25 mg Pediatric oral solution	Pediatric oral solution: 80/20 mg per mL (contains 42.4% alcohol by volume)	Oral solution should be administered **with** food[2].	**No –** tablets must be swallowed whole. Do not crush or split tablets[2].	Store oral liquid in refrigerator but stable at room temperature for 2 months[2].
Nelfinavir (Viracept)[2]	Tablets: 250 mg, 625 mg Powder for oral suspension. Crushed tablets are preferred over the powder for solution due to difficulties with powder.	Powder for oral suspension: 50 mg per one level gram scoop full (200 mg per one level teaspoon) Dissolved tablets are usually better tolerated than pwdr for oral suspension[2].	For powder for oral suspension: powder **may** be mixed with water, milk, pudding, ice cream, or formula. Do **NOT** mix with acidic food/juice and do not add water to bottles of powder![2] Must use scoop provided with oral powder for measuring purposes[2].	Tablets can be dissolved in a small amount of water. Once dissolved, cloudy mixture should be taken immediately. Rinse glass several times with water and drink rinse. Tablets can also be crushed and administered with pudding[2].	Mixture of powder with water, milk, pudding, ice cream, and formula is stable for up to 6 hours[2].

TABLE 6F (4)

Drug	Dosage Forms Available	Liquid Formulation	Special Instructions for Liquid Formulations	Crush Tablet or Open Capsule	Stability of Tablet/Capsule or Liquid when Mixed
Protease Inhibitors (PIs) *(continued)*					
Ritonavir (Norvir)[2]	Capsules: 100 mg Oral solution	Oral solution: 80 mg/mL (contains 43% alcohol by volume)	Solution should be stored at room temperature. Do NOT refrigerate. Shake well before use. Oral solution may be mixed with milk, chocolate milk, vanilla or chocolate pudding, or ice cream[2].	No	If oral solution is mixed with milk or other food, take immediately.
Saquinavir (Invirase)[1]	Capsule: 200 mg Tablet: 500 mg	None		No data	
Tipranavir (Aptivus)[2]	Capsule: 250 mg Pediatric oral solution	Pediatric oral solution: 100 mg/mL	Oral solution contains 116 IU per mL of vitamin E.	No	Oral solution should be stored at room temp. Must use solution within 60 days after opening bottle.
Entry/Fusion Inhibitors					
Enfuvirtide (Fuzeon)[2]	Injection for SQ	None		N/A	Reconstituted vial should be allowed to stand until powder goes completely into solution. Do not shake. Once reconstituted, vial should be used immediately or kept refrigerated until use but no more than 24 hrs. Do not draw up in syringe until time for use!
Maraviroc (Selzentry)[2]	Tablets: 150 mg, 300 mg	None		No data	

TABLE 6F (5)

Drug	Dosage Forms Available	Liquid Formulation	Special Instructions for Liquid Formulations	Crush Tablet or Open Capsule	Stability of Tablet/Capsule or Liquid when Mixed
Integrase Inhibitors					
Dolutegravir	Tablet: 50 mg	50 mg/10 gm pediatric oral granule formulation and dispersible tablet formulations (in development)		No data	
Raltegravir (Isentress)[1,2]	Tablet: 400 mg	Chewable 100 mg scored and 25 mg tablets; Granules 100 mg for oral suspension		Chewable tablets can be chewed or swallowed whole; Oral suspension is provided with a kit that includes two mixing cups, two dosing syringes, and 60 foil packets. Each foil, single-use packet contains 100 mg of raltegravir, which will be suspended in 5 mL of water for final concentration of 20 mg/mL. Dose should be administered within 30 minutes of mixing; unused solution should be discarded	
Combination Agents					
Abacavir/Lamivudine (Epzicom)[1]	Tablet	None--Liquid formulations are available as individual agents		No	
Abacavir/Zidovudine/ Lamivudine (Trizivir)[1]	Tablet	None--Liquid formulations are available as individual agents		No	
Bictegravir/TAF/FTC	Tablet	None		No data	
Elvitegravir/Cobicistat/ TDF/Emtricitabine (Stribild)	Tablet 150 mg	None		No	
Emtricitabine/TDF/ Efavirenz (Atripla)[1]	Tablet	None		No (current studies to see whether Atripla may be crushed are on-going – no results yet)	
Emtricitabine/TDF (Truvada)[1]	Tablet	None		No	
Zidovudine/Lamivudine (Combivir)[1]	**Scored tablet**	None--Liquid formulations are available as individual agents		Tablets can be crushed and mixed with a small amount of food or water and taken immediately.	Tablets in solution should be administered immediately.

[1] Source: package inserts
[2] *Guidelines for the Use of Antiretroviral Agents in Pediatric HIV Infection, Mar 1, 2016, http://AIDSinfo.nih.gov*

TABLE 7A: ACUTE HIV INFECTION

FIGURE 5 Natural History and Staging of HIV Infection

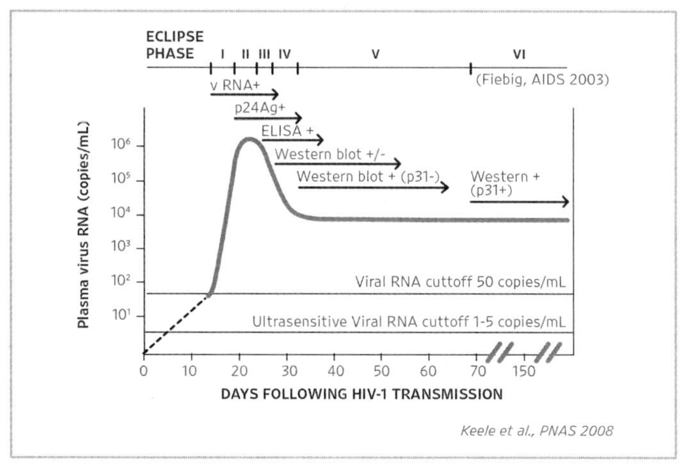

Acute (Recent or Primary) HIV Infection

- **Definition:** Initial burst of HIV viremia with undetectable anti-HIV antibody
- ART should be initiated immediately when HIV infection is recognized (even before resistance test results return). *(CID 60(11):1715, 2015);J Virol.88(17):10056, 2014*
- Perform genotype drug resistance testing (estimated 8% - 18% transmission of resistant virus)
- Use same regimens as recommended for treatment of chronic HIV infection, though preference for DTG- or BIC- containing regimen, since resistance to these drugs is uncommon. Combine with TAF-FTC, since HLA-B5701 testing not immediately available. Adjustment to this initial (urgent) regimen can be made once the baseline data have returned.
- Goal is suppression of viral load to below detectable limits
- **Once ART is started, therapy should continue for life**

Special Populations *(see www.aidsinfo.nih.gov)*

a. **Injection drug users.** Active drug use may compromise adherence. Potentially co-existing neuropsychiatric symptoms & ↑ prevalence of Hep B & Hep C add to risk of drug toxicities. Drug interactions may potentially cause ↑ or ↓ blood levels of ART drugs, & of methadone or drugs of abuse *(Mt Sinai J Med 67:429, 2000)*.

b. **Co-infection with Hep B &/or Hep C *(See Table 12, page 131)*.** Co-infection with HBV requires treatment with a TDF or TAF containing regimen. Lamivudine and emtricitabine have activity, but should not be used without TAF or TDF as components of the regimen. **Therefore the use of TAF/FTC and TDF/FTC or TDF/3TC are the nucleoside/nucleotide backbones of choice in HIV/HBV co-infected pts** because of concerns about emergence of HBV resistance when 3TC or FTC is used without tenofovir (TAF/TDF). When TDF cannot be used, entecavir should be added to the ARV regimen. If uncertain how to treat, seek expert consultation.

Severe hepatitis flare *(see Black Box warnings)* may occur in pts with chronic Hep B after stopping any anti-HBV drugs. In HCV/HIV co-infected pts, ↑ rate of progression to cirrhosis if HCV not treated. All patients with HIV/HCV coinfected should be treated for HCV, with cure of HCV expected in > 98% of treated patients. Start ARV Rx first, then treat for HCV once stable on ARV Rx.

Changes in ART drug elimination with hepatic dysfunction may necessitate dosing changes *(CID 40:174, 2005; see Table 15C)*. Therapeutic drug monitoring should be considered when there is significant liver dysfunction.

c. **Adolescents:** Adult guidelines for ARV use are generally appropriate for post-pubertal adolescents. Dosage should be prescribed according to Tanner staging of puberty and not on the basis of age. If Tanner Stage I and II, dose according to Pediatric dosing recommendations; if late puberty Tanner V, dose according to Adult dosing recommendations. Youth in a growth spurt should continue with pediatric dosing initially. Adherence to medication is particularly challenging in adolescent populations and need to be managed carefully. Efavirenz should be used with caution among female adolescents owing to potential teratogenicity concerns.

TABLE 7B: HIV EXPOSURE MANAGEMENT

A. HIV OCCUPATIONAL EXPOSURE

The decision to initiate post-exposure prophylaxis (PEP) is a clinical judgment made in concert with the exposed individual and is based on three factors:

1. Type of exposure
   a. Potentially infectious substances include: blood, unfixed tissues, CSF; semen and vaginal secretions (these have not been implicated in occupational transmission of HIV); synovial, pleural, peritoneal, ascitic, and amniotic fluids; other <u>visibly</u> bloody fluids.
   b. Fluids of low or negligible risk for transmission, unless visibly bloody include: urine, sweat, vomitus, stool, saliva, nasal secretions, tears, and sputum. **PEP is not indicated.**
   c. If the exposure occurred to intact skin, regardless of whether the substance is potentially infectious or not, and regardless of the HIV status of the source patient, **PEP is not indicated.**
   d. If the exposure occurred to mucous membranes (e.g., blood splash to the eye) or non-intact skin (e.g., abraded skin, open wound, dermatitis) or occurred percutaneously as a consequence of a needle stick, scalpel, or other sharps injury or cut, then **PEP may be indicated.** Human bites resulting in a break in the skin could theoretically transmit HIV, particularly if oral blood is present, although these have not been implicated in occupational transmission of HIV.

2. Likelihood that the source patient is HIV infected
   a. If the exposure constitutes a risk of HIV transmission as described above and the source patient is **known positive for HIV**, then **PEP should be instituted** immediately, within hours of exposure (Animal studies show PEP less effective when started >72h post-exposure but interval after which PEP not beneficial is unknown; initiation of PEP after a longer interval may be considered if exposure risk of transmission is extremely high).
   b. If exposure constitutes a risk of HIV transmission, and the HIV status is **unknown**, but patient is **likely to be HIV infected** or there is a **reasonable suspicion** for infection based on HIV risk factors, then **PEP should be initiated pending confirmation of the source patient's HIV status.**
      i. If a rapid HIV test of the source patient can be performed, it is reasonable to withhold therapy pending results of this test and initiating PEP if the test is positive.
      ii. If rapid testing cannot be performed, PEP should be initiated pending results of source patient testing and discontinued if the test returns negative.
      iii. NOTE: Antibody testing is sufficient to rule out HIV infection, unless the source patient has suspected acute retroviral syndrome, in which case HIV viral load testing is recommended.
   c. If the **source is unknown** or the source is known but status and risk cannot be determined, the decision to initiate PEP should be made on a case-by-case basis in **consultation with an expert** (PEPline at 1-888-448-4911 or *http://www.nccc.ucsf.edu/about_nccc/pepline/*), guided by the severity of the exposure and epidemiologic likelihood of HIV exposure.

3. Adverse effects and potential for drug interactions with the PEP regimen
   a. Newer agents are better tolerated and should allow a higher proportion of exposed healthcare providers to complete the prescribed four-week course of therapy. Doses of some agents may need to be adjusted based on renal function.
   b. Information about drug interactions is available at *https://www.hiv-druginteractions.org/checker*, in the package insert and on-line at *hivinsite.ucsf.edu.*
   c. Breast feeding and pregnancy are not contraindications to PEP.

FIGURE 6   PEP Algorithm

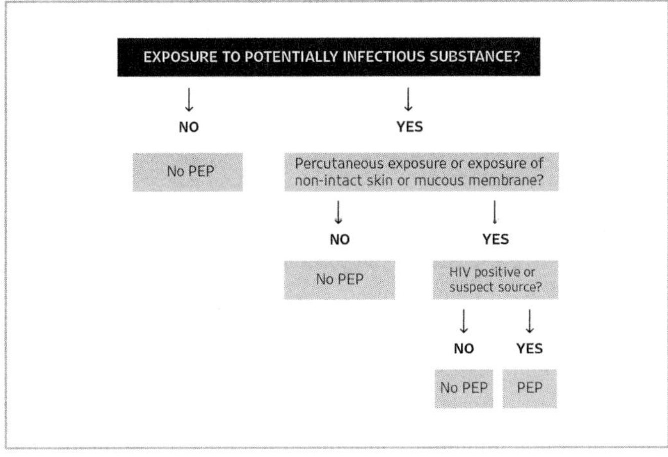

TABLE 7B (2)

REGIMENS FOR PEP: a 4-week course of 3 or more drugs now routinely recommended for all PEP

Preferred Regimen	**Descovy** (FTC 200 mg + TAF) (but not recommended if CrCl <30 mL/min) po once daily + (**Raltegravir** 1200 mg (two 600 mg tabs) once daily or **Dolutegravir** 50 mg orally daily) If Creatinine clearance < 30 mL/min: [**Tenofovir disoproxil fumarate** (TDF) 300 mg q72-96h + **Emtricitabine** (FTC) 200 mg q72-96h + (**Dolutegravir** 50 mg po once daily OR Raltegravir 400 mg po twice daily]
Alternative Regimens	**Descovy** po once daily + ([**Darunavir** 800 mg po once daily + **Ritonavir** 100 mg po once daily] or [Prezcobix (**Darunavir** 800 mg + **Cobicistat** 150 mg) one tab once daily]) OR
	Descovy po once daily + Lopinavir-Ritonavir 800/200 mg po once daily OR
	Creatinine clearance < 30 mL/min: Renally adjusted doses of **Zidovudine** + **Lamivudine** + **Darunavir** 800 mg po once daily + **Ritonavir** 100 mg po once daily

1. Abacavir, efavirenz, enfuvirtide, maraviroc should be used only in consultation with an expert
2. Didanosine, nelfinavir, tipranavir, stavudine (d4T) and nevirapine (contraindicated) are not recommended
3. If transmission of drug resistant virus is suspected, the regimen should be appropriately modified in consultation with an expert to include agents to which it is likely to be susceptible.
4. **Descovy is the preferred substitute for Truvada** given lower potential for renal injury and osteomalacia for TAF vs. TDF. Note that Descovy is not recommended for CrCl <30 mL/min.
5. Do not use dolutegravir in pregnancy. Efavirenz can be used with caution.

FOLLOW-UP
1. Complete blood count, renal and hepatic panels recommended at baseline and repeated at 2 weeks with further testing if results are abnormal.
2. HIV antibody testing to monitor seroconversion should be performed at baseline, 6 weeks, 12 weeks, and 6 months post-exposure.
3. If a 4th generation p24 antigen-HIV antibody test is used, testing may be terminated at 4 months.
4. Extended follow-up for 12 months is recommended if HCV conversion occurred upon exposure to an HIV-HCV co-infected patient.

B. HIV NON-OCCUPATIONAL EXPOSURE
- Risk of transmission of HIV via sexual contact or needle sharing may reach or exceed that of occupational needlestick exposure, thus HIV post-exposure prophylaxis (PEP) not later than 72 hours (and ideally within a few hours) of the exposure is recommended for HIV-negative persons non-occupationally exposed to blood or other potentially infected fluids from an HIV+ source.
- Substantial risk of HIV acquisition from HIV+ source
    - Exposure of vagina, rectum, eye, mouth, mucous membrane, non-intact skin, percutaneous contact
    - With blood semen, vaginal secretions, rectal secretions, breast milk, or any body visibly contaminated with blood
- Negligible risk of HIV acquisition regardless of HIV status for any exposure to
    - Urine, nasal secretions, saliva, sweat, or tears if not visibly contaminated with blood
- PEP not effective and not recommended if ≥73 hours after an exposure.
- 4-week course of 3 ARV drugs is recommended for PEP.

Preferred Regimens

Age	Regimen
Age ≥13 years (not pregnant women; avoid TAF and DTG with pregnancy. Use **TDF** 300 mg + **FTC** 200 mg instead of Descovy as part of regimen), CrCl ≥30 mL/min	**Descovy** (Emtricitabine [FTC] 200 mg + Tenofovir alafenamide fumarate [TAF]) + (**Dolutegravir** 50 mg po once daily OR **Raltegravir** 400 mg po twice daily) (*See comments;* not recommended if CrCl is <30 mL/min).
Age ≥13 years (in pregnancy use **TDF** 300 mg + **FTC** 200 mg instead of Descovy), CrCl <30 mL/min	**TDF** 300 mg q72-96h + **FTC** 200 mg q72-96h + (**DTG** 50 mg po once daily OR **RAL** 1200 po once daily)
Children aged 2-12 years	**TDF** + **FTC** + Raltegravir, each dose adjusted for age and weight
Children aged 4 weeks to <2 years	**Zidovudine** + **Lamivudine** + (**Raltegravir** OR **Lopinavir-Ritonavir**) each as an oral solution dose adjusted for age and weight
Children aged birth to 27 days	Consult a pediatric HIV specialist

Alternative Regimens

Age	Regimen
Age ≥13 years (includes pregnant women), CrCl ≥30 ml/min	**Descovy** (FTC 200 mg + Tenofovir alafenamide fumarate [TAF]) + **Darunavir** 800 mg po once daily + **Ritonavir** 100 mg po once daily (See comments; not recommended if creatinine clearance is <30 ml/min).
Age ≥13 years (includes pregnant women), CrCl <30 ml/min	Renally adjusted doses of **Zidovudine** + **Lamivudine** + **Darunavir** 800 mg po once daily + Ritonavir 100 mg po once daily
Children aged 2-12 years	**Zidovudine** + **Lamivudine** + (**Raltegravir** OR **Lopinavir-Ritonavir**) once daily each dose adjusted for age and weight OR **TDF** + **FTC** + (**Lopinavir-Ritonavir** OR [**Darunavir** + **Ritonavir**]) each dose adjusted for age and weight
Children aged 4 weeks to <2 years	**Zidovudine** + **FTC** + (**Raltegravir** OR [**Lopinavir-Ritonavir**]) each as an oral solution dose adjusted for age and weight

- **Descovy (FTC + TAF) is preferred over Truvada (FTC + TDF)** given lower potential for renal injury and osteomalacia for TAF compared to TDF. However, if subject is pregnant, use TDF with FTC (Truvada) as part of the regimen.
- If transmission of drug resistant virus is suspected, the regimen should be appropriately modified in consultation with an expert to include agents to which it is likely to be susceptible.
- Baseline testing and follow-up:
    - All patients initiating nPEP after potential HIV exposure should be tested for the presence of HIV-1 and HIV-2 antigens and antibodies ideally before nPEP initiation using a rapid test. Patients with existing HIV infection should not be started on nPEP. There should be no delay in initiation of nPEP which should be started while awaiting baseline HIV test results.
    - Click here for recommendations for laboratory evaluations of source and exposed persons.

PRE-EXPOSURE PROPHYLAXIS (PREP) FOR MEN WHO HAVE SEX WITH MEN (MSM)

Once daily **Truvada** (combination of FTC 200 mg + TDF 300 mg) resulted in a 44% decrease in incidence of HIV infection in one clinical trial *(NEJM 363:27, 2010)*. NB: It remains uncertain whether the newer formulation of tenofovir alafenamide fumarate (TAF) is effective as part of a PrEP regimen (though it seems likely to be effective). Therefore, TAF based regimens are not currently recommended for PrEP. Questions remain about cost-effectiveness overall. *(Ann Intern Med 156:541, 2012)*. PrEP is considered a key component in a comprehensive HIV prevention agenda globally, especially when used to prevent transmission among MSM. Recent data from the US indicates that the life-time risk of acquisition of HIV in MSM is 1:6; for black MSM, the risk is 1:2. *(Hess et al, CROI 2016, # 52; and http://www.cdc.gov/nchhstp/newsroomdocs/factsheets/lifetime-risk-hiv-dx-us.pdf)*. As demonstrated below, PrEP when used with more extensive and successful ARV Rx can reduce new infections in the US by 75%.

TABLE 8A: HIV/AIDS IN WOMEN/PREGNANCY

I. **General Aspects**
   A. Women represent half of persons with HIV/AIDS in the world. Among young people (15–24 yrs) in developing countries with HIV/AIDS, 64% are women. In 2014, 19% of new HIV diagnoses were among women.
   B. Heterosexual transmission is dominant mode of transmission worldwide. Among new HIV/AIDS diagnoses among women in the U.S. in 2014: 87% heterosexual contact, 13% IDU.
   C. Transmission of HIV from men to women occurs more readily than from women to men. Risk factors for male-to-female transmission: genital ulcers, partner with advanced disease, other STDs, trauma.
   D. Risk after several years of unprotected sex with same infected partner is 10–45%.
   E. Despite these aspects, relatively less is written about women's issues. Women are generally underrepresented in therapy trials.

II. **Initial Assessment:** *See Table 2*

III. **Clinical Manifestations** (Adapted from *Newman, MD, Global HIV/AIDS Medicine 2008*)
   A. **AIDS-defining diagnoses:**
   - Disease progression similar in women & men *(NEJM 333:751, 1995)*.
   - Survival is related to access to care, which may be worse for women.
   - Viral load at high CD4 counts tends to be lower in women *(CID 35:313, 2002)*.
   - Gender difference narrows as CD4 drops.
   B. **Human papillomavirus (HPV):**
   - HPV disease incidence increased! Cervical intraepithelial neoplasia (CIN) more prevalent in multiple studies. Prevalence increases with decreasing CD4 *(CID 38:737, 2004)*.
   - Aggressive course, with high rate of progression to cancer if immunosuppressed.
   - Pap smear recommended for HIV+ women. If initial Pap smear is neg, repeat in 6 mos. If both are negative, annual Pap smears adequate *(CDC Guidelines)*. We recommend every 6 mos for those with CD4 <200. Colposcopy recommended for any suspicious lesions. There are no contraindications to standard treatment modalities for CIN. Risk of recurrence higher after treatment.
   - Although many women with HIV are already infected with some HPV genotypes, there may be benefit to use of HPV vaccine according to recommendations for HIV negative women.
   C. **Recurrent/refractory vaginal candidiasis**
   - May be early manifestation although poorly predictive of HIV infection *(CD4 may be >500)*.
   - HIV diagnosis often missed because testing not offered.
   D. **Other conditions**
   - PID may be more severe, 7–17% require hospitalization; tubo-ovarian abscess more likely.
   - Menstrual disorders (41% HIV+ women had menstrual abnormalities vs. 24% in controls) include irregular periods, heavier or scantier periods, early menopausal symptoms, ↑ in premenstrual symptoms.

IV. **Family Planning.** 85% of women with AIDS are in child-bearing years. Contraceptive and pre-conceptional planning are essential components of care. Hormonal contraceptives are generally safe in HIV+ women and HIV+ women can use all forms of hormonal contraception including implants and IUDs. (AIDS 29:2353 2015) However, only condoms protect against STIs and HIV transmission. Be aware of interactions between ARV's and hormonal contraception, most significant for ritonavir. For interactions *https://aidsinfo.nih.gov/guidelines/html/3/perinatal-guidelines/152/overview*.

Method of Contraception	Failure Rate	Risks
Sterilization	0.4	No HIV protection
Latex condom	12-15	HIV and STI protection
Diaphragm	16	Potential vaginal abrasions
Sponge	9-32	Potential vaginal abrasions
Oral Contraceptive	3-8	Drug interactions with ART decrease efficacy or increase side effects
Injectable depot progestin	3	No significant ART interactions. May increase HIV shedding. Use condoms in addition
Copper IUD	<1	No HIV protection
Hormonal IUD	<1	No HIV protection. May lower amprenavir levels. Other ART may change estrogen level
Implant	<1	Progestin only no significant interactions
Vaginal ring	1-9	Effect of drug interactions on efficacy unknown

V. **Treatment Issues**
   A. **Inadequate gender-specific data!**
   B. **Theoretical issues**
   - Baseline anemia (iron deficiency)
   - Low mean body weight, higher body fat, different hepatic metabolism compared to men
   C. **Menstrual dysfunction**
   - Amenorrhea should be evaluated; start with pregnancy test
   - Premature menopause occurs frequently; consider short term hormone replacement therapy
   D. **Recommended treatment regimens currently identical for men & women**
   - Rates of some side effects different in women (↑ rash and hepatitis on nevirapine with CD4 >250, ↑ GI side effects on lopinavir/ritonavir)
   - **Efavirenz should be avoided in women who may become pregnant** [though not prohibited under new Guidelines *(DHHS and WHO)*]
   - Lactic acidosis more common in women, associated with d4T & ddI

TABLE 8A (2)

VI. **HIV in Pregnancy: Care of the Mother**
   A. **Pre conception counseling**
   - All HIV + women should be asked if they are or might consider becoming pregnant
   - For serodiscordant couples who want to conceive, several options are available including pre-exposure prophylaxis (PrEP). Maximal viral suppression of the HIV-infected partner is critical. For discussion, *see "Reproductive Options for HIV-Concordant and Serodiscordant Couples"* in Recommendations for Use of Antiretroviral Drugs in Pregnant HIV-1-Infected Women for Maternal Health and Interventions to Reduce Perinatal HIV Transmission in the United States 2014 available at *http://aidsinfo.nih.gov/guidelines/html/3/perinatal-guidelines/0*
   - HIV+ women who wish to become pregnant should achieve maximally suppressed viral load first
   - Recommend folate supplement or multivitamin during pre-conception period and pregnancy

   B. **Antepartum Care**
   - **All pregnant women should be offered HIV testing & counseling regardless of risk factors.** Include HIV in routine unless patient declines (opt-out testing)
   - Repeat HIV screening in the 3rd trimester for women with ongoing risk
   - Quantitative measure of **HIV RNA** initially 1 month after starting ART, then every 3 months
   - Obtain CD4 count and percent at outset & each trimester (some ↓ CD4 count in normal pregnancy)
   - **Screening tests** (HBsAg, RPR, chlamydia, gonorrhea) as in any pregnancy
   - Discourage illicit alcohol use, drug use, smoking, unprotected sex with multiple partners
   - Administer influenza, pneumococcal, Hep B, Hep A, and Tdap vaccines, as indicated *(MMWR 60 (RR 2, RR41), 2011)*
   - Assess need for OI prophylaxis

   C. **Use of antiviral therapy in pregnancy** *(www.aidsinfo.nih.gov)* (updated July 2012). Treatment of HIV in pregnancy requires attention to 2 separate but equal goals:
   - Provide optimal treatment to the woman and reduce viral load to <50 cps/mL
   - Prevent transmission to the infant without drug toxicity
      1. Risk factors for mother-to-child transmission (MTCT)
         - Maternal viral load (outset & at delivery are independent predictors *(JID 183:539, 2001)*
         - Maternal CD4 count (risk of transmission ↑ 3-fold if CD4 <400)
         - Lack of antiviral therapy (independent of other factors) *(JID 183:539, 2001)*
         - Prolonged rupture of membranes (rate doubled if >4 hours) *(NEJM 334:1617, 1996)*
         - Mode of delivery
         - Breastfeeding (additional 10–14% transmission) *(JAMA 282:744, 1999)*
         - Shorter duration of antepartum ART *(AIDS 22:973, 2008)*
      2. General principles
         - Preventing MTCT should be integrated with obstetrical & HIV medical care for the mother. The mother should be informed & involved in decisions
         - Combination antiretroviral therapy ↓ risk of MTCT regardless of viral load
         - ARV is generally safe for the mother (avoid use of ddI with d4T—↑ risk of lactic acidosis; Package insert continues to recommend avoiding EFV in 1st trimester but human data are reassuring.
         - Maximal viral suppression with combination therapy ↓ risk of resistance in mother & loss of future options, & is more effective than 1- or 2-drug regimens. **Preferred for all pregnant women**
         - Resistance testing recommended before beginning ART and if on therapy, but detectable viral load
         - Long-term safety of ART for infant exposed in utero is not fully known. Generally safe, although conflicting data on mitochondrial toxicity; myocardial function *(J Am Coll Cardio 57:76, 2011)*
         - Some data suggest ↑ rate of prematurity, low birth weight with PI use during pregnancy; given clear benefits, PIs should not be withheld
         - Optimal dosing in pregnancy has not been adequately studied for all agents
         - PI levels fall in third trimester (nelfinavir, indinavir, lopinavir/ritonavir, atazanavir). Consider obtaining levels
      3. **Combination therapy with 2 NRTIs and a potent third drug is preferred for all pregnant women regardless of CD4 count or viral load** *(see http://www.aidsinfo.nih.gov)*
         - Transmission 0.7-2.0% with 3 drug ART
         - Principles of regimen selection are generally the same for pregnant women as for non-pregnant women
         - Consider treatment experience, resistance, tolerability, comorbidities, convenience, drug interactions and experience in pregnancy
         - All pregnant women should be screened for Hep B and Hep C. TDF/FTC is the preferred NRTI backbone for Hep B/HIV co-infected women
         - Antepartum, intrapartum and post-natal ART for the infant are all important
         - Women on ART who become pregnant and are fully suppressed should continue regimen If they have detectable viremia, resistance testing and optimization of adherence and resistance testing follow principles for non-pregnant
         - **Design a 3 drug regimen regimen with at least one drug with high transplacental passage: Abacavir, 3TC, FTC, TDF, ZDV, NVP (if possible)**: *(See chart in the next page)*

TABLE 8A (3)

Preferred NRTI backbone + 3rd drug (treatment naïve patient)	• **ABC/3TC** or • **TDF/FTC** + (select one from next column) • **ZDV/3TC** is an alternative	*Preferred* • **ATV/r** or • **DRV/r** or • **Raltegravir** *Alternative* • **LPV/r** (twice daily only) or • **Rilpivirine** or • **NVP**
Notes: - **EFV** can be used after first 8 weeks of pregnancy. Recent meta analysis on teratogenicity reassuring but concern remains based on animal studies *(AIDS 28 Supl2:S123 2014)*. - Data for **DTG** is limited		

4. Severe skin rash, ↑ transaminases & rarely fulminant hepatitis can occur after starting nevirapine. Rates higher in non-pregnant women than in men, esp. with higher CD4 count. Monitor LFTs, instruct mother to seek care for nausea, abdominal pain. Check transaminases in any woman who develops rash. **Consider non-nevirapine containing regimens if CD4 count >250 unless benefits clearly outweigh risks**

D. **Intrapartum Care-Specific situations** (consider obtain HIV VL at 34-36 weeks to help)
1. **For pregnant women who have been on combination ART and have sustained viral suppression and HIV RNA <1000 copies/mL at or near delivery:** Continue oral combination ART during labor. Therapy can be continued preoperatively with sips of water even if caesarian section is planned. Intravenous zidovudine is not required.
2. **For pregnant women who have received antepartum combination ART but have suboptimal viral suppression near delivery.** Women who have HIV RNA >1000 copies/mL should be offered scheduled C-section at 38 weeks. Intravenous zidovudine should be given along with the other oral ART. Additional antiretroviral prophylaxis for the neonate should be considered *(see D.4 below)*
3. **Women in labor who have not received combination ART during pregnancy:** All HIV-infected women who present in labor who were not on therapy and those with a positive rapid HIV test should be immediately started on intravenous zidovudine. Additional antiretroviral prophylaxis should be given to the neonate.
4. **Postpartum antiretroviral prophylaxis for infants born to HIV-infected women**
   - All infants should receive postpartum prophylaxis with oral zidovudine for at least 4 weeks
   - A 4-week regimen can be considered for infants of women with consistent viral suppression during pregnancy and no concerns about maternal adherence. All other should receive 6 weeks *(see Table 8F for dose based on gestational age)*
   - **Infants born to women who were not on combination ART or who had suboptimal viral suppression benefit from additional antiretroviral prophylaxis.** In NICHD-HPTN 040/PACTG 1043 use of zidovudine plus 3 doses of nevirapine (birth, 48 hours after dose 1, and 96 hours after dose 2) reduced transmission from 4.9% to 2.2% *(NEJM 366:2368, 2012)*. No trial data exist by experts increasingly using 3 drug regimens for prophylaxis. Reasonable safety and PK data exist for ZDV, 3TC (2 mg/kg 2x/day) and nevirapine (6 mg/kg 2x/day). Anemia and neutropenia common. Raltegravir is under investigation.
   - **Prophylaxis for infants born to women with antiretroviral resistance must be individualized. Expert Consultation Recommended (National (US) Perinatal Hotline 1-888-448-8765)**
   - If an infant on antiretroviral prophylaxis is found to be HIV infected by HIV RNA or DNA PCR, prophylaxis should be stopped immediately and treatment should be initiated with combination ART
   - In high resource settings where formula and safe water are available, breast feeding should be avoided. Recommendations for combination ART for HIV-infected who breast feed in low resource settings include "option B+" – lifelong combination ART for the mother regardless of CD4 count and "option B"- combination ART for the mother for the duration of breastfeeding if treatment is not otherwise indicated. *(See WHO PMTCT guidelines http://www.avert.org/world-health-organisation-who-pmtct-guidelines.htm)*

E. **Elective C-section before the onset of labor** ↓ transmission by 50% for women on no therapy or ZDV monotherapy *(NEJM 340:977, 1999)*. However, in recent cohorts on 3-drug therapy with suppressed HIV RNA, no apparent additional benefit of C-section was observed *(AIDS 22:973, 2008)*.
- This should be discussed with the woman & she should be involved in the decision.
- Elective C-section (before 38 weeks) should be considered if:
  - Maternal viral load >1000 at delivery despite ART. Possible benefit if >50 copies.
- Unknown viral load at delivery
  - Mother received less than 3-drug therapy
  - Mother presents late in pregnancy
  - Obstetrical indications or maternal preference
- Elective C-section is not cost-effective in resource-poor settings
- Cefazolin prophylaxis recommended for C-section.
- AROM, fetal scalp electrodes, operative delivery (forceps, vacuum extractor) and episiotomy should be avoided unless clear obstetric indications exist.

F. **Pneumocystis pneumonia (PJP) prophylaxis:** Recommended for women with CD4 count <200 or on prophylaxis. PJP during pregnancy can be more severe.
- **TMP/SMX** may be used, although use in last trimester may be associated with ↑ bilirubin. Risk of kernicterus unknown but very small. TMP/SXZ reduced maternal & infant mortality among mothers with CD4 <200 in resource poor setting. 1st trimester exposure might be related to small increase in birth defect rate.
- **Dapsone:** no known adverse effects, although experience limited.
- **Aerosolized pentamidine.** Little systemic absorption, although less effective in advanced disease. Effect of ventilation changes due to pregnancy on distribution is unknown. Can be used in 1st trimester.

TABLE 8B: HIV IN THE FETUS & NEWBORN

GENERAL:

- In 2011, about 200 children <13 were diagnosed with HIV infection in the U.S. Only 55 new perinatal infections were reported. Almost 11,000 people were living with perinatally acquired HIV. The number of new perinatal infections has also decreased significantly worldwide, and will continue to decline Worldwide, an estimated 2.5 million children are living with HIV.
- In the US in 2011, African Americans accounted for 77% of HIV diagnoses in children (age <13 yrs) but only 14% of the population. Hispanics/Latinos accounted for 13% of HIV diagnoses; Caucasians accounted for 15% of HIV diagnoses, but 58% of the population.
- Thus, the success of HIV testing and treatment of pregnant women dramatically ↓ HIV infection in children. **Universal testing & counseling must be offered to all pregnant women.**
- In 2006, an estimated 8700 infants were born to HIV-positive mothers in the US. This number has increased substantially *(JAIDS 57:218, 2011)*.
- An increasing number of children with HIV in the U.S. are foreign born and at increased risk of TB, non-subtype B infection and intrapartum nevirapine resistance.

TRANSMISSION:

- **Over 90% of HIV+ children in U.S. acquired infection from their mothers perinatally:** in utero, during delivery, or postpartum through breastfeeding. Risk of transmission 13–40% *(http://aidsinfo.nih.gov/guidelines)*.
- **Time of transmission:**
    - In utero: HIV has been identified in fetal tissues as early as 8 weeks. Probably in the majority, in utero transmission occurs late in pregnancy *(Lancet 345:518, 1995)*.
    - Intrapartum: 50–70% of transmissions believed to occur through exposure to mother's blood, cervical secretions or amniotic fluid during delivery.
    - Postpartum acquision rare in developed countries, important in developing countries. Breast-fed infants have a 10-14% add'l risk of becoming infected. In mothers seroconverting during lactation, risk is 1/3 *(Lancet 342:1437, 1993)*.

DIAGNOSIS: *(See Table 8C, next page)*

- HIV can be diagnosed in most infants by 1-2 mos & all infants by 6 mos of age by demonstration of virus by viral RNA PCR or DNA PCR. Viral culture is not used for routine diagnosis.
- HIV DNA PCR is sensitive and specific by 2-4 weeks of age (>90% sensitive). Quantitative RNA PCR assays are at least as sensitive and may better detect non-subtype B virus and provide viral load data. Low viral loads (<5000 copies/mL) must be repeated and confirmed *(http://aidsinfo.nih.gov/ guidelines, JID 175:707, 1997; J AIDS 32:192, 2003)*. HIV RNA assays may theoretically be falsely negative in infants receiving combination therapy for post partum prophylaxis. Some experts perform both assays. Others use HIV RNA PCR to confirm positive HIV DNA PCR.
- Maternal anti-HIV IgG crosses the placenta & persists until 9–15 mos, so infants born to HIV-infected mothers may test positive for up to 15 mos regardless of infection. Assays for p24 antigen are less sensitive & less specific than PCR.
- PCR should be performed:
    - By age 48 hrs (not on cord blood) (In children at high risk of perinatal infection e.g. acute HIV infection during pregnancy, detectable viral load at delivery, no ARV or ARV at delivery only).
    - At 2–3 wks
    - At 4–8 wks
    - Repeat at 4–6 mos if initial tests negative
- Consider repeat testing 2-4 weeks after end of prophylaxis for infants at high risk of transmission. Any pos test should be repeated immediately along with quantitative HIV RNA PCR (viral load) before treatment begun.
- **Presumptive evidence of in utero infection is PCR positive in 1st 48 hours of life.** Intrapartum infection defined by negative test in 1st 48 hours followed by positive test *(NEJM 275:606, 1995)*.
- If PCR is not available, HIV can be diagnosed by persistence of HIV antibody after 18 months of age.
- HIV infection can be presumptively excluded by 2 negative PCRs; one at >14 days and one at >1 month; HIV is definitively excluded (in absence of breast feeding) by at least 2 negative PCR tests; one at >1 month and one at >4 months.

NATURAL HISTORY:

- Bimodal distribution. Approximately 20-35% will be rapid progressors with onset of symptoms by median 8 months & median survival of <2 yrs.
- Median survival, untreated, for non-rapid progressors was 66 mos. Survival has greatly ↑ in the era of ART, & many perinatally infected children are reaching adolescence & young adulthood and transitioning to adult care.

TABLE 8C: HIV INFECTION IN CHILDREN

1. HIV-Infected
   - Child <18 mos with positive virologic assays (HIV RNA or DNA PCR) on 2 separate determinations from one or more: HIV DNA PCR, HIV RNA PCR.
   - Child ≥18 mos born to HIV+ mother or infected by blood products, sexual contact who is HIV antibody + by ELISA & Western blot or + PCR (2 separate samples).
2. Perinatally Exposed: A child who does not meet criteria above but
   - is HIV seropositive & <18 mos of age.
   - unknown antibody status but born to HIV+ mother.
3. HIV-uninfected (definitive): Child with 2 or more HIV PCR assays which are neg: 1 after 1 month and 1 after 4 mo of age, or HIV antibody negative after 6 months (2 separate specimens).

HIV Infection Stage Based on Age-Specific CD4 Cell Counts or Percentage

Stage	Age of Child					
	<12 mos		1–5 yrs		6–12 yrs	
	CD4/µL	(%)	CD4/µL	(%)	CD4/µL	(%)
	≥1,500	(≥34)	≥1,000	(≥30)	≥500	(≥6)
	750–1,499	(26-33)	500–999	(22-29)	200–499	(14-25)
	<750	(<26)	<500	(<22)	<200	(<14)

REVISED WHO STAGING SYSTEM FOR HIV INFECTION & DISEASE IN CHILDREN
(See http://www.who.int/HIV/paediatric/infants2010/en)

Clinical Stage 1:	Asymptomatic
Clinical Stage 2:	Mild
Clinical Stage 3:	Advanced
Clinical Stage 4:	Severe

TABLE 8D: CHILDREN: INITIAL EVALUATION, INITIATION OF ANTIRETROVIRAL THERAPY, PJP PROPHYLAXIS & SUPPORTIVE THERAPY

A. **Initial evaluation of the HIV-infected child**
   1. Document actual HIV infection
   2. History
      - General well-being
      - Infections and HIV-related conditions
      - Disclosure status
      - Growth and Developmental status, educational level, school performance
      - Psychiatric history
      - Medications (including over-the-counter and other supplements/complementary meds)
      - Social history including parent/caregiver's health, drug use, insurance
      - Sexual and drug use history
      - Risk factors for opportunistic infections including places of residence, travel, pets
      - Immunization history and documentation
   3. Comprehensive Physical Exam
      - Plot height, weight, BSA
      - Attention to lymph nodes, cardiac, dermatologic, developmental, neurologic exams
   4. Baseline Laboratory Evaluation
      - Complete blood count
      - Complete metabolic panel including BUN, creatinine, LFT's, cholesterol and lipid profile
      - RPR, TB testing (eg. QuantiFERON TB Gold), CMV antibody, Hepatitis B surface antibody (HBsAb), HBsAg, HBcAb Hepatitis C antibody, perhaps vitamin D level
      - For adolescents, chlamydia/gonorrhea nucleic antibody testing
      - HLA-B*5701 testing
   5. HIV staging
      - CD4 count and CD4 percent, quantitative HIV RNA, genotypic resistance testing
   6. Initial Health Maintenance
      - HIV risk reduction as age appropriate. Include contraception and safer sex for adolescents. Long acting reversible contraception should be considered for contraception with condoms to prevent disease transmission.
      - Psychosocial support
      - Immunization update *(See Table 19)*

TABLE 8D (2)

3. **Pneumocystis pneumonia (PJP)—Revised Guidelines**
   1. In infants with perinatally acquired HIV, PJP occurs most frequently at 3–6 mos, often acute in onset with poor prognosis. HIV+ infants <1 yr of age at risk even with CD4 ≥1500.
      - Identify infants born to HIV+ mothers promptly (screen mothers during pregnancy), obtain PCR as described above.
      - Begin PJP prophylaxis at 4-6 wks in infants born to HIV-infected mothers who are HIV positive or who remain indeterminate.
      - Stop prophylaxis in children found to be presumptively HIV-negative (e.g., 2 negative PCRs; one obtained after 14 days and one after 1 mo of age).
      - Continued PJP prophylaxis in HIV-infected children until 1 year of age. Continue if CD4 <500 cells/µL or <15% for kids 1-6 years. In resource poor settings, WHO recommends for all HIV-exposed children age <2 yr, WHO Clinical Stage 2, 3 or 4, or CD4% <25%.
   2. Drug Regimens for PJP Prophylaxis in Children ≥4 wks of Age:
      - **TMP/SMX (150 mg TMP/M2/day)** po divided twice daily 3x/wk on consecutive days (i.e., Mon., Tues., Wed.). Alternatives: same daily dose 1x/day. Once-daily regimen may be best for adherence.
      - If TMP/SMX not tolerated:
         - **Dapsone 2 mg/kg po 1x/day** or 4 mg/kg po q wk
         - **Aerosolized pentamidine (children ≥5 yrs) 300 mg** via Respirgard II inhaler monthly
         - **Atovaquone 30 mg/kg po q24h** for children 1–3 mos old. Atovaquone 45 mg/kg po q24h for children 4–24 mos.

4. **Antiretroviral Therapy (ART) in Children**
   1. **When to start:** Data specific to outcomes in children are limited, & clinical trial data do not address when to start. Natural history studies in children & extrapolation from adult studies are used to derive guidelines. Most factors argue for early treatment in children:
      - 25–35% of HIV-infected children will be rapid progressors
      - Viral load & CD4 are associated with rapid progression but cannot accurately identify all rapid progressors in first year of life
      - The CHER study in South Africa demonstrated improved survival in asymptomatic infected infants when therapy was started at <12 months compared to waiting for symptoms *(4th AIDS Conference on HIV Pathogenesis, Treatment and Prevention 2007 Sydney Abstract LB WES103)*
      - Immune control of virus limited in first year of life
      - HIV encephalopathy, other neurological disease & cardiac involvement may occur at young age
      - **Trials in adults have shown clear benefits to early treatment. (NEJM 373:795 2015). Therefore, ART is now recommended for all children regardless of disease stage**

      Some factors, nonetheless, are different in children:
      - Slow progressors may maintain good immune function for many years without treatment
      - Limited number of drugs with liquid formulation
      - Difficulties with adherence are common & lead to drug failure
      - Children still have somewhat more limited treatment options

TABLE 8D (3)

Three sets of guidelines have been developed. They share several features. In infants who are known to be HIV-infected, they favor starting therapy in all infants, due to the inability to identify rapid progressors. In older children, the guidelines favor treatment, especially when the child shows immune deterioration. All emphasize the need for education to ensure adherence, & routine monitoring for efficacy & safety:

RECOMMENDATIONS FOR BEGINNING TREATMENT IN INFANTS & CHILDREN

Age Group	DHHS 2016	PENTA 2015	WHO 2013
<12 months	**Treat** All (AI) Urgent	**Treat** All	**Treat** All (strong recommendation, moderate quality evidence)
12-<24 months	**Treat** • CDC stage 3-defining OI (AI) **Urgent** • CDC stage 3 immunodeficiency: CD4 <500 cells/ µL(AI) Urgent • CD4 500-999 cells/µL (AII) • Moderate HIV-related symptoms (AII) • HIV RNA >100,000 copies/µL (AII) • Asymptomatic or mild symptoms and CD4 ≥1000 cells/µL (BI)	**Treat** • CD4 ≤1000 cells/mL • CD4% ≤25% • WHO stage 3/4 • CDC stage B or C • HIV RNA >100,000 copies/µL **Consider** • All	**Treat** All children with HIV (conditional recommendation, very low-quality evidence)
24-<36 months			
36 months <5 years		**Treat** • CD4 ≤750 cells/mL • CD4% ± 25% • WHO stage 3/4 • CDC stage B or C **Consider** • HIV RNA ≥100,000 copies/mL	
>5 years	**Treat** • CDC Stage 3-defining OI (A1) **Urgent** • CD4 <200 cells/µL (AI) **Urgent** • CD4 cells 200-499/µL • Moderate HIV-related symptoms (AII) • HIV RNA >100,000 copies/µL (AII) • Asymptomatic or mild symptoms <u>and</u> • CD4 ≥500 cells/µL (BI)	**Treat** • CD4 <350 cells/mL • WHO stage 3/4 • CDC stage B or C **Consider** • HIV RNA ≥100,000 copies/mL • CD4 cells ≤500 cells/µL	**Treat** • WHO Stage 3 or 4 • CD4 <500 cells/µL • CD4 cells <350 cells/µL priority strong recommendation, moderate-quality evidence

DHHS: Panel on Antiretroviral Therapy and Medical Management of HIV-Infected Children. Guidelines for the Use of Antiretroviral Agents in Pediatric HIV Infection. March 5, 2016. Available at *http://aidsinfo.nih.gov/ContentFiles/PediatricGuidelines.pdf*
PENTA: PENTA Steering Committee. PENTA 2015 guidelines for the use of antiretroviral therapy in pediatric HIV-1 infection. HIV Medicine (2015), *www.ncbi.nlm.nih.gov/pubmed/25649230*
WHO: WHO. Consolidated ARV guidelines June 2013. Available at *http://www.who.int/hiv/pub/guidelines/arv2013/art/statartchildren/en/*
(The strength of the recommendation [A-C] and the strength of the evidence (I-III] is shown for the DHHS recommendations)

* Excludes LIP or single episode of serious bacterial infection

2. **Recommended therapy**

    Combination therapy with at least 3 antiretroviral drugs is recommended for all children started on therapy. Choice of drugs depends on supporting data, age of the patient, local availability, & need for liquid formulation. WHO guidelines emphasize initial use of NNRTI-based regimens because of costs, local availability, & to complement adult guidelines. U.S. & European guidelines recommend regimens shown below, but recognize the risk of NNRTI-resistant virus being transmitted from mother to child *(see below)*.

    If available, resistance testing should be obtained for children before starting ART, especially if an NNRTI is being considered. If the local prevalence of resistance is known, it may influence the need for resistance testing.

    If abacavir therapy is being considered, HLA B*5701 screening can virtually eliminate risk of hypersensitivity reaction and should be obtained if available.

TABLE 8D (4)

RECOMMENDED FIRST-LINE THERAPY FOR HIV-INFECTED INFANTS & CHILDREN

	DHHS 2015	PENTA 15	WHO 2013
Preferred	**Infants birth to <14 days:** 2 NRTIs plus nevirapine **Neonates/infants aged ≥42 weeks postmenstrual and ≥14 days postnatal and children <3 years:** 2 NRTIs[1] **plus** lopinavir/ritonavir **Children ≥3 to <6 years:** 2 NRTIs[1] plus atazanavir + low dose ritonavir **or** twice daily darunavir + low dose ritonavir **or** raltegravir **Children ≥6 years to <12 years:** 2 NRTIs plus atazanavir + low dose ritonavir or dolutegravir **Children ≥12 years and not sexually mature[2]:** 2 NRTIs **plus** atazanavir + low-dose ritonavir **or** dolutegravir or once daily darunavir + low dose ritonavir **or** elvitegravir + cobicistat **Children ≥12 years who are sexually mature:** refer to adult guidelines *Table 6A*	**Infants <1 years:** 2 NRTIs **plus** lopinavir/ritonavir **or** 2 NRTIs **plus** nevirapine **Children 1-3 years:** 2 NRTIs **plus** lopinavir/ritonavir **or** 2 NRTIs **plus** nevirapine **Children 3-6 years:** 2 NRTs plus lopinavir/ritonavir **or** efavirenz **Children 6-12 years:** 2 NRTs plus atazanavir/ritonavir **or** efavirenz **Children ≥12 years:** 2 NRTs plus atazanavir/ritonavir **or** efavirenz or darunavir/ritonavir	**Children <3 yrs:** 2 NRTIs **plus** lopinavir/ritonavir **Children ≥-10 yrs:** 2 NRTIs plus efavirenz **Adolescents:** TDF + 3TC (or FTC) + efavirenz
Preferred NRTIs	**Infants <3 months:** zidovudine + 3TC or FTC **Children >3 months to <12 years:** abacavir[1] + 3TC or FTC **or** zidovudine + 3TC or FTC **Children ≥12 years and not sexually mature:** abacavir[1] + 3TC or FTC or TAF + FTC **Adolescents tanner 4 or 5:** refer to *Table 6A* (Adult ART)	**Children <3 years:** abacavir[1] + 3TC (+zidovudine if nevirapine and high viral load) **Children 3-12 years:** abacavir[1] + 3TC **Children >12 years:** tenofovir + FTC or abacavir[1] + 3TC (if VL <100,000 copies/µL)	**Children <3 years:** abacavir[1] + 3TC or zidovudine + 3TC **Children ≥3-9 yrs:** abacavir[1] + 3TC **Children ≥10 yrs (>35 kg):** tenofovir + 3TC or FTC
Alternative NRTIs	**Children aged ≥2 weeks:** zidovudine + ddi or ddi + 3TC or FTC **Children aged ≥3 months:** zidovudine + abacavir **Children aged ≥13 years:** zidovudine + 3TC or FTC **Children and adolescents Tanner 3:** Tenofovir + 3TC or FTC	**Children 0-12 years:** zidovudine + 3TC **Children 3-12 years:** Tenofovir + 3TC or FTC	**Children ≥3-9 yrs:** tenofovir + 3TC or FTC **Children ≥10 yrs:** Zidovudine + 3TC
Alternative Regiments	**Children >14 days to <3 years:** 2 NRTIs + nevirapine **Children aged ≥3 months to <3 years and ≥10 kg:** 2 NRTIs +atazanavir + low-dose ritonavir **Children aged ≥4 weeks and <2 years and ≥3 kg:** 2 NRTIs + raltegravir **Children aged ≥3 years to <6 years:** 2 NRTIs **plus** EFV **or** lopinavir + low dose ritonavir **Children aged ≥6 years to <12 years:** 2 NRTIs **plus** darunavir + low dose ritonavir **or** EFV **or** lopinavir + low dose ritonavir **or** raltegravir **Adolescents aged ≥12 years and not sexually mature:** 2 NRTIs **plus** efavirenz **or** raltegravir **or** rilpivirine	**Children 3-12 years:** 2 NRTIs + darunavir/ritonavir **or** nevirapine **Children >12 years:** 2 NRTIs + lopinavir/ritonavir **or** raltegravir **or** dolutegravir	2 NRTIs + nevirapine

HLA-B* 5701 genetic testing should be performed and abacavir should not be used if a child tests positive for HLA-B* 5701

Co- formulated products may be appropriate for older children who meet appropriate weight guidelines (and are Tanner stage 4-5 if tenofovir-containing) and may improve compliance. Examples include but are not limited to TDF/FTC/EFV; TDF/FTC/elvitegravir/cobicistat(COBI); TDF/FTC/rilpivirine; ABC/3TC/dolutegravir(DTG); DTG/CCBI; ATZ/COBI

DHHS: Panel on Antiretroviral Therapy and Medical Management of HIV-Infected Children. Guidelines for the Use of Antiretroviral Agents in Pediatric HIV Infection. March 5, 2015. Available at *http://aidsinfo.nih.gov/ContentFiles/PediatricGuidelines.pdf*

PENTA: PENTA Steering Committee. PENTA 2015 guidelines for the use of antiretroviral therapy in paediatric HIV-1 infection. HIV Medicine (2015), *www.ncbi.nlm.nih.gov/pubmed/25649230*

WHO: WHO. Consolidated ARV guidelines June 2015. Available at *http://www.who.int/hiv/pub/arv/policy-brief-arv-2015/en/*

TABLE 8D (5)

3. **Monitoring of children on antiretroviral therapy (ART)**
    Children should be monitored at 1-2 weeks after beginning a new antiretroviral regimen to check for adherence and adverse effects. When nevirapine is started, serum transaminases should be monitored at 2 and 4 weeks and then monthly for 3 months.
    Children on antiretroviral therapy should be followed at regular intervals, usually every -4 mos.
    Clinical parameters:
    *   Weight & height growth
    *   Nutritional status (including Vitamin D levels)
    *   Developmental milestones & neurological symptoms
    *   Adherence & side effects
    *   No consensus on bone mineral density testing by DEXA but considered by some experts especially if on TDF before puberty

    Laboratory monitoring should include: CBC with differential, CD4 % & count. If available, viral load, liver enzymes, creatinine, glucose, electrolytes, & total cholesterol should be monitored. Laboratory monitoring can be reduced to every 6 months after 2-3 years if normal CD4, suppressed VL, no concerns about adherence. Periodic testing for sexually transmitted infections for sexually active adolescents.

4. **Therapeutic drug monitoring**
    Age-related changes in drug metabolism & wide interpatient variability of drug levels suggest that therapeutic drug monitoring may be very useful for PIs & NNRTIs after unexpected failure or for unusual regimens. In some European countries, therapeutic drug monitoring has become routine. Information on laboratories & on laboratory participation in quality assurance programs is available at *www.hivpharmacology.com.* Target minimum trough concentrations in *Table 6F* and in the *DHHS Guidelines for the Use Antiretroviral Agents* at *www.aidsinfo.nih.gov.*

5. **When to change antiretroviral therapy**
    The goal of initial therapy is to suppress viral load to the lowest level possible, usually below the limits of quantification, & to allow the immune system to reconstitute. For children who are fully suppressed, it may become desirable to change regimens as the child grows and becomes able to swallow pills to simplify regimen, allow once daily dosing, and improve adherence.

    For children whose regimen has failed *(see below)*, **the goal of subsequent regimens is to re-establish maximal viral suppression.** With the availability of newer agents in pediatric formulations, it has become possible to construct regimens for many treatment-experienced children when viral suppression cannot be achieve, the goal is to prevent immunologic deterioration while limiting the development of additional resistance mutations.

    Poor adherence is the most common cause of ART failure. Starting a new regimen without addressing behavioral or social causes of non-adherence will lead to development of additional resistance. Inadequate dosing, poor absorption, and viral resistance can also lead to failure. The decision on when to start a new regimen will depend on addressing adherence, remaining options, clinical status, family preference, & family situation.

    Considerations on when to change are divided into virologic, immunologic, & clinical. Most decisions are based on virologic failure.

Virologic failure	• **Incomplete response:** Less than a minimally acceptable virologic response after 8–2 wks of therapy (defined as a <10-fold (1.0 log$_{10}$) decrease from baseline HIV RNA levels • HIV RNA not suppressed to <200 copies after 4–6 mos of antiretroviral therapy • **Viral Rebound:** Repeated detection of HIV RNA >200 copies in children who initially had undetectable levels in response to antiretroviral therapy. Consider observation and repeat testing if rebound temporary adherence problem.
Immunologic failure	• **Incomplete immunologic response to therapy:** Failure of a child with severe immune suppression (CD4 percentage <15%) to ↑ CD4 at least above the age-specific cutoff for severe immunosuppression.
Clinical failure	• Progressive neurodevelopmental deterioration* (2 or more of: impaired brain growth, cognitive decline, or motor dysfunction) • Growth failure: persistent decline in weight-growth velocity despite adequate nutritional support & without other explanation* • Severe or recurrent infection or illness – Recurrence or persistence of AIDS-defining conditions or other serious infections*
Toxicity	• It may be desirable to control some side effects (e.g., diarrhea dyslipidemia or GI upset) rather than changing therapy. If a single drug can be associated with the toxicity, it is acceptable to change the offending agent

* Criteria marked with asterisk are from WHO guidelines (& may overlap with DHHS recommendations). These may be particularly helpful in the resource-limited setting.

6. **What to use as alternate therapy** *(see also Table 6F)*
   There are limited data on sequencing antiviral therapy in HIV-infected children. Several general principles are useful (See also *TABLE 5B* - failure in adults):
   a. When treatment failure occurs, always assess adherence to the treatment
   b. Try to address adherence problems before changing regimens
   c. If adherence has been good, assume viral resistance has developed, but it may not have developed to all agents. Viral resistance testing, if at all possible, should be performed. If possible, obtain viral resistance testing while on failing regimen. Without testing, all 3 drugs should be changed if possible
   d. Take into account predicted cross-resistance
   e. Avoid dose reduction for toxicity unless levels can be measured
   f. Treatment failure may occur due to inadequate absorption or drug levels
   g. Consider enrolling in clinical trial
   h. **The use of at least 2 new active drugs with non-overlapping resistance best predicts response. Never add a single drug to a regimen that is clearly failing**
   i. **Consider likelihood of availability of (or ability to use) new drugs in near future and try and construct regimen with 2-3 active drugs**
   j. If regimen with 2 active drugs cannot be constructed or adherence cannot be assured and clinically stable, consider waiting and maintaining partially suppressive regimen, e.g., lamivudine monotherapy
   k. If adherent patient is failing in absence of severe resistance, consider measuring drug levels and addressing pharmacokinetic issues

). **Supportive Treatment & Prophylaxis**

   1. Intravenous gamma globulin (IVIG)
      a. Not routinely used. Recommended for infants & children with evidence of humoral immune defects (hypogammaglobulinemia or documented failure to form specific antibody responses) IVIG 400 mg/kg q28 days is recommended.
      b. Thrombocytopenia (<20,000/mm^3) on antiretroviral therapy: IVIG 0.5–1 gm/kg/dose x 3–5 days
         (See Table 21 for WinRho®)
   2. Immunization: *See Table 19*
   3. Pneumocystis jirovecii: *See above, Section A*
   4. Mycobacterium avium complex: prophylaxis recommended for advanced immune suppression *https://aidsinfo.nih.gov/contentfiles/lvguidelines/oi_guidelines_pediatrics.pdf.* Begin if CD4 <50 for children ≥6 yrs; 2–6 yrs, if CD4 <75; 1–2 yrs if CD4 <500; <1 yr CD4 <750. Clarithromycin 7.5 mg/kg po q12h or azithromycin 20 mg/kg po once weekly is preferred. Rifabutin now used as 3rd-line, 5 mg/kg po once daily (only for children ≥6 yrs). Dose of rifabutin should not exceed 300 mg/day. Can discontinue MAC prophylaxis if stable viral suppression for ≥6 mos and CD4 count above target for prophylaxis ≥3 mos.
   5. Psychosocial support *(see Am Acad Pediatrics, Red Book, 1994):* School attendance, child/foster care, adolescent education

TABLE 8E: CLINICAL SYNDROMES, OPPORTUNISTIC INFECTIONS IN INFANTS & CHILDREN, WHICH DIFFER FROM ADULTS

In HIV-infected infants & children, disease progression is manifest by decrements in growth & delayed neurodevelopment as well as opportunistic infections as occur in adults

(J Ped 128:58, 1996)

CLINICAL SYNDROME	INFANT/CHILD	ADULT	CLINICAL FEATURES (in children)/COMMENTS
Central Nervous System			
Encephalopathy			General: HIV encephalopathy is a syndrome that includes motor & cognitive dysfunction seen in pts with advanced HIV. Administration of ARV therapy has been shown to be beneficial in treating children with HIV encephalopathy.
Static course	Common	0	25% children show cognitive & motor deficits. Most have head circumference in 10–25th percentile. Problems with verbal expression, attention deficits, hyperactivity. Mild ↑ reflexes in legs to spastic diplegia. IQ stable.
Plateau course	Uncommon	0	Infant's or child's gain of cognitive or motor skills plateaus. Motor deficits are common. IQ usually only 50–79.
Subacute progressive course	Uncommon	AIDS dementia common	Gradual progressive decline in motor, language, adaptive function. Early, child is alert, wide-eyed, with a paucity of facial movements. Endstage: mute, dull-eyed, quadriparetic. CSF: mild pleocytosis, ↑ protein, may be + for HIV antibody & virus. CT: atrophy, progressive calcification in basal ganglia (most common in infants & young children).
Focal brain diseases: seizures, focal neurologic deficits			
Infections			
Toxoplasmosis	V. rare	Common	Toxo is uncommon in infants & children since it is most often due to reactivation.
Progressive multifocal leuko-encephalopathy (JC virus)	V. rare	Common	PML is uncommon in infants & children since it is most often due to reactivation.
Endocrine			
Failure to thrive & growth retardation	Common	Wasting syndrome common	33/36 HIV+ children showed failure to thrive, not purely related to diarrhea & malnutrition. Known causes of growth failure are growth hormone deficiency, hypothyroidism, & glucocorticoid excess. 1/3 of HIV+ children have abnormal thyroid function (↑ thyrotropin, ↑ TBG) which correlates with disease progression *(J Ped 128:70, 1996)*. Inc rate of delayed puberty.
Eye			
Cytomegalovirus retinitis	Uncommon	Common	CMV chorioretinitis in 1.6% children vs. 10–20% in adults *(Arch Ophthal 107:978, 1989)*. In children, it usually occurs with generalized CMV infection, viremia & multiple organ involvement. When present, ocular lesions are same as in adults, *Table 11A, page 92.*
Retinal depigmentation, on ZDV	~5%	0	Asymptomatic peripheral retinal depigmentation (dosages >300 mg/M²/day).
HIV-associated "cotton wool" spots	Rare	Common	Seen only in children >8–10 yrs, while seen in 60–70% of adults.
Gastrointestinal Tract			
Mouth			
Kaposi's sarcoma	V. rare	Common	More prevalent in HIV+ children in areas of Africa.
Esophagus			
Dysphagia, odynophagia	Uncommon	Common	When pain/difficulty occur, children more likely to refuse to eat. CMV—odynophagia, Candida—dysphagia.
Diarrhea	Common	Common	Most common agents: rotavirus 24% (more common in inpatient setting), salmonella (19%), campylobacter (8%) (more common in outpatients). Presence of blood &/or WBC in stool has high positive predictive value for salmonella or campylobacter *(PIDJ 15:876, 1996)*.

CLINICAL SYNDROME	INFANT/CHILD	ADULT	CLINICAL FEATURES (in children)/COMMENTS
Heart	Common	Common	Abnormal ECG changes (ventricular hypertrophy & non-specific ST-T changes) in 55–93% HIV+ children.
Cardiomyopathy	Common	Uncommon	Left ventricular dysfunction 29–74% (most important cardiac change). 20% transient or chronic congestive failure. Unexpected cardiorespiratory arrests in 8/81 *(JAMA 269:2869, 1993)*. Pericardial effusions & tamponade have been noted frequently in children *(PIDJ 15:819, 1996)*.
Hematologic			
Hypergammaglobulinemia	**Common**	**Uncommon**	By age 6 mos, almost all HIV+ children have ↑ gamma-globulins.
Protein S (coagulation inhibitor)	Common	Common	19/26 children had ↓ levels, but risk of thrombosis low *(Ped IDJ 15:106, 1996)*. Adults, ↑ protein S in 27–73%, thrombotic complications in 12%.
Hepatobiliary	Rare	Common	Very few reports relating to children. Etiologies such as AIDS cholangiopathy, peliosis hepatis (bacillary angiomatosis) not reported. 2 cases of fatal hepatic necrosis associated with adenovirus reported *(Rev Inf Dis 12:303, 1990)*.
Lung			
Tuberculosis	Uncommon	Common	Virtually all are primary infections. Clinical: fever, cough. X-ray: often focal infiltrates with hilar adenopathy, cavitation uncommon.
Lymphocytic interstitial pneumonitis (LIP)	Common	V. rare	LIP occurs in 40% of children with perinatally acquired HIV. HIV & EBV antigens have been demonstrated in lung tissue. Usually diagnosed in children >1 yr as compared with PJP which is most common in first year. LIP has better prognosis than PJP. Median survival is ~5x shorter in children diagnosed with PJP than in children with LIP *(Lancet 348:866, 1996)*. Clinical: slowly progressive tachypnea, cough, wheezing, hypoxemia. Rales are infrequent. Clubbing of digits is characteristic. Generalized lymphadenopathy, hepatosplenomegaly & parotid swelling. X-ray: diffuse reticulonodular infiltrates associated with hilar lymphadenopathy. Bacterial suprainfection is common. Diagnosis by lung biopsy. Rx: steroids may be of some benefit.
Cryptococcosis	Uncommon		Disseminated infection or localized process of the lungs. Intermittent fever is most common presenting manifestation. All pts have low CD4, history of previous OIs, & onset of cryptococcosis most commonly in 2nd decade of life *(PIDJ 15: 796, 1996)*.
Congestive heart failure	Common	Uncommon	*See Heart, above*
Leiomyosarcoma	Rare (but ↑)	V. rare	EBV demonstrated by PCR in tumors *(NEJM 332:12, 1995)*
Renal			
Nephropathy	Common	Rare	Nephropathy observed in 29% children with perinatal AIDS *(Kidney 31:1167, 1987)*. In children may present with nephrotic syndrome with a course of 12–18 mos *(NEJM 321:625, 1989)*. Steroid rx may be of value.
"Sepsis"	Common	Uncommon	25% of symptomatic HIV+ children will have bacteremic episodes, most due to bacteremic pneumonia or bacteremia without a focus *(Pediatric AIDS, Eds. P.A. Pizzo, C.M. Wilfert, Ch. 13, page 199, 1991)*.
Fungemia (a nosocomially-acquired infection)			Risk factors: central venous catheter (>90 days), prior antibiotic therapy (>3 different antibiotics, parenteral ↑ risk), parenteral hyperalimentation, hemodialysis, prolonged neutropenia, colonization by Candida species *(CID 23:515, 1996)*
Skin			
Impetigo	Common	Uncommon	Due to Staph. aureus or Group A strep. Clinical: areas of erythema with "honey crusting". May be widespread & evolve into "cellulitis". Increasing incidence of MRSA skin & soft tissue infections.

TABLE 8F: SELECTED DRUGS COMMONLY USED IN CHILDREN WITH HIV INFECTION

INDICATION/DRUG	DOSAGE	FORMULATIONS	COMMENTS
Antifungal Drugs			
Amphotericin B	0.5–1 mg/kg/day IV	Same as adult	
Ampho B lipid complex	5 mg/kg/day IV as for adults		
Caspofungin	75 mg/M^2 IV q24h loading dose, then 50 mg/M^2 IV q24h	Same as adult	
Fluconazole		Oral suspension (orange-flavored), 50 mg/5 mL (teaspoon)	**Adult Dose** **Pediatric Equivalent** 100 mg 3 mg/kg 200 mg 6 mg/kg 400 mg 12 mg/kg (not to exceed 600 mg/day)
Oral/esophageal candidiasis	6–12 mg/kg/day		
Systemic candidiasis	12 mg/kg/day IV or po		
Cryptococcal meningitis			
Treatment	12 mg/kg po 1st day, then 6 (to 12) mg/kg/day po		
Suppression	6 mg/kg/day po		
Itraconazole	3 mg/kg po q24h (capsules) 5 mg/kg po q24h (suspension)	Oral suspension 10 mg/mL	Efficacy & safety not established Extensive drug-drug interactions Bioavailability of capsules is low & variable Administer suspension on empty stomach with 4–6 oz of Coca-Cola.
Voriconazole	6 mg/kg q12h x 2, then 4 mg/kg q 12h (FDA approved but 8-9 mg/kg may be needed)	Capsules 50 mg, 200 mg Oral suspension 40 mg/mL	Extensive drug-drug interactions Reversible visual disturbance in 20% Measure trough level: goal is 1-6 mcg/mL
Anti-HIV Drugs[1]			
Nucleoside analogue reverse transcriptase inhibitors (NRTIs)			

Abacavir (Ziagen)	Age ≥3 mos: 8 mg/kg 2x/daily not to exceed 300 mg
	Neonatal dose unknown
	Wt-based dosing:
	  14<20 kg: ½ tablet po qAM; ½ tablet po qPM
	  ≥20 - <25: ½ tablet po qAM; 1 tablet po qPM
	  >25 kg: 300 mg (1 tablet) po 2x/day
	Adolescent/adult dose: 300 mg 2x/day or 600 mg 1x/day
		Solution 20 mg/mL
		300 mg tablets , generic 300 mg tablets
		Fixed combination 600 mg with 300 mg lamivudine (Epzicom)
		Fixed combination 300 mg with 300 mg zidovudine & 150 mg lamivudine (Trizivir)
		Fixed combination 600 mg with 300 mg lamivudine and 50 mg dolutegravir (Triumeq)
			Hypersensitivity reaction in ~5%, may be difficult to recognize. Rechallenge may be fatal.
			Hypersensitivity associated with HLA B✱5701. Screening for HLA B✱5701 virtually eliminates hypersensitivity reactions and should be obtained before starting if available.

Didanosine (ddI, Videx)	120 mg/M^2 q12h not to exceed 200 mg per dose.
	240 mg/M^2 q24h not to exceed 400 mg per dose if >3 and treatment naïve
	  Body weight 20-25 kg: 200 mg once daily
	  Body weight 25-60 kg: 250 mg once daily
	  Body weight >60 kg: 400 mg once daily
	Neonatal dose (2 weeks-<3 months): 50 mg/M^2 q12h
	Infant dose (age 3-8 mos): 100 mg/M^2 q12h
		Pediatric powder (when reconstituted with antacid): 10 mg/mL
		Delayed-release capsules (enteric-coated bead-lets): Videx EC 125, 200, 250, 400 mg
		Generic delayed-release capsules 125, 200, 250, 400 mg
		Tablet for oral suspension: 100, 150, 200 mg
			Dose on empty stomach.
			Reduce didanosine dose if combined with tenofovir.
			Do not administer with ribavirin
			Increased risk of pancreatitis. Risk higher if co-administered with tenofovir or stavudine.
			Tablets for oral suspension may be chewed or added to ≥1 oz of water

[1] Adolescents ≥ Tanner 4 should be dosed according to adult dosing (*see Table 6B*)

TABLE 8F (2)

INDICATION/DRUG	DOSAGE	FORMULATIONS	COMMENTS
Anti-HIV Drugs/Nucleoside analogue reverse transcriptase inhibitors (NRTIs) *(continued)*			
Emtricitabine (Emtriva) (oral solution)	Neonatal aged 0 to ≤3 months 3 mg/kg 1x/day 6 mg/kg 1x/day 3 months of age to 17 years or 33 kg 200 mg 1x/day if >33 kg Adolescent/adult dose 200 mg 1x/day	Solution 10 mg/mL Tablet 200 mg Fixed combination 200 mg with 300 mg tenofovir (**Truvada**) Fixed combination 200 mg with 300 mg tenofovir, 600 mg efavirenz (**Atripla**) Fixed combination 200 mg with 300 mg tenofovir, 25 mg rilpivirine (**Complera**) Fixed combination 200 mg with 300 mg tenofovir, 150 mg elvitegravir, 150 mg cobicistat (**Stribild**) Fixed combination 200 mg with 25 mg TAF (**Descovy**) Fixed combination 200 mg with 25 mg TAF, 150 mg elvitegravir, 150 mg cobicistat (**Genvoya**) Fixed combination 200 mg with 25 mg TAF, 25 mg rilpivirine (**Odefsey**)	Screen for HBV infection before starting. Oral solution stable for 3 months at up to 77F/25C.
Lamivudine (3TC, Epivir)	4 mg/kg 2x/day (>30 days max 150 mg 2x daily) Neonatal dose (<30 days): 2 mg/kg 2x/day Wt based recommendations for tablet Body weight 14-20 kg: 75 mg po 2x/day >20-25 kg: 75 mg AM/150 mg PM >25 kg: 150 mg po 2x/day Adolescent/adult dose (weight >30 kg) 150 mg 2x/day or 300 mg once daily	Solution 10 mg/mL (Epivir) 5 mg/mL (Epivir HBV) Tablets 150 (scored), 300 mg Fixed combination 150 mg with 300 mg ZDV (**Combivir**) Fixed combination 150 mg with 300 mg ZDV, 300 mg abacavir (Trizivir) Fixed combination 300 mg with 600 mg Abacavir (**Epzicom**) Fixed combination 600 mg with 300 mg lamivudine and 50 mg dolutegravir (**Triumeq**)	Screen for HBV infection before starting. Consider switching to 8-10 mg po once daily if >3 years and undetectable viral load (max 300 mg po 1 x day)
Stavudine (d4T, Zerit)	Body weight <30 kg: 1 mg/kg 2x/day >30 kg: 30 mg 2x/day. Neonatal dose birth to 13 days 0,5 mg/kg 2x/day	Solution 1 mg/mL Capsules 15, 20, 30, 40 mg (Generic approved for sale in U.S.)	Better tolerated than zidovudine but more strongly associated with lipoatrophy, peripheral neuropathy, mitochondrial toxicity. Combination with ddl associated with increased risk of lactic acidosis
Zidovudine (ZDV, AZT, Retrovir)	180-240 mg/M² q12h Adolescent/adult dose 300 mg 2x/day Neonatal dose (age 35 weeks EGA to <6 wks) 4 mg/kg po q12h; 1.5 mg/kg IV q6h Premature infant 30-35 wks: 2 mg/kg po 2x/day or 1.5 mg/kg IV q12h. Increase to 3 mg/kg po q12h or 2.3 mg/kg IV at 14 days of age. Premature infant <30 weeks: 2 mg/kg po q12h or 1.5 mg/kg IV. Increase to 3 mg/kg po q12h or 2.3 mg/kg IV at 4 weeks of age Body wt based dose (once 8-10 weeks of age): 4-9 kg: 12 mg/kg 2x daily 9-<30 kg: 9 mg/kg 2x daily >30 kg: 300 mg 2x daily	Syrup 10 mg/mL Capsules 100 mg Tablets 300 mg Generic syrup 10 mg/mL & tablets 300 mg, 10 mg/mL IV Fixed combination 300 mg with 150 mg 3TC (**Combivir**, generic) Fixed combination 300 mg with 150 mg 3TC, 300 mg abacavir (**Trizivir**) Concentrate for IV use 10 mg/mL	

INDICATION/DRUG	DOSAGE	FORMULATIONS	COMMENTS
Anti-HIV Drugs *(continued)*			
Nucleotide reverse transcriptase inhibitor (NtRTI)			
Tenofovir disoproxil fumerate (TDF) (Viread)	8 mg/kg po once daily (age ≥2 yrs) maximum 300 mg 1 scoop powder = 40 mg Use tablets for children >17 kg who can swallow tablets Wt-based dosing: 17-22 kg: 150 mg once daily 22-<28 kg: 200 mg once daily 28-<35 kg: 250 mg once daily ≥35 kg: 300 mg once daily Adult dose 300 mg 1x/day Truvada dosing: 17-22 kg one FTC 100 mg/TDF 150 mg tablet 1x/day 22-≤28 kg one FTC 133 mg/TDF 200 mg tablet 1x/day 28-≤35 kg one FTC 167 mg/TDF 250 mg tablet 1x/day ≥35 kg one FTC 200 mg/TDF 300 mg tablet 1x/day	Tablets 150 mg, 200 mg, 250 mg, 300 mg Tablets dissolve in water, orange or grape juice Powder formulation 40 mg/gm Fixed combination 150 mg with 100 mg emtricitabine, 200 mg with 133 mg emtricitabine, 250 mg with 167 mg emtricitabine, 300 mg with 200 mg emtricitabine (**Truvada**) Fixed combination 300 mg with 200 mg emtricitabine and 600 mg efavirenz (**Atripla**) Fixed combination 200 mg with 300 mg TDF, 25 mg rilpivirine (**Complera**) Fixed combination 200 mg with 300 mg TDF, 150 mg elvitegravir, 150 mg cobicistat (**Stribild**)	Screen for HBV before starting. Monitor renal function. ↓ bone mineral density observed in young animals. ↓ BMD was prevalent in HIV-infected children before treatment; small ↓ in BMD in 5/15 at 1 yr in 1 study *(Pediatrics 116:e846, 2005)*. No change compared to controls at 1 yr in another *(JAIDS 40:448, 2005)*. Use with caution & decrease dose if any renal impairment. Decrease ddI dose if used with tenofovir. Consider Vitamin D level and Vitamin D supplement. Follow creatinine, urine glucose and protein while on therapy
Tenofovir alafenamide fumarate (TAF)	Adolescents ≥35 kg: 25 mg 1x/day (Descovy; Odefsey) When used with cobicistat (Genvoya) 10 mg 1x/day Not yet fully studied or approved for children <12 years	Tablets 25 mg with 200 mg emtricitabine (**Descovy**) Tablets: 10 mg with 150 mg elvitegravir, 150 mg cobicistat, 200 mg emtricitabine (**Genvoya**) Tablets: 25 mg with 25 mg rilpivirine, 200 mg emtricitabine (**Odefsey**)	Fewer changes in BMD and renal function than tenofovir DF. Observe for renal dysfunction. Not recommended for patients with CrCl ≤30 mg/mL/ Cobicistat is inhibitor of CYP 3A4. Check drug interactions for Genvoya
Non-nucleoside reverse transcriptase inhibitors (NNRTIs)			
Efavirenz (Sustiva)	10–15 kg, 200 mg; 15–20 kg, 250 mg; 20–25 kg, 300 mg; 25–32.5 kg, 350 mg; 32.5–40 kg, 400 mg; >40 kg, 600 mg—all 1x/day Neonatal dose unknown/not approved for infants Adult dose 600 mg 1x/day	Capsules 50, 200 mg Tablets 600 mg Fixed combination 600 mg with TDF 300 mg/Emtricitabine 200 mg (**Atripla**) Liquid preparation used in PACTG 382 (contact BMS to check on availability)	Give at night to reduce CNS side effects. Capsules can be opened & added to food or liquid but contents have peppery taste. Atripla should be administered on an empty stomach. Minimum weight for Atriplia 40 kg. Lowers concentration of unboosted PIs, LPV/ritonavir, voriconazole. Increase dose of EFV if given with RIF. Pregnancy Class D. Avoid if possibility of pregnancy
Etravirine (Intelence)	Age >6 to 17 yrs: Wt-based dosing: ≥16-<20 kg: 100 mg 2x/day 20-<25 kg: 125 mg 2x/day 25-<30 kg: 150 mg 2x/day ≥30 kg: 200 mg 2x/day	Tablets 25 mg, 100 mg, 200 mg	Administer with food. Tablets disperse in water. Glass should be rinsed with water and the rinses swallowed to ensure consuming the entire dose. Do not co-administer with efavirenz, atazanavir or tipranavir due to interactions. Multiple other drug interactions.

INDICATION/DRUG	DOSAGE	FORMULATIONS	COMMENTS
Anti-HIV Drugs/Non-nucleoside reverse transcriptase inhibitors (NNRTIs) *(continued)*			
Nevirapine (Viramune)	<8 yrs of age, 7 mg/kg 2x/day or 200 mg/M^2 ≥8 yrs of age, 4 mg/kg 2x/day or 120-150 mg/M^2 **Note:** Initiate dosing once daily x 14 d; if no rash, ↑ to 2x/day. **Dosing by M^2 preferred** Neonatal dose 6 mg/kg 2x/day, no lead in 34-37 weeks 4 mg/kg 2x/day for one week then 6 mg/kg 2x/day Adolescent/adult dose 200 mg 1x/day x 14 d then 200 mg 2x/day Neonata prophylaxis: 2 mg/kg at birth 34-37 weeks 4 mg/kg 2x/day for one week then 6 mg/kg 2x/day and 96 hours after second dose	Suspension 10 mg/mL Tablets 200 mg, 400 mg extended release Generic: suspension 10 mg/mL, 200 mg immediate release, 400 mg extended release	Do not dose-escalate in presence of rash. If rash is associated with fever, oral lesions, conjunctivitis, blistering, or hepatitis, stop medication immediately. Severe cholestatic hepatitis & Stevens-Johnson syndrome are rare but life-threatening complications that may occur in the 1st 6 wks. In adults, risk of severe toxicity increased in women with CD4 >250 & men with CD4 >400. Lowers concentration of LPV/ritonavir. Risk of rash and hepatoxicity higher when CD4% >15%.
Rilpivirine (Edurant)	Not approved in children age <12 yrs. No PK or dosing data available. Adolescent/adult dose: 25 mg once daily with food	Tablets 25 mg Fixed combination 25 mg with TDF 300 mg/ emtricitabine 200 mg (**Complera/Eviplera**). Fixed combination 25 mg with 200 mg with TAF 25 mg/ emtricitabine 200 mg (**Odefsey**)	Administer with food. Metabolized by CYP3A. Do not administer with rifampin, rifabutin, rifapentine, PPIs.
Protease Inhibitors			
Atazanavir (Reyataz)	Age ≥3 months: (Powder) 5 kg to <15 kg: ATV 200 mg (4 packets) + RIT 80 mg once daily 15 kg to <25 kg: ATV 250 mg (5 packets) + RIT 80 mg once daily Age>6 yrs: (Capsules) 20 kg-<32 kg: ATV 200 mg + RIT 100 mg once daily 32 kg-<40 kg: ATV 250 mg + RIT 100 mg once daily ≥40 kg: ATV 300 mg + RIT 100 mg once daily Neonatal use not recommended Adolescent/adult dose 400 mg 1x/day or 300 mg + 100 mg ritonavir both 1x/day	Capsules 150, 200 mg, 300 mg Powder packet: 50 mg/packet Fixed combination: 300 mg with cobicistat 150 mg (**Evotaz**)	Administer with food. Mix powder with at least one tablespoon of food, e.g., yogurt. Wide variability in levels in children with unboosted atazanavir. Ritonavir-boosted atazanavir may give more consistent levels. If using unboosted atazanavir in adolescents, consider TDM. Avoid in infants due to ↑ bilirubin. Avoid use with proton pump inhibitors if possible. If PPI must be used, no more than 20 mg omeprazole should be given, 12 hrs after atazanavir/ ritonavir. Boost with ritonavir if co-administered with tenofovir or efavirenz. **Do not co-administer with nevirapine.**

TABLE 8F (5)

INDICATION/DRUG	DOSAGE	FORMULATIONS	COMMENTS
Anti-HIV Drugs/Protease Inhibitors (continued)			
Darunavir (Prezista)	FDA approved for age >3 yrs: Wt-based dosing: For children weighing 10-15 kg, dosing is based on darunavir (DRV) 20 mg/kg + ritonavir (RIT) 3 mg/kg 2x/day: 10-<11 kg: DRV 200 mg (2 mL) + RIT 32 mg (0.4 mL) 11-<12 kg: DRV 220 mg (2.2 mL) + RIT 32 mg (0.4 mL) 12-<13 kg: DRV 240 mg (2.4 mL) + RIT 40 mg (0.5 mL) 13-<14 kg: DRV 260 mg (2.6 mL) + RIT 40 mg (0.5 mL) 14-<15 kg: DRV 280 mg (2.8 mL) + RIT 48 mg (0.6 mL) For children >15 kg who can swallow tablets: 15-29 kg: darunavir 375 mg + ritonavir 50 mg 2x/day 30-39 kg: darunavir 450 mg + ritonavir 60 mg 2x/day >40 kg: Adult dose Adult/adolescent dose 600 mg + ritonavir 100 mg 2x/day (treatment experienced) 800 mg + ritonavir 100 mg (treatment naïve adults only) once daily 800 mg + cobicistat 150 mg once daily	Tablets 75 mg, 150 mg, 400 mg, 600 mg Oral suspension 100 mg/mL Fixed combination: 800 mg + cobicistat 150 mg (**Prezcobix**)	Administer with food. Active against many strains with extensive protease inhibitor resistance. Potential for many drug-drug interactions. Review other medications. May substitute ritonavir 100 mg tablets for children 20-40 kg instead of ritonavir liquid. Do not use in children < age 3 years weighing <10 kg because of concerns related to seizures and death in infant rats. Do not use once daily in children age <12 years.
Fosamprenavir (Lexiva)	2-5 yrs naïve only: 30 mg/kg 2x/day (not to exceed adult dose of 1400 mg 2x/day). Not recommended 6-18 naïve only unboosted 30 mg/kg (not to exceed 1400 mg) 2x daily All 2 x day: <11 kg: FPV 45 mg/kg + RIT 7 mg/kg 11-<15 kg: FPV 30 mg/kg RIT 3 mg/kg 15-<20 kg: FPV 23 mg/kg + RIT 3 mg/kg 20 kg FPV 18 mg/kg + RIT 3 mg/kg (not to exceed adult dose of 700 mg + 100 mg ritonavir 2x/day) Neonatal use not recommended Adolescent/adult dose: Antiretroviral naïve: 1400 mg 2x/day (>47 kg) 700 mg + 100 mg ritonavir 2x/day 1400 mg + 100 or 200 mg ritonavir 1x/day Antiretroviral experienced: 700 mg + 100 mg ritonavir 2x/day	Tablet 700 mg (equivalent to 600 mg amprenavir) Oral suspension 50 mg/mL	Administer tablets with or without food if used alone. Administer solution with food and when boosting with ritonavir. Once daily dosing is not recommended for children. FDA approved for children as young as 4 weeks but DHHS panel does not recommend for children <6 months.
Indinavir (Crixivan)	500 mg/M^2 q8h (not approved) Adolescent/adult dose 800 mg q8h or 800 mg + ritonavir 100 or 200 m g 2x/day	Capsules 100, 200, 333, 400 mg	Response associated with C_{min} (AAC 44:1029, 2000). Consider measuring C_{min} if available & adjusting dose. Nephrolithiasis in 20% of children. Ensure hydration.

TABLE 8F (6)

INDICATION/DRUG	DOSAGE	FORMULATIONS	COMMENTS
Anti-HIV Drugs/Protease Inhibitors *(continued)*			

Lopinavir/Ritonavir (Kaletra)	Age 14 days - 12 months:
	  300 mg lopinavir/75 mg r/M^2 2x/day
	Age 12 months - 18 years:
	  230 mg lopinavir/57.5 mg r/ M^2 2x/day if not taking efavirenz, nevirapine or fosamprenavir. Increase to 300 mg/75 mg/ M^2 2x/day if taking above drugs but many prefer this dose for all children.
	Alternate wt based for oral soln:
	  <15 kg: 12 mg/3 mg/kg 2x/day
	  15-40 kg: 10 mg/2.5 mg/kg 2x/day
	  >40 kg Adult dose
	Tablet Dosing:
	  15-20 kg: 2 tablets (100 mg lopinavir/25 mg r) 2x/day
	  20-30 kg: 3 tablets 2x/day
	  30-45 kg: 4 100/25 mg tab or 2 200/50 mg tab 2x/day
	  >45 kg Adult dose
	Adult adolescent dose:
	  400 mg lopinavir/100 mg r 2x/day if not receiving NVP, EFV, fosamprenavir. Increase dose in patients on NVP, EFV, FPV
		Pediatric solution 80 mg lopinavir/20 mg ritonavir per mL (contains alcohol and polyethylene glycol)
		Tablets 100 mg lopinavir/25 mg ritonavir
		200 mg lopinavir/50 mg ritonavir
			Administer tablets with or without food. Do not split or crush. Oral solution should be administered with food. Oral solution should be refrigerated but stable up to 2 months at room temp. For adults who are treatment naïve, tablets can be dosed as 400 mg/100 mg once daily in naïve PI naïve patients; this has not been evaluated in adolescents who might have more rapid clearance. Higher doses (eg 300 mg/M^2 or 600 mg/140 mg 2x/day should be considered in treatment-experienced patients with PI resistance mutations. Standard dose of 230 mg/M^2 gives trough lower than target associated with response in treatment experienced adults (5.7 mcg/mL *CROI 2008 abstr 574)*. Crushed tablets give lower exposure: not recommended ***(CROI 2010 abst 871).***
			Life threatening events including heart block reported in premature infants. Should not be used in premature infants until 2 weeks beyond due date or in term infants 14 days unless benefits clearly outweigh risks.

Nelfinavir (Viracept)	Age 2-13 yrs: 45–55 mg/kg q12h *(8th CROI, 2001, Abst. 250)*. Approved dose of 30 mg/kg q8h may lead to inadequate levels.
	Neonatal wt-based dosing:
	  1.5-2 kg 100 mg 2x/day
	  2-3 kg: 150 mg 2x/day
	  >3 kg: 200 mg 2x/day
	Adolescent/adult dose 1250 mg q12h
		Powder for oral suspension 50 mg/level scoop
		Tablets 250, 625 mg
			Take with meal to ↑ absorption. Large variability in levels. Crushed or dissolved tablets more reliably absorbed. Consider measuring C$_{min}$ if available & adjusting dose. Maintaining C trough > 0.8 mcg/mL associated with improved response in one study.

Ritonavir (Norvir)	350-400 mg/M^2 2x/day (NOT RECOMMENDED) Used as pharmacologic enhancer	Solution 80 mg/mL Capsules 100 mg Tablets 100 mg	Full dose ritonavir is rarely used and not recommended. Use lower dose as pharmacokinetic enhancer. Solution is unpleasant tasting. Refrigerate capsules; stable 30 days at room temperature.

TABLE 8F (7)

INDICATION/DRUG	DOSAGE	FORMULATIONS	COMMENTS
Anti-HIV Drugs/Protease Inhibitors *(continued)*			
Saquinavir (Invirase) Note: Soft-gel capsules no longer available.	Under study: Not approved in infants or children, but Saquinavir Wt based dose (limited data): 5-15 kg: 50 mg/kg + ritonavir 3 mg/kg 2x daily 15-40 kg: 50 mg/kg + ritonavir 2.5 mg/kg 2x daily >40 kg: 50 mg/kg + ritonavir 100 mg 2x daily Adolescent/adult dose: 1000 mg + 100 mg ritonavir 2x/day With Lopinavir/ritonavir: Saquinavir 1000 mg + Lopinavir/ritonavir 400 mg/100 mg both 2x/day	Hard-gel capsules 200 mg Film-coated tablets 500 mg	Consider measuring C_{min} if available & adjusting dose. (C_{min} >100 ng/mL associated with response). Should only be used with ritonavir enhancement. Not recommended for children with prolonged QT interval.
Tipranavir (Aptivus)	Not approved in 2 yrs of age. 375 mg/M^2 + ritonavir 150 mg/M^2 2x/day wt-based: 14 mg/kg + ritonavir 6 mg/kg 2x/day Adolescent/Adult dose: 500 mg with 200 mg ritonavir 2x/day	Capsule 250 mg Solution 100 mg/mL with 116 IU Vit E/mL	Administer with food. Active against many virus strains with extensive PI resistance, & used only in patients with extensive prior experience. Most effective when given with other active agents, such as enfuvirtide. Activity and tolerability in PACTG1051 similar to adult trials *(Intl AIDS Conf 2006 Abstr WEAB0301)* Induces metabolism of other PIs & should not be co-administered with them. Possible association with intracranial hemorrhage
Fusion Inhibitors			
Enfuvirtide (Fuzeon)	6–16 yrs 2 mg/kg 2x/day, maximum dose 90 mg (1 mL) injected subcutaneously <6 yrs not approved Adolescent/adult dose 90 mg (1 mL) 2x/day injected subcutaneously	Injection: lyophilized powder for injection 108 mg of enfuvirtide, when reconstituted with 1.1 mL sterile water to deliver 90 mg/mL	

INDICATION/DRUG	DOSAGE	FORMULATIONS	COMMENTS
Anti-HIV Drugs (*continued*)			
CCR5 Inhibitors			

Maraviroc (Selzentry)	Not approved in neonates/infants
	≥2 years and ≥10 kg with CYP 3A inhibitors e.g. low dose ritonavir
	  10-<20 kg 50 mg 2x/day
	  20-<30 kg 75 mg 2x/day
	  30-<40 kg 100 mg 2x/day
	  >40 kg 150 mg 2x/day
	without a potent CYP 3A inhibitor
	  <30 kg not recommended
	  >30 kg 300 mg 2x/day
	Adolescent/adult doses:
	150 mg 2x/day when given with strong CYP3A inhibitors (with or without CYP3A inducers) including all PIs (except tipranavir/ritonavir)
	300 mg twice daily when given with NRTIs, enfuvirtide, tipranavir/ritonavir, nevirapine, raltegravir
	600 mg twice daily when given with CYP3A inducers, including efavirenz, rifampin, phenobarbital, etravirine, phenytoin, etc. (without a CYP3A inhibitor)
		Tablets 25 mg, 75 mg, 150 mg, 300 mg
		Oral solution 20 mg/mL
			Tropism assay should be used before prescribing to exclude X 4/dual tropic virus.
			Cytochrome P450 substrate. Do not use in patients with CrCl <30 mL/min who are receiving potent CYP3A4 inhibitors

Integrase Inhibitors			

Raltegravir (Isentress)	Investigational dose for neonates
	  0-7 days 1.5 mg/kg 1x/day
	  8-28 days 3 mg/kg 2x/day
	  >4 weeks 6 mg/kg 2x/day
	Age and Wt-based dosing:
	  6-12 yrs and >25 kg: 400 mg tablet 2x/day **or**
	  2-<12 yrs chewable tablet dosing:
	    11-<14 kg: 3 x 25 mg 2x/day
	    14-<20 kg: 1 x 100 mg 2x/day
	    20-<28 kg: 1.5 x 100 mg 2x/day
	    28-<40 kg: 2 x 100 mg 2x/day
	    >40 kg: 3 x 100 mg 2x/day
	Oral suspension for children ≥4 weeks and ≥3-20 kg
	    3 to <4 kg: 1 mL (20 mg) twice daily
	    4 to <6 kg:1.5 mL (30 mg) twice daily
	    6 to <8 kg: 2 mL (40 mg) twice daily
	    8 to <11 kg: 3 mL (60 mg) twice daily
	    11 to <14 kg: 4 mL (80 mg) twice daily
	    14 to <20 Kg: 5 mL (100 mg) twice daily
	Adolescent/adult dose 400 mg 2x/day
		Tablets 400 mg
		Chewable tablet 25 mg and 100 mg scored
		Granules 100 mg packet
			Give with or without food
			Chewable tablets may be chewed or swallowed whole
			Efavirenz and etravirine may decrease raltegravir concentrations

TABLE 8F (9)

INDICATION/DRUG	DOSAGE	FORMULATIONS	COMMENTS
Anti-HIV Drugs/Integrase Inhibitors (*continued*)			
Elvitegravir	No pediatric dosing currently for children <35 kg Adult and adolescent (>35 kg) dose 1 tablet once daily, *see Table 6A*	Tablet 85, 150 mg fixed dose combination Elvitegravir 150 mg, Cobicistat 150 mg, TDF 300 mg, FTC 200 mg (**Stribild**) Fixed combination: 150 mg with cobicistat 150 mg, TAF 10 mg, emtricitabine 200 mg (**Genvoya**)	Give with food
Dolutegravir (Tivicay)	Children 30–<40 kg 35 mg 1x/day Adults and children >12 years and >40 kg 50 mg po once daily if INSTI-Naïve 50 mg po bid if INSTI-experienced or with efavirenz, fosamprenavir/ritonavir, tipranavir/ritonavir or rifampin	Tablets 10 mg, 25 mg, 50 mg. Granules under study Fixed combination: 50 mg with lamivudine 300 mg & abacavir 300 mg (**Triumeq**)	Give with or without food Hypersensitivity has been reported. Separate from cation containing antacids or laxatives by 2 hours before or 6 hours after. Causes slight increase in serum creatinine but does not affect GFR
Antimycobacterial Drugs			
M. tuberculosis			
Ethambutol	15–25 mg/kg/day po	No pediatric formulation	Not approved in children <13 yrs but can be given. Monitor for closely for visual change
Isoniazid	Neonates: 10 mg/kg po q24h. Infants/Children: 10–20 mg/kg po q24h (maximum 300 mg/day).	50 mg/5 mL syrup	Can give IM
Pyrazinamide	20–40 mg/kg po q24h as 1 or more doses (maximum 2 gm/day)	No pediatric formulation	
Rifampin	10–20 mg/kg po q24h (maximum 600 mg/day)	No pediatric formulation. Ad hoc solution can be made by pharmacy	Can give po or IV. Do not use with protease inhibitors. Reduced dose rifabutin can be substituted
Streptomycin	10–20 mg IM q12h (max. 1 gm/day)		
MAC—Mycobacterium avium-intracellulare complex			
Azithromycin	5 mg/kg/day for treatment 20 mg/kg once weekly, not to exceed 1200 mg	Oral suspension 100 or 200 mg/5 mL, 250 mg, 600 mg capsules	
Clarithromycin	15 mg/kg/day divided q12h po (not to exceed 500 mg po q12h)	Granules for oral suspension (125 or 250 mg/5 mL) (DO NOT refrigerate suspension)	
Clofazimine	1–2 mg/kg/day po to max. of 100 mg/day	No pediatric formulation	
Rifabutin	10–20 mg/kg/day po (max 300 mg/day)	No pediatric formulation	↓ dose with protease inhibitors, inc with NNRTI's
Antifungal Drugs			
Pneumocystis pneumonia (PJP)			
Prophylaxis (*See Table 8D*)			
TMP/SMX OR	150 mg/M² TMP component po divided q12h on 3 consecutive days (M, T, W) each week. Abbreviated schedules: *Table 8D*	Oral suspension (cherry or grape flavored), 40 mg TMP/ 200 mg SMX/5 mL (teaspoon); 80 mg TMP/400 mg SMX tablet (single strength)	Breakthrough episodes of PJP: TMP/SMX 3%, dapsone 15% or higher, aerosol pentamidine 15%, IV pentamidine 25% (*J Ped 122:163, 1993*)
Dapsone OR	2 mg/kg/day po (not to exceed 100 mg)	No pediatric formulation	
Aerosolized pentamidine— only if ≥5 yrs old	300 mg with Respirgard II inhaler 1x monthly		Used as young as 8 mos (*PIDJ 12:958, 1991*)

TABLE 8F (10)

INDICATION/DRUG	DOSAGE	FORMULATIONS	COMMENTS
Antifungal Drugs/Pneumocystis pneumonia (PJP) *(continued)*			
Treatment			
Atovaquone suspension	30–40 mg/kg po q24h. Dosing interval not established	Not FDA-approved for pediatric use	Efficacy in children not established. CNS levels <1%.
Pentamidine isethionate	4 mg/kg/day IV or IM x 12–14 days		
TMP/SMX	Children >2 mos 20 mg TMP/100 mg SMX/kg/day divided q6h po or IV in same dose q6–8h		Start with IV in all but mildest cases
Antiviral Drugs—other than anti-HIV			
Cytomegalovirus			
Cidofovir Induction Maintenance	No studies in children. 5 mg/kg once a week for two doses 5 mg/kg every 14 days	IV solution only	Must follow guidelines for hydration & probenecid. Dose adjust for renal disease
Foscarnet Induction Maintenance	180 mg/kg/day divided q8h 90–120 mg/kg IV q24h		No studies reported in children. Deposited in teeth & bone of growing animals. Dose adjust for renal disease
Valganciclovir Induction Maintenance	7 mg x m^2 x CrCl 2x/day induction (max 900 mg) 900 mg po 2x/day for 21 days 900 mg po q day	Tablets 450 mg Solution 50 mg/5 mL	Dose adjust for renal diseases
Ganciclovir Induction Maintenance	5 mg/kg IV q12h 5 mg/kg IV q24h	Adult capsule or IV solution	Has potential carcinogenicity Dose adjust for renal disease
Herpes simplex virus			
Acyclovir	30 mg/kg IV q8h (age <12 yrs) 15 mg/kg IV q8h (age >12 yrs)	200 mg/5 mL oral suspension (banana flavored) available if appropriate	Daily urine output should be 1 mL/1.3 mg of acyclovir
Influenza			
Oseltamivir	<1 year: 3 mg/kg po q12h ≥1 year and ≤15 kg: 30 mg po q12h 16-23 kg: 45 mg po q12h 24-40 kg: 60 mg po q12h >40 kg: 75 mg po q12h	30, 45, 75 mg capsule and oral suspension 12 mg/mL	
Varicella zoster (<2 yrs old)			
Acyclovir	500 mg/M^2 IV q8h		

For additional data on drugs for pain &/or nutritional management, see www.aidsinfo.nih.gov/guidelines, Supplements to Pediatric Guidelines Mar 2008.

TABLE 8G: PROPHYLAXIS FOR FIRST EPISODE OF OPPORTUNISTIC DISEASE IN HIV-INFECTED INFANTS & CHILDREN

PATHOGEN	INDICATION	PREVENTIVE REGIMENS*	
		FIRST CHOICE	**ALTERNATIVES**
Pneumocystis pneumonia (PJP)	HIV-infected or HIV-indeterminate infants aged 1–12 mos	**TMP/SMX** 150/750 mg/M^2/day in 2 div. doses po 3x/wk on consecutive days (A2)	Aerosolized pentamidine (children aged ≥5 yrs) 300 mg 1x monthly via Respirgard II nebulizer (C3); dapsone (children aged ≥1 mo.) 2 mg/kg (max 100 mg) po q24h (C3); Atovaquone 30 mg/kg po q24h for 1–3 mos old & >24 mos old; 45 mg/kg po q24h for 4–24 mos old; IV pentamidine 4 mg/kg every 2–4 wks if other options are unavailable (C3)
	HIV-infected children aged 1–5 yrs with CD4 count <500 or CD4 percent <15%	Acceptable alternative dosage schedules: (A2) Single dose po 3x/wk on consecutive days or daily	
	HIV-infected children aged 6–12 yrs with CD4 <200 OR CD4 percent <15%	2 div. doses po q24h; 2 div. doses po 3x/wk on alternate days	
Mycobacterium tuberculosis Isoniazid-sensitive	TST reaction ≥5 mm OR prior positive TST result without treatment OR contact with case of active tuberculosis	**Isoniazid** 10–20 mg/kg (max. 300 mg) po OR IM q24h x 9 mos. (A1) OR 20–40 mg/kg (max. 900 mg) po 2x/wk x 9 mos. (B3)	**Rifampin** 10–20 mg/kg (max. 600 mg) po or IV q24h x 12 mos. (B2) (Rifampin duration of rx is 4–6 mos. according to 1999 USPHS guidelines).
Isoniazid-resistant	Same as above; high probability of exposure to isoniazid-resistant tuberculosis	**Rifampin** 10–20 mg/kg (max. 600 mg) po OR IV q24h x 12 mos. (B2)	Uncertain
Multidrug (isoniazid & rifampin)-resistant	Same as above; high probability of exposure to multidrug-resistant tuberculosis	Choice of drug requires consultation with public health authorities	None
Mycobacterium avium complex	For children aged ≥6 yrs, CD4 <50; 2–6 yrs, CD4 <75; 1–2 yrs, CD4 <500; <1 yr, CD4 <750	**Clarithromycin** 7.5 mg/kg (max. 500 mg) po q12h (A2) OR **azithromycin** 20 mg/kg (max. 1200 mg) po 1x/wk (A2)	Children aged ≥6 yrs, **rifabutin** 300 mg po q24h (B1); <6 yrs, 5 mg/kg po q24h when suspension becomes available (B1); azithromycin 5 mg/kg (max. 250 mg) po q24h (A2)
Varicella zoster virus	HIV-infected children who are asymptomatic & not immunosuppressed	Varicella zoster vaccine	
	Significant exposure to varicella with no history of chickenpox, shingles, or varicella vaccine	Varicella zoster immune globulin (VZIG), 1 vial (1.25 mL)/10 kg (max. 5 vials) IM, administered ≤96 hrs after exposure, ideally within 48 hrs (A2)	None

* See Table 4A for HIV classification

TABLE 9: HIV-HCV CO-INFECTION

- Screen all HIV patients for presence of Hepatitis C (HCV) antibody
- ART benefits host defense against HCV
    - **Start ART in all HIV-HCV coinfected patients prior to initiation of anti-HCV therapy.**
    - Choose a regimen that has low risk of drug-drug interactions; specifically a DTG-, BIC- or RAL- based regimen.
- Avoid the following:
    - **Ribavirin-containing HCV treatment regimens with ART regimens**
- HCV treatment recommendations are changing rapidly with the advent of new direct-acting agents (DAAs). For current treatment options, *see The Sanford Guide to Viral Hepatitis Therapy; webedition.sanfordguide.com* or *www.hcvguidelines.org*
- Monitoring response to HCV therapy
    - HCV RNA should be measured at baseline, then at End of Therapy, and at 12-24 weeks after therapy has been completed (SVR or 'cure')

TABLE 10: PRIMARY PROPHYLACTIC ANTIMICROBIAL AGENTS AGAINST OPPORTUNISTIC PATHOGENS IN ADOLESCENTS & ADULTS

Prevention of First Episode of Disease (for 2nd, *see Table 12*). See *http://aidsinfo.nih.gov/guidelines*

Lowest CD4 Count	Pathogen	Preventive Regimens		Comments
		Primary	Alternative	
All patients regardless of CD4 level	**Mycobacterium tuberculosis:** TST[1] ≥5 mm or prior untreated pos. TST or contact with case of active TB. Positive gamma interferon gamma release assay. Rule out active TB.	[**INH** 5 mg/kg/day po, maximum 300 mg po + **pyridoxine** 50 mg po q24h x 9 mos.] or [**INH** 900 mg po + **pyridoxine** 100 mg po 2x/wk x 9 mos.]	**RIF**✳✳ 600 mg po q24h or **RFB**✳✳ 300 mg po q24h x 4 mos.[2] OR **INH** 900 mg + **RFP** 900 mg + **Pyridoxine** 50 mg once weekly for 12 wks	*See Table 11A, page 102.* Regimens are adult doses. INH + RFP can be administered either self-administered or directly observed, including those on antiretroviral therapy. No significant drug interactions between rifapentine and efavirenz or raltegravir *(MMWR Vol. 67 No. 25 page 723 and http://www.who.int/tb /publications/2018/executivesummary_ consolidated_guidelines_ltbi.pdf)*
	As above but high probability of exposure to INH-resistant TB	**RIF**✳✳ 600 mg po q24h or **RFB**✳✳ 300 mg po q24h x 4 mos.		
	Exposure to multi-drug resistant TB	Consultation recommended		
CD4 <200/mm³	**Pneumocystis pneumonia (PJP):** *(See Table 11A page 103)* **DC prophylaxis when CD4 count >200 for >12 wks in response to ART.**	**TMP/SMX-DS** one tab po q24h or 3x/week or **TMP/SMX-SS** one tab po q24h or **Dapsone** 100 mg po q24h	**Aerosolized pentamidine** 300 mg q month via Respirgard II nebulizer (if toxo pos., *see below)* OR **Atovaquone** suspension 1500 mg po q24h.	TMP/SMX superior to other rx in actual practice (incidence of failure 0.0002/100 person yrs) vs. dapsone or inhaled pentamidine or atovaquone (0.001/100 person yrs). Atovaquone = pentamidine but had ↑ rx-limiting adverse events.
CD4 <100/mm³	**Toxoplasma gondii:** (in pts with + IgG toxo, antibody titer). DC primary prophylaxis in toxo Ab+ pts with CD4 >200 for >12 wks in response to ART.	**TMP/SMX-DS** one po q24h.	**Dapsone** 100 mg po q24h + **pyrimethamine** 50 mg po q week + **leucovorin** (folinic acid) 25 mg po q week	Another option: Atovaqone 750 mg po q6–12h + pyrimethamine 25 mg q24h + leucovorin 10 mg po q24h.
	Histoplasmosis: Not routinely recommended. Can be considered for patients at high risk because of occupational exposure or residence in a hyperendemic region for histoplasmosis (≥10 cases/100 patient-years).	Itraconazole 200 mg **twice daily**		If used, primary prophylaxis can be stopped once CD4 >150 for 6 months for patients on ART and restarted if CD4 falls below 150.

✳✳ See Table 12, pg 114, for options regarding concurrent use of protease inhibitors & RIF or RFB.

[1] TST = tuberculin skin test (Mantoux).
[2] Interaction with protease inhibitors to be considered; *see Table 12, pg 114.*

TABLE 10 (2)

Lowest CD4 Count	Pathogen	Preventive Regimens		Comments
		Primary	Alternative	
CD4 <50/mm³	**Mycobacterium avium-intracellulare**³ **(MAC):** *(See Table 11A, page 106).* **DC prophylaxis when CD4 count >100 sustained for 3 mos. in response to ART**. Restart if CD4 drops <50–100/mm³.	[**Clarithromycin** 500 mg po q12h or **azithromycin** 1200 mg po weekly (both assoc. with emergence of resistant respiratory flora)].	**Rifabutin** 300 mg po q24h⁴ or Azithro 600 mg po 2x/wk	*See Table 12, page 118.*
	Cytomegalovirus (CMV): *(See Table 12, page 129).* Preemptive rx of pts with CMV viremia without evidence of organ involvement generally not recommended. May safely **dc CMV preventive therapy** when CD4 count >100-150 per mm³ and HIV viral load has been suppressed on ARVs for >6 mos. Restart if CD4 drops ≤100–150/mm³.	Chronic suppression: **Valganciclovir** 900 mg po q24h *(see Comment)* Best prevention is ART that ↑ CD4 to >100 cells/mL	Oral **ganciclovir** 1 gm po q8h	*See Table 12, page 129, primary prophylaxis.* If plasma PCR for CMV pos., 43% risk of disease (↓ to 26% on oral ganciclovir); if PCR neg., 14% (↓ to 1% on oral ganciclovir). Therefore, some use prophylaxis in gay males when PCR pos.
	Candida species, cryptococcus: Not routinely recommended prior to 1st fungal infection.		Patients with positive CRAG, even with low titers, but other evidence of disease should be treated for cryptococcal infection	

✳✳ See Table 12, pg 114, for options regarding concurrent use of protease inhibitors & RIF or RFB.

³ Authors think it reasonable to observe pts closely, rx strongly suspected or active MAC, then institute chronic suppression *(see Table 12, page 115).*

⁴ Interaction with protease inhibitors to be considered; *see Table 12, page 114.*

TABLE 11A: DIAGNOSIS & DIFFERENTIAL DIAGNOSIS OF CLINICAL SYNDROMES, OPPORTUNISTIC INFECTIONS & NEOPLASMS

(For Treatment, see Table 12)

CLINICAL SYNDROME, ETIOLOGY, EPIDEMIOLOGY	CLINICAL PRESENTATION, DIAGNOSTIC TESTS, COURSE
Acute HIV infection (primary HIV infection, acute retroviral syndrome) Differential diagnosis includes: EBV mononucleosis, CMV mononucleosis, toxoplasmosis, rubella, viral hepatitis, syphilis, primary HSV, drug reactions **Think acute HIV when mononucleosis suspected but serological tests for mono are negative.** NOTE: During acute retroviral syndrome, individuals have very high plasma & genital secretion viral titers and **are highly infectious both from sexual activity & needle sticks.** Drug-resistant virus (to at least one drug) commonly isolated in 15-20% of patients with acute retroviral syndrome.	**Symptoms:** Occur in 50–90%, others have asymptomatic seroconversion; diagnosis made in <10% Time from exposure to sx usually 2–6 wks.

Symptoms	Frequency (%)	Symptoms	Frequency (%)	Lab Abnormalities	Frequency (%)
Fever	>95	Headache	33	↑ ALT, AST	50
Adenopathy	75	Hepatosplenomegaly	15	↓ platelets	45
Pharyngitis	75	Neuropathy	6	↓ lymphs (CD4)	35
Macular or papular rash	70	Oral/genital ulcers	<5	Atypical lymphs	35
Myalgias/arthralgias	80	Esophageal ulcers	<5	(↑ CD8)	
N, V, or diarrhea	30–60	Palpable purpura	<5		
		Conjunctivitis	<5		

Up to 50% have neurological manifestations from severe headache to signs of meningitis or encephalitis. Those with acute neurologic syndromes have 10x higher CSF viral loads than those without neurologic symptoms. OIs are rare.

Course/Prognosis: symptoms usually resolve in 1–2 wks & rarely up to 10 wks among untreated individuals. ART recommended immediately; reduces symptom burden rapidly. The occurrence of the acute retroviral syndrome, a short incubation period to symptoms (fever, fatigue, myalgias), & duration of illness >14 days correlate with more rapid progression to AIDS.

TABLE 11A (2)

CLINICAL SYNDROME: ETIOLOGY, EPIDEMIOLOGY	CLINICAL PRESENTATION, DIAGNOSTIC TESTS, COURSE

Central Nervous System CNS invasion occurs early in HIV infection. ART produced ↓ CNS AIDS- defining events *(Eur J Neurol 18:527, 2011)* but mortality is high when these occur and other CNS conditions may be increasing (immune reconstitution leukoencephalitis, chronic "burnout" VZV encephalitis, toxoplasma or PML).

Cognitive Disorders, Diffuse Brain Dysfunction

Declining mental acuity with preservation of alertness

HIV-1 associated dementia (HAD or HIVD), also known as AIDS dementia complex (ADC), multinucleated giant cell encephalitis, or HIV-1-associated cognitive/motor complex. Frequency: 1/3 of adults, ½ children with AIDS. Most common cause of dementia worldwide in adults <40 years of age

Stage 0: normal
Stage 1: mild, can work
Stage 2: moderate but cannot work
Stage 3: severe, cannot work, major intellectual disability
Stage 4: vegetative **(In AIDS dementia complex, a "vegetative" patient can be aroused to a level of alertness. This is an important distinction between AIDS dementia complex & many other potential etiologies)**

Overview: *Topics Antiviral Med 22:594, 2014*

Impaired short-term memory, ↓ concentration, clumsiness, slowness, apathy, irritability, & personality changes. Process is slowly progressive, weeks to months (usually occurs after AIDS defining diagnosis) **& CD4 count usually <200/mm³.**

Degree of intellectual impairment & stage of ADC correlates with CSF HIV RNA. Higher levels of HIV RNA in CSF predict progression of neuropsychological impairment & postmortem evidence of HIV encephalitis.

Neuro exam: non-focal	Early	Late
Cognition	Inattention ↓ concentration Forgetfulness, slowing of thought processing	Global dementia
Motor	Slowed movements Clumsiness Ataxia	Paraplegia
Behavior	Apathy Blunting of personality Agitation	Mutism

CSF: Normal 30–50%, ↑ WBC (monos) 5–10% [CSF abnormalities: pleocytosis, ↑ protein or ↑ immunoglobulin levels reported in 30% asymptomatic HIV+ individuals].

MRI scan: Early is typically normal. **Cerebral atrophy, occ. with diffuse fluff ("spilled milk"), edema of antral white matter & basal ganglii, best seen on T-2 weighted imaging.** No mass effect. Normal gadolinium rules out most cases of primary brain lymphoma & toxo but does not rule out other infections (neurosyphilis, cryptococcal meningitis, MAC encephalitis).

Pts receiving antiretroviral therapy (ART) have fewer cognitive abnormalities than untreated pts, & when impaired may show marked improvement with rx. Symptoms of acute meningoencephalitis may reflect failure of ART with ↑ CSF HIV viral load & may respond to change in ART.

Declining mental acuity with concomitant depression of alertness (without focal findings)

AIDS dementia complex (ADC) *(as above, Stage 3 or 4)*

Cryptococcal disease *(see meningitis, page 70; Eye, page 68)*

Toxoplasmic encephalitis

Progressive multifocal leukoencephalopathy (PML) *(see page 87)*

Primary CNS lymphoma *(see page 87)*

Depression of alertness occurs only in advanced disease.

Late stage: ARVs with high levels of CNS penetration did not protect against dementia *(Neurology 83:109 & 134, 2014).*

Often assoc. with ↑ CSF pressure

Usually focal findings

Pts usually alert in early stages of disease; can become depressed later

Rare without focal findings, occurs when deep structures in brain involved

TABLE 11A (3)

CLINICAL SYNDROME, ETIOLOGY, EPIDEMIOLOGY	CLINICAL PRESENTATION, DIAGNOSTIC TESTS, COURSE
Central Nervous System/Cognitive Disorders, Diffuse Brain Dysfunction/Declining mental acuity with concomitant depression of alertness *(continued)*	
Cytomegalovirus (CMV) encephalitis (CD4 <50/mm3)	
Frequency not well defined. Overall CMV ~20%, clinical encephalitis occurs in ~1% of CMV cases. **Diagnosis made by detection of CMV DNA by PCR in CSF.** Response to rx variable. CMV can cause apoptosis of neuronal, glial, & endothelial cells of the CNS *(J. Clin Viro 32:218, 2005).*	Onset subacute: delirium/confusion 90%, apathy & withdrawal 60%, focal neurologic signs 50%. Antecedent CMV disease is common. Metabolic abnormalities, hyponatremia, hyperkalemia, hypo-osmolality, hypernatremia secondary to dehydration. **Non-specific CSF:** no cells or mildly ↑ **cells,** or mildly ↑ **protein, mild ↓ glucose.** Typical neuropathologic feature is ventriculoencephalitis with periventricular necrotic lesions. Micronodular encephalitis with microglial nodules involving parenchyma, cerebellum, spinal cord also occurs; meninges may be involved. **MRI with contrast: meningeal enhancement, focal ring-enhancing lesions, or periventricular enhancement with gadolinium; lacks sensitivity and may be normal despite advanced CMV disease. PCR for CMV DNA ~90% sensitive & 90% specific.**
Tuberculosis. *See meningitis, page 70.*	Always consider in 3rd World (esp. Africa) or immigrant from a region with a high prevalence of TB with symptoms of altered mental status, headache, lethargy or coma.
Neurosyphilis (general paresis, meningovascular)	Serum VDRL & FTA/ABS + in >90%. Diagnosis established by presence of CSF lymphocytic pleocytosis, high protein or positive CSF serology in presence of compatible clinical syndrome and/or + FTA-ABS in serum. CSF VDRL sensitivity ranges from 10–89%. CSF FTA-ABS highly sensitive in HIV- cases (>95%), with similar sensitivity likely in HIV+ cases. MRI: cortical infarcts. *(Clin Radiol 61:393, 2006).* Indications for CSF examination: neurologic, ophthalmic, or otologic symptoms; evidence of acute tertiary syphilis; treatment failure (4-fold increase in nontreponemal serology after treatment or lack of 4-fold decrease within 12 mo. after treatment) Routine CSF examination does not improve outcome. CSF examination indicated for those with serological evidence of syphilis and neurological symptoms, isolated ophthalmic syphilis, or <4-fold decrease in RPR titers after treatment *(MMWR 59/RR-12, 2010 and CID 53:S110, 2011).*
Herpes simplex virus (HSV) encephalitis Frequency & role still undefined but probably no more common than in non-AIDS population *(Clin Raiolo 61:393, 2006).*	Clinical presentation: confusion, fever & headache, anxiety & depression, memory loss, aphasia. CSF: virus seldom cultured from CSF. Definitive dx requires brain biopsy or CSF PCR test for HSV DNA (98% sensitive during 1st wk of disease). HSV2 encephalitis also reported *(AIDS Reader 17:67, 2007)*
Focal brain dysfunction: seizures &/or focal neurologic findings (hemiparesis, cerebrovascular abnormalities, blindness).	Risk of focal brain lesions ↓ with ART but most dramatic ↓ with primary CNS lymphoma & toxo, PML slight ↑.
Abrupt onset Cerebrovascular events: transient ischemic attack (TIA), cerebrovascular accident (stroke, CVA); risk of ischemic/hemorrhagic stroke may be increasing in ART era.	Causes of ischemic events include atherosclerosis, embolism, vasculitis, hypercoagulable state *(Neurol 17:1257, 2007).* Exclude meningovascular syphilis, VZV, lymphoma, cryptomeningitis, cocaine use with vasospasm ischemic events. ↑ life expectancy & metabolic side effects leading to atherosclerosis from ART; expect ↑ incidence of strokes.
Subacute course (days)	
Toxoplasmic encephalitis (TE). Common in untreated AIDS and frequent AIDS-defining illness, even during ART era. Frequency ↓ with use of TMP/SMX prophylaxis vs. *P. jirovecii* and ART. Seroprevalence varies widely among countries: from 10-20% to 50% or higher, especially in African countries.	Symptoms: Headache 50–70%, altered mental status 70%, hemiparesis &/or other focal signs 60%, seizures 30%. Fever, confusion, coma also seen. Symptoms may recur with immune reconstitution from ART even with successful rx for toxo. **Lab: CD4 <100/mm³ in 80%.** Toxoplasma serum IgG is + in essentially all pts who develop TE (frequency 85–99%) & titer predictive of development of disease: Relative risk ↑ with >150 intl units/mL IgG and CD4 <200. Specific prophylaxis is protective. **Scan:** MRI more sensitive than CT. **Multiple spherical ring-enhancing lesions,** corticomedullary junction, basal ganglia, thalamus often involved and mass effect common. Lesions often identified even without concomitant neurologic findings. **Course:** >85% will respond to specific anti-toxo treatment *(Cochrane Database System Rev Jul19:CD005420, 2006),* most within 7 days. **If no improvement after 7–10 days of rx–biopsy.** Primary CNS lymphoma common in "non-responsive" cases. Brain biopsy indicated earlier (in <7 days) in patients with CD4 >100 or if negative toxo antibody titer, single lesion & progression of symptoms on antitoxo rx. If improvement, biopsy not required. Neurologic deficits often persist *(Clin Microbiol Infect 13:510, 2007).*

TABLE 11A (4)

CLINICAL SYNDROME, ETIOLOGY, EPIDEMIOLOGY	CLINICAL PRESENTATION, DIAGNOSTIC TESTS, COURSE
Focal Brain Dysfunction/Subacute course *(continued)*	
Primary CNS lymphoma ↓ incidence from 8.0/1000 person-years pre-ART to 2.3/1000 person-yrs post-ART. Epstein-Barr virus DNA present in nearly all.	Symptoms: Usually afebrile; headache, confusion, focal neurologic deficits, seizures. Often alert, but with mass effect may have more global mental dysfunction. **Lab:** CSF: Normal 30–50%, protein 10–150 mg/dl, cells (monos) 0–40/mm^3, cytology + in <5%. CSF PCR for detection of **EBV DNA has sensitivity >90%, but lacks specificity and may have a poor positive predictive value** *(CID 38:1629, 2004)*. **Scan:** White matter more often involved than gray matter. One or a few weakly enhancing irregular lesions, typically in periventricular region with mass effect. Biopsy necessary for definitive diagnosis. **Course:** median survival time poor (<3 mo); improved survival with ART.
Tuberculous/non-tuberculous mycobacterial brain abscess *(see meningitis, page 70)-tuberculoma*	Uncommon.
Cryptococcoma *(see meningitis, page 70)* May coexist or be confused with toxo encephalitis	Usually concomitant with cryptococcal meningitis, CRAG of CSF & serum positive, but with an isolated cryptococcoma, CRAG (serum & CSF) may be negative.
Varicella zoster virus (VZV) encephalitis *(AIDS Reader 17:64, 2007)* Less common complication of dermatomal zoster with ART.	Often associated with dermatomal zoster or vesicular rash. Signs and symptoms: headache, altered mental status, seizures, seizures, cranial nerve palsies. CSF: 0-300 WBCs, predom. lymphs, mild ↑ in protein. **PCR detection of VZV DNA sensitive & specific.** Scan: nonspecific with multifocal white matter lesions. >50% recovery with antiviral therapy.
Aspergillosis • ↑ in pts with ↓ WBC & rx with corticosteroids • Direct extension from sinuses or orbits—also from lung	Nonspecific neuro symptoms including headache, cranial or somatic nerve weakness or paresthesias, altered mental status & seizures. High mortality; medical rx usually unsuccessful. Scan—CT reveals hypodense lesions.
Herpes simplex virus (HSV) encephalitis	*See page 86.*
Bartonella henselae, with neurologic complications	Encephalitis, dementia. Scan: Contrast-enhancing mass lesion.
Nocardia brain abscess	Rare; can be confused with tuberculosis.
Chronic course (weeks)	
Progressive multifocal leukoencephalopathy (PML) Frequency 4–7% of AIDS patients. Caused by JC virus (a papovavirus), which infects oligodendrocytes, the myelin-producing cells of the CNS. CD4 usually ≤100/mm^3. Prolonged survival & remission reported with highly effective antiretroviral rx but not consistently. Although typically non-inflammatory, inflammatory lesions from immune reconstitution syndrome upon institution of ART may worsen and lead to a fatal outcome *(Scand J Infect Dis 39:347, 2007)*.	**Symptoms: Develops insidiously with a single focus** (limb weakness 1/3, ataxia 13%, visual defects 1/3, altered mental status 1/3) but afebrile & arousable (preservation of alertness until late into disease course). With progression, multiple foci occur. Seizures found in 20% in one series. **Lab:** CSF: Normal (pleocytosis in 20%, ↑ protein 30%). CSF **JC IgM antibody & PCR of CSF for JCV 82% sensitive, 100% specific.** If CD4 <100, JC viral load in CSF predictive of disease state & progression but true not in patients Rx with ART *(CID 40:738, 2005)* on ART with CD4 >100. **MRI Scan: Multiple fluffy or diffuse hypodense non-contrast enhancing lesions in subcortical white matter, no mass effect.** High signal intensity on T-2 images in hemispheric white matter, ill-defined margins (CT/MRI—clinical dissociation, images worse than pt. symptoms). May become contrast-enhancing with immune reconstitution assoc. with ART. Occ. inflammation present without ART. Brain biopsy is definitive diagnostic procedure (demyelination, JCV on electron microscopy), sensitivity 40–96%, but not required if MRI is characteristic & CSF JC PCR is positive. **Course:** Death usual within 6 mos but spontaneous sustained remissions occur in 5–10. **Immune reconstitution with ART may have serious consequences due to** ↑ inflammatory changes in area of PML lesion. **No clear consensus on management of PML currently exists.**

CLINICAL SYNDROME, ETIOLOGY, EPIDEMIOLOGY	CLINICAL PRESENTATION, DIAGNOSTIC TESTS, COURSE
Central Nervous System *(continued)*	
Most Common Peripheral Nerve Syndromes in HIV Disease by Stage	
Peripheral neuropathies are common (6–13%) in HIV/AIDS. They most commonly affect the sensory nerves & are caused by either HIV, opportunistic infections, drugs or are idiopathic. They present as part of several discrete syndromes & vary according to stage of disease.	
Acute retroviral syndrome Neuropathy (6–8%)	*See Acute retroviral syndrome, page 84.* Headache/retro-orbital pain, often ↑ with eye movement (30%), photophobia. Myelopathy, peripheral neuropathy, brachial neuritis, facial palsy, cauda equina & Guillain-Barré syndrome. **Course: Usually self-limited, but persistence reported.**
Early (asymptomatic HIV: CD4 >200)	
Inflammatory demyelinating polyneuropathy (IDP) (occurs <5%) *(see below)*	
Subacute (Guillain-Barré syndrome) or acute inflammatory demyelinating polyradiculoneuropathy (AIDP).	Ascending paralysis with preservation of sensory function—global limb weakness. Probably represents autoimmune phenomenon. Nerve conduction studies show demyelinating features. One pt with CMV-associated Guillain-Barré responded to ganciclovir + ART. May be associated with immune reconstitution.
Chronic (chronic inflammatory demyelinating polyneuropathy) (CIDP or IDP) (may also occur late)	Progressive weakness in arms & legs, paresthesias with minor sensory loss, may be asymmetrical, absent DTRs Demyelinating polyneuropathy, CSF ↑↑ protein, mild to moderate lymphocytic pleocytosis (10–50 cells/mm³), EMG shows demyelination.
Mononeuritis, multiplex (MM) (also occurs late) (rare)	Facial weakness, foot or wrist drop EMG, multifocal axonal neuropathy, multifocal cranial & peripheral neuropathies, thought to be immune mediated or vasculitis
Multiple sclerosis-like syndrome (rare) *(Neurologist 13:154, 2007).*	Waxing & waning course, multifocal defect, may rarely represent immune reconstitution inflammatory syndrome (IRIS).
Late (symptomatic HIV), CD4 <200	
Weakness/spasticity:	
Vacuolar myelopathy (occurs in as many as 40% of patients at autopsy) & is the most common form of spinal cord disease in HIV-infected individuals; under-recognized clinically. Infectious causes of myelopathies: HTLV-1, herpesviruses (VZV, HSV2, CMV), enteroviruses, *T. pallidum*, TB, various fungi, & parasites.	Progressive painless gait disturbance with ataxia & spasticity. Also rarely occurring in upper extremities. CSF normal or ↑ protein, 5–10 cells/mm³. Imaging usually normal. Use of somatosensory-evoked potentials in pts with absent ankle DTRs valuable dx tool in differential dx of myelopathy from neuropathy.
CMV, Progressive lumbosacral polyradiculopathy/myelitis (DDx: VZV, syphilis, spinal lymphoma)	Subacute onset. Back & radicular pain, ascending weakness, areflexia, bladder & sphincter dysfunction, variable sensory loss but may produce "saddle anesthesia." May progress rapidly to flaccid paralysis. CMV PCR in blood and CSF positive.
Mononeuritis multiplex due to CMV	Multifocal sensory & motor deficits in major peripheral or cranial nerves (esp. laryngeal nerves & upper > lower extremities—acute onset over 1 mo), usually painful. CD4 <50. CMV PCR in blood and CSF positive.

TABLE 11A (6)

CLINICAL SYNDROME, ETIOLOGY, EPIDEMIOLOGY	CLINICAL PRESENTATION, DIAGNOSTIC TESTS, COURSE
Central Nervous System/Most Common Peripheral Nerve Syndromes in HIV Disease by Stage/Late *(continued)*	
Numbness/burning: Distal sensory loss with neuropathic pain (most common neuropathy). Symptoms: pain (often described as excruciating unremitting pain), paresthesias, ↓ ankle reflexes, ↓ vibratory or pinprick sensation.	
Distal predominantly sensory symmetrical polyneuropathy (DSP) (occurs in up to 50% of pts with late-stage HIV) *(Neurology 66:1679, 2006)*. Risk factors include age >40, diabetes, white race, nadir CD4 <50 & 50–199, VL >10,000 copies/mL at 1st measurement plus ETOH abuse, drugs (vincristine, INH & thalidomide & ribavirin) *(CID 40:148, 2005; Neurology 66:1679, 2006)*. ↓ incidence with ART *(CID 40:148, 2005)*.	Hyperesthesia, **"burning" feet,** distal numbness with ↓ ankle DTR, stocking/glove sensory loss. Severity of symptoms (pain) correlates with plasma HIV-1 RNA levels. Suppression of HIV may improve symptoms.
Toxic neuropathy from antiretroviral drugs (TNA) (ddI > d4T >3TC) (occurs >5%) but has been reported to occur in up to 30% of pts on ddI. Frequency associated with dose & duration of exposure: d4T in combination with ddI doubles risk. FDA warning for ribavirin + ddI ± d4T assoc. with mitochondrial toxicity. Disease progression & host factors (mitochondrial haplogroup & age) all predispose individuals to neurotoxic effects of antiretroviral drugs *(CID 40: 148, 2005)*. Protease inhibitors may also potentiate neuronal damage & toxic neuropathy *(Ann Neurol 59:816, 2006)*. Etiology associated with NRTI selective inhibition of γ-DNA polymerase leading to depletion of mitochondrial DNA & degeneration of mitochondria of neurons & Schwann cells.	**Aching feeling of feet, burning sensation.** ↑ serum lactate levels discriminated d4T neuropathy from DSP neuropathy (90% sensitivity, 90% specificity). **EMG:** axonal neuropathy; symptoms (pain) may worsen for up to 4 wks after discontinuation of rx. Some pts able to continue drugs with full or reduced dose & neuropathy may improve or resolve; however, substantial. Substantial portion of pts continue to experience debilitating pain. **Lamotrigine** (an anticonvulsant drug) ↓ pain vs. placebo in 227 pts. Rash a common side effect. Results confirmed in 92 pts receiving ART. No difference from placebo in 135 pts with DSP without ART. Coenzyme Q actually ↑ pain. Rx with acetyl-l-carnitine (1500 mg q12h po) up to 33 mos. assoc. with ↓ symptoms & peripheral nerve regeneration in 21 HIV+ pts with TNA *(HIV Clin Trials 6:344, 2005)*.
Weakness/myalgias:	
Myopathy due to drugs: H V, zidovudine [ZDV + ddC > ZDV + ddI]	Weakness without sensory finding, DTRs intact with myalgias. EMG: irritative myopathy, ↑ CPK, muscle biopsy, myofibril degeneration + inflammation.

TABLE 11A (7)

CLINICAL SYNDROME, ETIOLOGY, EPIDEMIOLOGY	CLINICAL PRESENTATION, DIAGNOSTIC TESTS, COURSE
Endocrine System	

Adrenal gland (the most commonly affected endocrine gland)
Primary adrenal failure; causes include: Too little steroid:
• CMV adrenalitis (found in 33–88% of AIDS pts at autopsy)
• HIV infection of adrenal
• Infiltration by Kaposi's sarcoma, lymphoma or infection (MAC, crypto, histo, pneumocystis)
• Drug-induced: ketoconazole (impairs steroid synthesis), fluconazole (1 report: 800 mg q24h x 68 days, *J Microbiol Immun Inf 37:250, 2004*); 6 cases of overt Addison's diseases on withdrawal of inhaled corticosteroids (fluticasone) with ritonavir *(J Clin Endocrinol Metab 90:4394, 2005)*, megestrol (prolonged use) *(AnIM 122:843, 1995)*
• Pituitary insufficiency *(see above)*
Too much steroid:
• Iatrogenic Cushing's Syndrome
  o Use of glucocorticosteroids with ritonavir boosted protease inhibitors *(J Asthma 47:830, 2010)*
  o Avascular necrosis of bone reported with ritonavir and even inhaled steroids *(Int J STD AIDS:458, 2014)*
	Addison's disease: fever, hypotension, abdominal pain, hyponatremia, hyperkalemia.
	Overt Addison's disease is uncommon, although blunted responses to ACTH are common. Addisonian crisis may be precipitated by excessive stress or ketoconazole. CMV antigenemia assoc. with adrenal insufficiency. If suboptimal response to ACTH stimulation & ↓ stress cortisol serum levels should receive stress doses of corticosteroids where there is infection, trauma, etc.

Pancreatitis
Etiology of pancreatitis correlates with CD4 count.
• CD4 count ≤200:
  o Disseminated infection or tumor infiltration predominate.
  o Infection: CMV, Crypto, Mycobacteria
  o Tumor: KS or lymphoma
	• CD4 >200:
	  o Infection less common
	  o Medication-induced pancreatitis major concern, e.g., didanosine, stavudine, pentamidine, ritonavir & sulfonamides. Mechanism postulated as mitochondrial toxicity
	  o Other etiologies are similar to non-HIV patients, e.g., stones, stricture, alcohol, hypertriglyceridemia

Hypogonadism in Males: *J Clin Endocrin Metab 95:2536, 2010.* • Primary hypogonadism results from testicular disease; secondary hypogonadism results from pituitary or hypothalamic dysfunction. In patients on ART, secondary is more common. With early ART, prevalence is lower. • In men age >49 yrs, lower testosterone levels were associated with viral load, not CD4 count *(CID 41:1794, 2005)*. In men with ART-controlled HIV, lower testosterone levels may be due to obesity and insulin resistance (Nat Rev Endocrin 5:673, 2009), HCV, alcohol, opiates (including methadone), marijuana and psychotropic medications. • Testosterone level normally decreases with age. Some evidence of accelerated decrease in younger men despite effective ART *(PLoS One 6:e28512, 2011)*	• Can present with some combination of decrease in facial & body hair, reduced muscle strength, low libido, testicular atrophy and gynecomastia. • **Screening test is total serum testosterone level; <300 ng/dL is abnormal; can confirm with free testosterone level.** Draw testosterone levels at 8:00 am. • **If low** serum testosterone present, suggest LH and FSH levels *(J Clin Endocrin Metab 92:405, 2007)*. • **If elevated**, consistent with primary hypogonadism. Ultrasound of testicles indicated. • **If normal or low**, consistent with secondary hypogonadism. Consider MRI of pituitary and hypothalamus. **Indications for testosterone replacement therapy:** • Low libido, low bone density, weight loss despite low levels of circulating HIV • Testosterone can be given transdermally (patch or gel) or by injection *(J Clin Endocrin Metab 95:2536, 2010)* • Do not use in those with prostate or breast cancer *(Endocrinol Metab Clin North Am 43:709, 2014)* • Replacement may increase cardiovascular risk *(Hosp Pharm 52:712, 2016)*

TABLE 11A (8)

CLINICAL SYNDROME, ETIOLOGY, EPIDEMIOLOGY	CLINICAL PRESENTATION, DIAGNOSTIC TESTS, COURSE
Eyes: Ocular disease occurs in 45% of HIV patients (higher % in AIDS pts). Clinical complaints range from red eye to painful globe and loss of vision. It is convenient to divide the clinical syndromes anatomically: anterior eye structures (lids, conjunctiva, cornea & anterior uveal tract), posterior eye structures (posterior uveal tract and retina) &retrobulbar (retinal nerve) problems. Selected common problems are summarized in rough order of frequency. Syphilis, which can affect virtually any part of the eye, is increasingly recognized *(MMWR 64:1150, 2015; Curr Inf Dis Rep 18:36, 2016).*	
Anterior Eye Syndromes:	
Varicella zoster: Vesicular eruption in dermatomal distribution involving eyelid skin, conjunctiva & potentially cornea. Most common anterior problem in HIV pts with ocular disease *(Int Ophthal 32:145, 2012).*	Acute onset of painful vesicles. Diagnosis: clinical presentation diagnostics; 2/3 pts develop keratitis; iritis in 2/5. Need ophthalmology consult, systemic antivirals, topical corticosteroid drops.
Blepharitis: red itchy eyelids. Can be on outer or inner surface.	Outer blepharitis often due to Staph. aureus. There is also seborrheic blepharitis that acts like dandruff. Inflammation of the inner surface is due to dysfunction of the meibomian glands.
Keratoconjunctivitis sicca (KCS) (dry eye syndrome). Multifactorial dysfunction of the tear film. More common in HIV pts. Often co-exists with blepharitis.	KCS presents as scratchy dry eyes. Can document by measuring tear production. Responds to artificial tears. In Ethiopian study, KCS did not correlate with CD4 counts *(BMC Ophthalmol 13:20, 2013).*
Conjunctivitis: Red eye with/without exudate. Can be due to bacteria, virus or allergy. Often history of contact with persons with pink eye. Rarely, in AIDS, etiology is microsporidiosis.	Diagnose by clinical appearance. If uncertain, can culture exudate. If associated pain, need to evaluate for corneal involvement: keratitis. Adenovirus is most common etiology of pink eye.
Herpes simplex type 1 (HSV-1) keratitis: No more common in HIV, but more severe. Presents with red, painful eye and decreased visual acuity.	HSV-1 keratitis: Fluorescein staining demonstrates dendritic ulcer. Confirm with HSV-1 PCR. Treatment: topical antivirals. Some require concomitant steroids. Need ophthalmologic consult. Can cause significant scarring of the cornea.
Anterior uveitis (iris &ciliary body): Pain, redness, variable loss of vision. Can be associated with posterior uveitis (choroid & retina): visual impairment is more prominent symptom.	Many etiologies: OIs, drug toxicities, IRIS: Need ophthalmologic consult.
Posterior Eye Syndromes:	
HIV retinopathy/HIV microangiopathy: Causes visual impairment. More common in AIDS. Often associated cognitive impairment.	On exam: cotton wool spots, ischemic microangiopathy, retinal hemorrhages, microaneurysms. HIV-neuroretinal degeneration associated with subtle changes *(AIDS Patient Care STDs 29:519, 2015).* Increased macular retinal thickness and decreased cone density in HIV compared with controls *(PLoS One 10:e0132996, 2015).*
Cytomegalovirus (CMV) retinitis: Severity correlates with degree of immunodeficiency. Large decrease in prevalence with ART. Variable degrees of reduced visual acuity. Early symptoms include "floaters", flashings, scotoma. Silent CMV retinitis can flare with initiation of ART (IRIS).	Often starts in peripheral areas of retina, then advances toward macula and/or optic disc. Involved area appears white with associated hemorrhages ("cottage cheese" and "ketchup"). Retinal detachment can occur. Globe is not red or painful. Diagnosis: clinical appearance and detection of CMV DNA in serum by PCR. Risk of permanent visual field loss *(Ophthal 118:895, 2011).*
Herpes zoster/Varicella zoster retinitis: Primarily seen in AIDS. Can cause rapidly progressive necrosis of peripheral retina associated with occlusive vasculopathy plus inflammation of vitreous and anterior chambers. Can also occur as IRIS syndrome after starting ART.	Progressive outer retinal necrosis can quickly spread to central structures with complete loss of vision. Diagnosis: appearance of retina; also Varicella PCR on vitreous aspirate.
Toxoplasma chorioretinitis: Mostly in AIDS. More common in Europe, especially France. In South America, Tg strains are more virulent and more frequently associated with symptomatic disease. Presents with red, painful eye. May have associated inflammatory foci in brain.	Inflamed uveal tract. Retinal lesions may be single or multiple; perivascular. Variable degrees of impaired vision. Many have associated toxoplasma encephalitis. Diagnosis: Serum toxoplasma antibody titers may be low or only positive with undiluted samples; Inflamed uveal tract toxoplasma PCR on vitreous aspirate. Usually responds to toxoplasma treatment + ART.
Ocular Syphilis: Ocular syphilis more severe in HIV. Can involve uveal tract, retina and/or optic nerve. Wide variety of clinical syndromes: pain, blurry vision, red eye, scotomata. Think syphilis if uveitis in HIV. If retrobulbar neuritis, only symptom may be loss of vision.	Eye may/may not be red. Can cause necrotizing retinitis that could resemble CMV exudate. Diagnosis: Anti-treponemal serum antibody/RPR. Penicillin generally beneficial, but relapses can occur *(CID 51: 468, 2010).* Cluster of ocular syphilis reported among MSM *(MMWR 64: 1150, 2015).*

TABLE 11A (9)

CLINICAL SYNDROME, ETIOLOGY, EPIDEMIOLOGY	CLINICAL PRESENTATION, DIAGNOSTIC TESTS, COURSE
Eye *(continued)*	
Posterior Segment Infections:	
Cytomegalovirus (CMV) retinopathy: Rx: *See Table 12, page 130* **ART markedly improves survival & success of anti-CMV rx.** but vision loss from immune recovery uveitis (epiretinal membrane, cystoid macular edema or cataract) occurs. Rates of 2ⁿᵈ eye involvement ↓ with ART but not if CD4 stays <50/mm³ *(Ophthalmology 111:2232, 2004).*	**Peripheral retinitis, CD4 count is <50/mm³.** Course: Usually begins with unilateral "floaters" to ↓ visual acuity to blindness. **Ophthal. exam: Findings are usually initially in the periphery, moving centrally until macula &/or optic disc involved. Lesions are large creamy to white areas with granular borders & perivascular exudates & hemorrhages ("cottage cheese & ketchup" appearance) with little overlying vitreous reaction. If redness or pain of the eye, photophobia or irregular-shaped pupil develops, suspect infection other than CMV retinopathy.** Dx: Based on clinical features, CMV DNA+ in serum; ↓ with effective anti-CMV rx *(CID 15:1756, 2001).* ↑ CMV-specific CD4 &/or CD8 cells predict prevention of recurrence after ART *(AIDS Res Hum Retrovir 17:1749, 2001; (JID 184:256, 2001),* while failure to ↑ CMV-specific CD4 response assoc. with multiple relapses *(JID 183:1285, 2001).*
Primary CMV papillitis	**Rapid ↓ in visual acuity.** Swelling of optic nerve head, atrophy within 4 wks. Treatment with systemic ganciclovir or foscarnet (Ophthalmol 103: 1476, 1996); consider pulsed systemic steroids *(Am J Ophth 108: 691, 1989)* Dx & rx: *See CMV peripheral retinitis, above, & Table 12, page 130.*
Herpes zoster/simplex virus (VZV) retinitis (mean CD4 24)	**May not be associated with cutaneous zoster.** (1) **Acute retinal necrosis (ARN) syndrome:** rapidly progressive necrosis of peripheral retina (often 360°) with occlusive vasculopathy, marked vitreous & anterior chamber inflammation, optic neuritis & scleritis. Complete visual loss in involved eye. May be associated with retrobulbar optic neuritis *(Am J Neuroradiol 25:1722, 2004).* (2) **Progressive outer retinal necrosis (PORN):** Ill-defined areas of peripheral retinal whitening without granular borders, minimal vitreous reaction, no pain or foveal lesions (confused with CMV). Report of progressive outer retinal necrosis treated with ART, systemic, and intra-vitreal anti-virals *(J Clin Virol 38:254, 2007).* PORN typically occurs at very low CD4 counts, but has also been described after starting ARV therapy (e.g., VZV-positive rapidly progressive necrosis with no vitreal inflammation, 2 months after starting therapy when CD4 was 127) *(J Med Assoc Thai 92; Suppl 3: S52, 2009).*
HIV-associated "cotton wool" spots (CWS) CWS occurs in about 50% of patients with non-infectious microvascular retinopathy. Nonspecific findings & seen in many other conditions *(Med 82:187, 2003)*	Usually asymptomatic but occur more in late-stage disease. Ophthal. exam: Small fluffy white lesions with indistinct margins without exudates or hemorrhages. Lesions do not progress & usually regress spontaneously, do not require treatment. CWS may indicate ↑ risk for onset of CMV retinitis.
Iritis secondary to cidofovir *(CID 25:337, 1997; CID 28:156, 1999)*	Common with intravitreal injection but recurrent episodes with IV also reported.
Retinal depigmentation	5% of children on didanosine (ddI) usually at >300 mg/M²/day developed retinal depigmentation. Chorio-retinal atrophy reported in adults *(JAMA Ophthalmol 12: 255, 2013)*
Rifabutin-associated uveitis 1–2% pts on 600 mg/day. Also rarely on 300 mg/day.	↑ common with use of protease inhibitors (↑ rifabutin serum levels)
Syphilis: iridocyclitis, vitreitis, optic neuritis, chorioretinitis, or combinations of these. **Uveitis in HIV: Think syphilis** *(Int J STD AIDS 12:754, 2001)* Uveitis was bilateral in 80%; evidence of optic neuritis was detected in 50% of eyes. Focal anterior scleritis with retinitis caused by syphilis uncovered with immune reconstitution *(Clin Exp Ophthalmol 32:526, 2004).*	**In HIV+, syphilitic ocular disease is more common, more severe & often bilateral.** Sx may include blurred or ↓ vision, scotomata, redness, pain *(Amer J Med 119:448. 2006).* **Necrotizing retinitis with hemorrhage may be confused with CMV. Cream-colored posterior plaques may be seen with mucocutaneous lesions in 2° syphilis. May present as bilateral exudative retinal detachment** *(Ocul Immunol Inflamm 13:459, 2005).* CSF examination indicated to r/o neurosyphilis. Lab: Positive syphilis serologies. Course: Rx failures or relapses reported with penicillin used intravenously for 2-week courses *(CID 51:468, 2010).* Response usually good but depends on visual acuity at start of therapy *(Invest Ophthalmol Vis Sci 57:404, 2016).*

CLINICAL SYNDROME, ETIOLOGY, EPIDEMIOLOGY	CLINICAL PRESENTATION, DIAGNOSTIC TESTS, COURSE
Eye/Posterior Segment Infections (*continued*)	
Toxoplasmic chorioretinitis Ocular involvement uncommon in AIDS. Lesions may be single or multifocal, usually discrete, perivascular in location.	Pre-existing chorioretinal scars usually absent. Hemorrhages are absent or minimal. Vitreitis & iridocyclitis (red, painful eye) are common. May occur without intracranial lesions. Lab: PCR for toxo DNA in vitreous fluid may be of value *(Ophthal 106:1554, 1999; Ophthal 111:716, 2004)*. Course: Response to rx usually good, prolonged suppression required. Oral steroids not used.

Fever of Unknown Origin: *Infect Dis Clin N Amer 21:1013, 2007; Eur J Int Med 20:474, 2009.*

Definition: In HIV/AIDS:
- o Temperature >38.3 C (100.9 F) on multiple occasions x 4 weeks (outpatient) or >3 days (inpatient)
- o No diagnosis after 3 days of investigation

Variables that influence distribution of infectious etiologies:
- o Degree of immune deficiency
- o Country of exposure
- o Antibiotic prophylaxis
- o Degree of immunodeficiency

Differential Diagnosis:
- Infection (82-91%):
  - o Mycobacteria: *M. tuberculosis* or MAC; local or disseminated; most common etiology (46%)
  - o Pneumocystis pneumonia (PJP) (5-13%)
  - o CMV (5%)
  - o Endemic mycoses: Histoplasmosis (7%) or Coccidiomycosis (less common)
  - o Visceral leishmaniasis (southwest Europe)
  - o Cryptococcosis, Penicillium marneffei, Toxoplasmosis, Bartonella (Bacillary angiomatosis), Nocardia, Rhodococcus, Babesiosis, neurosyphilis
  - o Primary HIV
  - o IRIS
- *Neoplasia (8%):* ^{18}F-FDG PET/CT helpful *(Nucl Med Comm 37:57, 2016)*
  - o Non-Hodgkin's lymphoma
  - o Visceral Kaposi's sarcoma
- *Drug-related:*
  - o TMP/SMX, Isoniazid, Rifampin, Pyrazinamide
  - o ART drugs: Abacavir, AZT, Nevirapine
- *Other:*
  - o Multi-centric Castleman's Disease
  - o St. Louis Encephalitis
  - o Factitious
- No identifiable etiology in 6-14%
- Diagnosis: varies by patient
- **Diagnostic methods:** vary by patient; not all tests for every patient
- **Suggested evaluations:**
  - o Complete history & physical exam
  - o Review of all medications
  - o Blood cultures: standard & mycobacterial
  - o Serum cryptococcal antigen
  - o Blood CMV PCR
  - o Toxoplasma antibody
  - o Sputum or BAL for pneumocystis; PCR
  - o Urine antigen for histoplasmosis (perhaps)
  - o CT scans: chest, abdomen
  - o Fluordeoxyglucose PET scan *(Am J Roentgenol 197:248, 2011)*(in selected cases)
  - o Biopsy: skin, lymph nodes, liver, bone marrow
  - o Echocardiogram

TABLE 11A (11)

CLINICAL SYNDROME, ETIOLOGY, EPIDEMIOLOGY	CLINICAL PRESENTATION, DIAGNOSTIC TESTS, COURSE
Gastrointestinal Tract (Review: *Gut 57:861, 2008*)	
Mouth (*Bull World Health Organ 83:700, 2005, Top HIV Med 13;143, 2006; Adv Dent Res 19:63 & 57, 2006*). Oral manifestations very common in HIV-infected persons worldwide.	
Oral lesions without soreness (or mild soreness)	
Acute retroviral syndrome	Oral ulcerations (aphthous ulcers), enanthems and oral candidiasis.
Candidiasis (majority have CD4 <200)	Response to ART with ↑ CD4 assoc. with ↓ oropharyngeal candidiasis.
Kaposi's sarcoma (100% had CD4 <200)	Red to purple macules, papules or nodules, occasionally the same color as adjoining tissue, on tongue, palate or buccal mucosa. Usually asymptomatic but may become painful with ulceration & inflammation. Lab: Biopsy necessary for dx since bacillary angiomatosis may have similar appearance.
Hairy leukoplakia (HLP) (majority have CD4 <200) Epstein-Barr virus can be detected by immunochemistry, in situ hybridization or EBV-DNA by PCR in nearly 100% of lesions (*J Oral Pathol Med 29:118, 2000; Am J. Clin Pathol 114:395, 2000*).	**Lesions usually asymptomatic. White thickening of oral mucosa &/or lateral tongue margins with vertical folds or corrugations.** Lesions range from few mm to covering entire dorsal surface of the tongue. ↑ frequency in smokers (*J AIDS 21:236, 1999*). Cannot be scraped off. **Lab: Biopsy; epithelial hyperplasia with thickened parakeratin layer with hair-like projections & vacuolated prickle cells.**
Warts [human papillomavirus (HPV)] Oral warts may ↑ in size & frequency in response to ART.	Usually asymptomatic. Present as single or multiple papilliform warts with multiple white spike-like projections, or as pink cauliflower masses, or as flat lesions resembling focal epithelial hyperplasia. Lab: Biopsy. Types 7, 13 & 32, but usually not 6, 11, 16 & 18 which are associated with anogenital warts. Optimal therapy unknown; surgery often needed (*aidsinfo.nih.giv/contentfiles/lvguidelines/adult_oi.pdf*). Rx with topical cidofovir gel 1% was successful in 1 recalcitrant case (*Cutis 73:191, 2004*).
Secondary syphilis (often multiple) (*Med Oral 9:33, 2004*)	Dx by syphilis serology and RPR, and/or biopsy.
Lymphoma	Poorly demarcated swelling on alveolar ridges &/or discrete oral masses. Lab: Biopsy. May be EBV+ (*Oral Oncol 38:96, 2002*). Plasmablastic lymphoma often presents with oral lesions (*Am J Hematol 83:804, 2008*).
Carcinoma, squamous cell: ↑ risk.	Squamous cell carcinoma of tongue reported in HIV disease. Lab: Biopsy.
Cytomegalovirus (CMV) oral ulcers	A rare manifestation of CMV. Usually with disseminated infection. Lab: Biopsy & immunohistochemistry.
Histoplasmosis, Geotrichosis, Cryptococcosis, Penicillium marneffei, Leishmaniasis.	Rare in occurrence. Lesions painless, clean ulcerations on palate, gingiva, tongue and/or oropharynx. Lab: Biopsy; organism identified on culture & stains.
Sore mouth without discrete lesions	
HIV-associated gingivitis & periodontitis: Common with advanced HIV. Pts at all stages of HIV infection have ↑ numbers of PMNs & mast cells throughout the gingiva & ↑ macrophages below the gingival epithelium (*AIDS 16:235, 2002*). Chronic periodontitis assoc. with ↑ cells with ↑ expression of HIV receptors/co-receptors/α defensins perhaps ↑ susceptibility of HIV infection via oral route (*J Dent Res 83:371, 2004*). Response to Rx improved with ART (*Eur J Med Res 11:232, 2006*).	Marked halitosis, spontaneous bleeding & deep-seated gingival pain are usual. Gingiva show fiery red margins with necrosis & ulceration of interdental papillae. May rapidly progress to loss of gingival soft tissue & destruction of supporting bone leading to loss of teeth & necrotizing stomatitis. Is similar to noma (gangrenous stomatitis). Consider in the differential of oral disease due to methamphetamine use (Xerostomia, extensive caries, periodontal disease, pain) (*Oral Dis 15:27, 2009*). Dx: Based on clinical features. Cultures not helpful. Rx: Start with curettage/debridement, followed by topical povidone-iodine (Betadine) irrigation, then chlorhexidine gluconate (Peridex) mouthwash + oral antibiotics effective against anaerobes (metronidazole, clindamycin, AM/CL).

TABLE 11A (12)

CLINICAL SYNDROME, ETIOLOGY, EPIDEMIOLOGY	CLINICAL PRESENTATION, DIAGNOSTIC TESTS, COURSE
Gastrointestinal Tract/Mouth (*continued*)	
Oral lesions, painful	
Recurrent aphthous ulcers (RAU) More common in HIV disease, last longer & produce more painful symptoms than in immunocompetent persons.	Recurrent crops of superficial painful ulcers (1 mm to 1 cm) on non-keratinized oral or oropharyngeal mucosa. Lab: Biopsy; shows only non-specific inflammation. *See Table 12, page 133.*
Herpes simplex virus (HSV)—*See rx, page 131* HSV-1 most common cause, rarely HSV-2; both can be shed in oral secretions (*Sex Trans Inf 80:272, 2004*).	Recurrent crops of small painful vesicles that ulcerate, usually on palate or gingiva. Usually heal but tend to recur. Herpetic geometric glossitis extremely tender longitudinal fissures occur, heal with acyclovir IV. Lab: Smears from lesions reveal multinucleate giant cells, + for HSV on immunofluorescent staining.
Xerostomia (dry mouth)	
Sjögren's-like syndrome—may be drug-associated	Clinical: Dry mouth occurs in 2% of patients on didanosine (ddI). PI-based ART was a risk factor for ↓ saliva and salivary gland enlargement in HIV-positive women (*Oral Dis 15:52, 2009*). *See Salivary gland enlargement, below.* Rx: Saliva substitutes (electrolytes in carboxymethylcellulose base) & nasal spray may help.
Salivary gland enlargement	
Benign parotid lymphoepithelial lesions (diffuse infiltrative CD8 lymphocytosis syndrome or DILS; *may have systemic features*) (*ArthrRheum 55:466, 2006*) CD4 counts 200–500/mm³ ↑ prevalence in Africans with HIV infection reported	Presents as painless (80%) bilateral parotid swelling due to infiltration with CD8 + T lymphocytes. Submandibular glands not involved. 80% have generalized lymphadenopathy, bilateral cervical. Resembles Sjögren's syndrome with sicca symptoms (dry mouth & eyes). Associated findings may include lymphocytic interstitial pneumonia (60%), aseptic meningitis. Most black pts were HLA-DR5. In contrast to Sjögren's, none had anti Ro/SS-A or anti La/55-B antibodies, rheumatoid factor usually negative. Dx based on fine needle aspiration. More common in children.
Other possibilities: CMV (17%), candida, PJP, mumps, parainfluenza, adenovirus, lymphoma, Kaposi's sarcoma, tuberculosis; 10 cases reported (*J Oral Pathol Med 34: 407, 2005*). MAC, sarcoid	Uni- or bilateral painful parotid swelling. KS present as painless mass in parotid or submandibular region.
Esophagus. Esophageal motility disorders common (16/18, 88%) with or without symptoms of dysphagia or odynophagia (*Dig Dis Sci 48:962, 2003*)	
Dysphagia (difficulty swallowing with a sensation of food sticking)	
Candidiasis Frequency 50–70%; decline in ART era (*Am J Gastro 100:1455, 2005*) The most common cause of dysphagia in HIV+ patients (42–79% of pts).	For therapy, *see Table 12, page 121*. If no response to therapy for candida, then endoscope to r/o CMV, HSV or aphthous ulcers. X-ray: Barium swallow; typically evidence of plaques & ulceration ("moth-eaten" appearance). Findings supportive but not diagnostic. Endoscopy: Large yellow-white plaques usually seen throughout the esophagus. Biopsy/brushing: Will show tissue-invasive pseudomycelia. Secondary prophylaxis: Recurrence rates (20–80%) in 45–90 days if ART not successful. *See Table 12, page 121.*
Odynophagia (pain on swallowing) or esophagospasm (retrosternal episodic pain without swallowing)	
Cytomegalovirus (CMV) esophagitis	Symptoms are odynophagia, usually without dysphagia, weight loss. Endoscopy: Large solitary (>10 cm² in surface area), shallow, superficial ulcers especially in distal esophagus. Histology necessary to establish diagnosis. If no inclusions and neg. immunohistochemical stain, rx as aphthous ulcer.
Idiopathic (aphthous) esophageal ulceration	Pts present with odynophagia. Differential diagnosis: CMV, HSV, drug-induced ulcers. Endoscopy: Large discrete ulcers. May respond to ART alone. Rx: Prednisone 40 mg po q24h, taper by 10 mg/wk, total course 4 wks. Thalidomide (200 mg po q24h x 14 d). Not FDA-approved indication. *See Black Box warnings.* MUST exclude pregnancy. (*ref JID 180: 61, 1999*).

TABLE 11A (13)

CLINICAL SYNDROME, ETIOLOGY, EPIDEMIOLOGY	CLINICAL PRESENTATION, DIAGNOSTIC TESTS, COURSE
Gastrointestinal Tract/Esophagus/Odynophagia (pain on swallowing) or esophagospasm *(continued)*	
Herpes simplex virus (HSV) esophagitis	Clinical: Acute onset, intense pain, widespread involvement. May be associated with oral herpes *in pts with CD4 < 100.* Occasionally seen in non-immunocompromised individuals. Endoscopy: Shallow erosive ulcers (like reflux esophagitis). Rx: Acyclovir.
Esophageal ulcers associated with acute HIV infection	Clinical: Acute retroviral syndrome (fever, myalgia, macular or papular rash) *(page 84)* + odynophagia or dysphagia. Lesions heal spontaneously. Pts are not predisposed to recurrent esophageal ulceration. Endoscopy: One or more discrete ulcers. On biopsy: retroviral virions. Rx: Viscous lidocaine may ↓ symptoms.
Other: Lymphoma, Kaposi's sarcoma, squamous cell carcinoma, histoplasmosis, leishmaniasis. Non-infectious causes include Crohn's, Behçet's, drugs (bisphosphonates, tetracyclines).	
Abdominal pain, acute onset *(J Emer Med 23:111, 2002)*	
See **Pancreatitis**	Predictive outcome similar to pancreatitis in non-HIV infected populations.
Bowel perforation/peritonitis Most common cause is CMV in advanced HIV infection (AIDS)	AIDS pts with perforation usually febrile, with rigid abdomen, rebound tenderness. Perforations most common in large bowel. Also lymphoma, typhlitis, KS, tuberculosis, salmonellosis. Immune reconstitution from ART assoc with perforation of ileocecal TB *(Dis Col Rect 15:977, 2002).*

Small bowel disease: cramping paraumbilical abdominal pain, weight loss, large volume diarrhea

Diarrhea is a common complication and presenting feature of HIV infection. Diarrhea lasting more than 5 days should be evaluated by microscopic exam (wet mount for Isospora and E. histolytica, modified acid fast for cryptosporidia and cyclospora, modified trichrome for microsporidia); cultures for salmonella, shigella, campylobacter, and enteropathogenic E. coli; PCR or toxin assay for C. difficile; stool antigen for giardia, cryptosporidium and E. histolytica. If studies are negative consider upper endoscopy and colonoscopy for CMV, MAC, KS, lymphoma. Non-infectious causes include antiretroviral therapy, protease inhibitors in particular, HIV enteropathy, pancreatic insufficiency *(CID 55:860, 2012).*

Acute infectious diarrhea *(for specific treatment, see Table 12)*

Agent	Prevalence/CD4 Stage	Clinical Features	Diagnostic Clues/Comments
Campylobacter jejuni, C. coli.	Any CD4	Watery or bloody diarrhea, fever, ± fecal WBC	Stool culture with selective media.
Clostridium difficile	**Most common cause of bacterial diarrhea regardless of CD4 count**	Watery diarrhea, fecal WBC, fever, leucocytosis, cramps, hypoalbuminemia; disease spectrum: nuisance diarrhea, colitis, megacolon. Endoscopy usually shows pseudo-membranous colitis but may be normal. PCR for C. difficile toxin is now test of choice. CT scan shows colitis with thickened mucosa. May present with leukemoid reaction.	Antibiotic exposure: most common—cephalosporins, clindamycin, FQs, ampicillin; rare—TMP/SMX, ZDV, albendazole, rifampin. Proton-pump inhibitors also a risk factor.
Enteric viruses: Noro, rota, adeno, corona, astro, picorna, & calicivirus	4–15% Any CD4 Adults presenting with acute gastroenteritis, comprehensive detection methods identified norovirus (26%) and rotavirus (18%) as the most frequent pathogens *(JID 205:1374, 2012).*	Acute watery diarrhea but 1/3 becomes chronic.	PCR for norovirus widely available. Rotavirus antigen detection tests available.

TABLE 11A (14)

Agent	Prevalence/CD4 Stage	Clinical Features	Diagnostic Clues/Comments
Gastrointestinal Tract/Diarrhea/Acute infectious diarrhea (*continued*)			
Enteroadherent E. coli Enteroaggregative E. coli & enteroinvasive E. coli.	Any CD4	Watery diarrhea, weight loss, ↓ D-xylose absorption, acute but may be chronic, usually in right colon, most pts on TMP/SMX prophylaxis. A large outbreak of infection occurred in Europe in 2011 due to E coli O104:H4, an enteroaggregative strain that also produced Shiga-toxin, with an unusually high proportion of cases with HUS (*NEJM 365:1771, 2011*).	Can detect Shiga toxin in stool by PCR. Identification of Enteroaggregative E. coli available in some commercial systems.
Idiopathic	25–40%. Variable CD4. Non-infectious causes; rule out drugs, diet, inflammatory bowel disease, anxiety, food poisoning.	Chronic, watery diarrhea most common but may mimic infectious causes.	Negative studies include culture, ova & parasites, C. difficile toxin assay.
Salmonella S. enteritidis S. typhimurium	5–15% 100x ↑ when compared to general population, any CD4 count, more common with lower CD4.	Watery diarrhea, fever, ± fecal WBC.	Blood culture, stool culture (sensitivity approx. 90%).
Shigella	2% ↑ in HIV+, MSM, direct oral-anal contact & foreign travel (*CID 44:327, 2007*). Any CD4	Watery or bloody diarrhea, fever, fecal WBC.	Stool culture. 20% of isolates from NYC (2013-15) had reduced susceptibility to azithro (MIC ≥32 mcg/mL) (*Emerg Inf Dis 23:332, 2017*).

Certain parasites may also cause acute diarrhea, including Isospora belli & Entamoeba histolytica/dispar (*Int J STD AIDS 14:487, 2003*).

Chronic infectious diarrhea
10% of pts with CD4 <200—unchanged frequency with ART but with change in etiology: ↓ OI (53 to 13%) & ↑ non-infectious causes (30 to 70%)

Agent	Prevalence/CD4 Stage	Clinical Features	Diagnostic Clues/Comments
Cryptosporidia Appear spread sexually between men who have sex with men.	CD4 <150	Enteritis; watery diarrhea, noninflammatory diarrhea (fecal WBC neg.), afebrile, malabsorption, wasting, large stool volume with abdominal pain, remitting symptoms for months, years.	Water-borne, low infectious dose, (in healthy adults only 132 oocysts). AFB smear of stool to show **oocyst 4–6 μm.** DFA available. In pts with CD4 >180/mm³, C. parvum cleared spontaneously in 7–28 days; with CD4 <180, 87% persisted. Rx: *See Table 12.*
Cyclospora cayetanensis	US <1%, Haiti 11% CD4 <100	Enteritis, watery diarrhea, up to 18x q24h for 10 mos.	Stool AFB smear, oocyte 8–10 μm, resembles cryptosporidia.
Cytomegalovirus (CMV) Usually colorectal infection.	13–20% CD4 <100	Fever, fecal WBC, ± blood, enteritis, colitis, perforation with toxic megacolon, solitary rectal ulcer, small bowel mass. Most common cause of lower GI bleeding.	Sigmoidoscopy with rectal biopsy (best initial invasive test), 10–30% of CMV colitis will affect only right side, further steps include colonoscopy with biopsy, including terminal ileum if available. CT segmental lesions or pancolitis. Rx: *See Table 12.*

TABLE 11A (15)

Agent	Prevalence/CD4 Stage	Clinical Features	Diagnostic Clues/Comments
Gastrointestinal Tract/Diarrhea/Chronic infectious diarrhea (continued)			
Entamoeba histolytica	1–3%. Any CD4 count.	Colitis, bloody stool, cramps, pos. fecal WBC, most are asymptomatic carriers. Course may be protracted.	Travel history (Latin America, SE Asia). Stool ova & parasites. Metronidazole or tinidazole were 97% effective in treating invasive amoebiasis (IA). Hep C antibody positivity associated with risk of recurrence of IA; newly diagnosed syphilis tended to be associated with recurrence, suggesting possibility of acquisition of new infection (PLoS Negl Trop Dis 5:1318 2011).
Giardia	1–5%. Any CD4 count	Enteritis, watery diarrhea, flatulence, bloating, malabsorption.	History of drinking mountain stream water. Stool ova & parasites; DFA available.
Idiopathic	More common with lower CD4 (<200).	Watery diarrhea, malabsorption, no fecal WBC.	Biopsy shows villous atrophy, crypt hyperplasia, no identifiable cause despite endoscopy with biopsy & electron microscopy for microsporidia.
Isospora belli	U.S. 1.5%, developing countries 10–12%. CD4 <100	Enteritis, watery diarrhea, wasting, noninflammatory diarrhea (no fecal WBC), no fever.	AFB stool smear, **oocysts 20–30 μm,** or seen on biopsy or exam of intestinal secretions.
Microsporidia Septata intestinalis Enterocytozoon bieneusi hellum	20% CD4 <50	Enteritis; watery diarrhea, noninflammatory diarrhea (fecal WBC neg.), fever is uncommon, remitting disease over years, malabsorption, wasting common. Pts improve with response to ART. May disseminate to kidneys, brain, lungs, etc.	Food/water-borne infection **spores 1–2 μm,** fluorescence with calcofluor (excellent screening test), confirmation with Giemsa stain. Special trichrome stain also diagnostic. Complications: disseminated disease, biliary disease.
Mycobacterium avium complex (MAC) (cause & effect for diarrhea not always clear)	10% CD4 <50	Enteritis, watery diarrhea, no fecal WBC, common fever & wasting (Curr Opin Gastroenterol 22:18, 2006), diffuse abdominal pain in late stage.	Stool culture unreliable, colonization may occur without diarrhea. Diagnosis: positive blood cultures, biopsy may show changes like Whipple's disease, hepatosplenomegaly, adenopathy, thickened small bowel.

CLINICAL SYNDROME, ETIOLOGY, EPIDEMIOLOGY	CLINICAL PRESENTATION, DIAGNOSTIC TESTS, COURSE
Gastrointestinal Tract *(continued)*	
Colorectal disease	
Cytomegalovirus (CMV)	Endoscopy—focal ischemic colitis with submucosal hemorrhages & discrete ulcers in distal colonic mucosa. Ganciclovir is effective in most patients. Rx: *See Table 12.*
Herpes simplex virus (HSV) Types 1 & 2	Painful recurrent small to persistent progressive large necrotizing ulcers in perirectal area. Emergence of acyclovir-resistant strains on rx can occur. Lab: Smears from lesions reveal multinucleate giant cells, + for HSV by PCR or DFA.
Histoplasmosis *(Diag Microbiol Infect Dis 55:193, 2006)*	Diarrhea, fever, abdominal pain & wt loss. Most commonly involving colon or cecum. Bx of lesions + 89%, blood or other site culture + 72%. Median CD4 34.
Mycobacterium tuberculosis	Tuberculosis in ileocecal area & colon may be seen in HIV patients without evidence of pulmonary TBc on chest x-ray.
Other considerations: Idiopathic inflammatory bowel disease (ulcerative colitis), Kaposi's sarcoma, lymphoma, epidermoid carcinoma & other neoplasms	Kaposi's sarcoma may be confined to the rectum & present as hemorrhagic rectocolitis.
Proctitis: differential diagnosis: Neisseria gonorrhoeae Herpes simplex virus Syphilis, primary or secondary Lymphogranuloma venereum (LGV) Chlamydia trachomatis (non-LGV immunotypes) Human papillomaviruses Cytomegalovirus Enteric pathogens, e.g., Shigella, Entamoeba histolytica, Campylobacter	Lab: Numerous PMNs on smear of exudate. Specific diagnosis depends on laboratory studies. Urine NAAT for GC & chlamydia. NAAT testing for rectal chlamydia recommended *(MMWR 64 (RR-3): 1, 2015).* Also consider herpes & syphilis. Note that treatment of LGV requires 3-week course of doxycycline *(MMWR 59 (RR-12): 1, 2C10).*
Genital Tract/Sexually Transmitted Diseases *[See CDC guidelines in MMWR 64(RR-3) 1, 2015]*	
Cervicitis/Urethritis: N. gonorrhoeae and/or C. trachomatis If treatment failure, consider treating for M. genitalium Assume dual infection. Ref: *CID 61: S774, 2015*	**Males:** Painful urination and purulent urethral discharge; gram stain sensitive (>95%) and specific (>99%). **Females:** May not have cervical discharge. Gram stain less reliable. **For both males and females:** NAAT on urine, urethral swab and/or cervical swab for both N. gonorrhea and C. trachomatis.
Genital ulcers (For H. simplex, *see genital vesicles*) **Chancroid:** H. ducreyi: Discrete outbreaks; cofactor for HIV transmission; 10% coinfected with syphilis or HSV	**Painful** genital ulcer + tender suppurative lymphadenopathy. Do darkfield to rule out syphilis. Even with special culture media, culture sensitivity is <80%. Retest for syphilis 3 months after treatment. All sex partners of pts with chancroid should be examined and treated if they have evidence of disease or have had sex with index pt within the last 10 days.
Granuloma inguinale (donovanosis): Klebsiella (Formerly Calymmatobacterium) granulomatis. Rare in US	**Painless** progressive ulcerative lesions without regional lymphadenopathy. Ulcers bleed easily. Hard to culture; rely on visualization of Donovan bodies on biopsy. Rule out syphilis.
Lymphogranuloma venereum: C. trachomatis C. trachomatis serovars L1, L2 or L3. NAAT test for C. trachomatis will be positive *(CID 61:S865, 2015)*	Unilateral inguinal/femoral lymphadenopathy. Self-limited papule/ulcer at site of inoculation. Rectal exposure leads to proctitis (rectal discharge, pain, constipation, fever and/or tenesmus) *(Dis Colon Rectum 52:507, 2009).* Can result in fistulas or stricture. **Diagnosis:** Based on serology; biopsy contraindicated because sinus tracts can develop.

CLINICAL SYNDROME, ETIOLOGY, EPIDEMIOLOGY	CLINICAL PRESENTATION, DIAGNOSTIC TESTS, COURSE
Genital Tract/Sexually Transmitted Diseases *(continued)*	
Pelvic Inflammatory Disease (PID): Acute: N. gonorrhoeae and C. trachomatis – esp. 1st episode Acute or recurrent: vaginal flora (anaerobes, enteric gm-neg bacilli, Streptococcus agalactiae). *NEJM 372:2039, 2015.*	Any combination of **endometritis, salpingitis, tubo-ovarian abscess** and **pelvic peritonitis.** Early diagnosis and treatment important to avoid scarring of upper genital tract with sequelae (infertility, dyspareunia). **Diagnosis:** Tender with cervical motion or uterine palpation or adnexal bimanual exam. Majority have mucopurulent cervical discharge. Urine nucleic acid amplification test for N. gonorrhoeae and C. trachomatis.
Perihepatitis (Fitzhugh-Curtis syndrome): Either N. gonorrhoeae and C. trachomatis	Right upper quadrant pain. Do NAAT for N. gonorrhoeae and C. trachomatis on urine and/or cervical swab.
Proctitis, proctocolitis: **Proctitis:** N. gonorrhoeae, C. trachomatis, to include LGV, T. pallidum & HSV **Proctocolitis:** Campylobacter, shigella, E. histolytica & rarely LGV **AIDS pts:** add CMV, MAI, cryptosporidium, microsporidia and isospora	Proctitis: Anorectal pain, tenesmus and/or rectal discharge. Proctocolitis: Proctitis plus diarrhea and abdominal cramps. Try to make a specific diagnosis: Urine NAAT for N. gonorrhoeae & C. trachomatis, stool C&S, stool ova & parasites, antigen detection for cryptosporidia, whole blood CMV-PCR.
Venereal (genital) warts: human papillomavirus (HPV)—multiple types, but type 6 & 11 most common; worry about oncogenic types.	Diagnosis is usually by appearance: flat, papular or pedunculated growth (condylomas) on genital mucosa. Can cause warts and/or malignancy at a variety of sites: cervix, vagina, vulva, penis, anus, oropharynx.
Hepatic Disease (↑ transaminase levels in 2–3.8% of asymptomatic HIV+ pts); reviewed in *Hepatology. 2015 Dec;62(6):1871-82*	
Drug-associated hepatic dysfunction (Avoid acetaminophen) Multiple drugs used in HIV patients are associated with abnormalities in LFTs: TMP/SMX (½ pts), acyclovir, nevirapine, didanosine (ddI), ZDV, ddC, all PIs, ganciclovir, foscarnet, ketoconazole, fluconazole, INH, rifampin *(see Table 12).* Most require dose reduction or discontinuation if abnormalities exceed about 5x normal values.	**Clinical:** Predictors of drug-induced hepatotoxicity: baseline ↑ aminotransferases, concomitant hepatotoxic medications, thrombocytopenia, renal insufficiency & Hep C coinfection (OR 2.7) *(J Acq Imm Def Synd 43:320, 2006).* **Inconsequential increase of indirect bilirubin in pts given atazanavir or indinavir.** Hepatic necrosis & death has been reported with nevirapine. **Nevirapine hepatotoxicity may be severe, esp. in pts with ↑ CD4 counts (CD4 >250 in women; >400 in men). Co-infection with Hep B & C, ↑ baseline ALT elevation & previous hx of parenchymal liver disease ↑ likelihood of drug toxicity.**
Bacillary Peliosis (bacillary angiomatosis). *Manifestation of Bartonella henselae in AIDS patients.*	**Clinical:** Fever, abdominal pain, weight loss, hepato- & splenomegaly. About ½ pts will have skin lesions (look like KS): painful, erythematous plaques or nodules. ½ have lymphadenopathy. 2/3 pts give history of cat bite or scratch. Lab: Alkaline phosphatase ↑ >hepatocellular tests. Etiologic agent: Bartonella henselae (usual), B. quintana (uncommon). Can be isolated from blood, 5–15 days of incubation and then lysis-centrifugation on blood agar under CO_2. Rx: *Table 12, page 115.*
Viral hepatitis **Hepatitis A** (HAV) Hep A in HIV-infected persons is clinically indistinguishable from Hep A in HIV-uninfected persons but viremia lasts longer and alkaline phosphatase is higher. *(CID 34:380, 2002).* Risk factors include homosexual activity, injection drug use, homeless populations. Hepatitis A and Hep B vaccine indicated for non-immune homosexual men.	**HIV/HBV co-infection & progression of liver disease/HIV:** • Co-infected patients have increased risk of cirrhosis. • No accelerated progression of HIV in co-infected pts. • Immune reconstitution inflammatory syndrome (IRIS); IRIS described in co-infected pts treated with ART. Can be life threatening if limited residual hepatic function. • Administer Hep A vaccine if non-immune

CLINICAL SYNDROME, ETIOLOGY, EPIDEMIOLOGY	CLINICAL PRESENTATION, DIAGNOSTIC TESTS, COURSE

Hepatic Disease/Viral hepatitis *(continued)*

Hepatitis B (HBV): *JAC 65:10, 2010; see Tables 9G-9J*

Diagnostic Issues: Tests & interpretation are same in HIV-infected and non-infected patients.

Isolated positive test for Anti HBc: *(JID 195:1437, 2007)*
- More common in HIV pts. especially if HBV/HCV coinfection.
- Unclear as to whether occult HBV viremia is occurring.
- Unclear whether to give HBV vaccine.

Pathogenesis & HIV:
- After recovery from acute disease, can detect HBV nucleic acid by PCR.
- HBV controlled by cellular & humoral immunity.
- Flares of HBV can occur with immunosuppression.
- HBV DNA levels and reactivation rates higher in HIV pts than pts with only HBV; HIV pts more likely to develop chronic infection.

Serologic markers and HBV DNA in response to HBV infection*							
HBsAg	HBeAg	IgM Anti-HBc	IgG Anti-HBc	Anti-HBs	Anti-HBe	HBV DNA	Interpretation
Acute Hep B:							
+	+	+				+++	Early infection
		+				+	"Core" window
			+	+	+	±	Recovery
Chronic Hep B:							
+	+		+			+++	Active replication
+			+		+	±	Low/non-replicative
+	±	+	+			+	Chronic HBV flare
+			+		+	++	Pre-core/core promoter mutants
			+			++/-	"Occult Hep B"

* Blank space means negative test. Hepatitis D not included.

HIV/HBV co-infection & ART associated liver toxicity:
Applies to HIV/HCV co-infection as well.

1) Cirrhosis and decreased cytochrome p450 activity leads to toxic drug levels; 2) IRIS can occur; 3) Withdrawal of any drug with HBV activity (e.g., TDF, TAF, 3TC, FTC, or entecavir) can lead to flare of hepatitis.

Hepatitis C (HCV)/HIV co-infection:
- HCV induced liver injury complicates treatment of HIV; concomitant HIV accelerates progression of HIV-induced liver injury *(LnID 9:775, 2009)*.
- Liver ultrasound every 6-12 months to check for hepatocellular carcinoma.
- Determine HCV quantitation, genotype, and liver fibrosis stage.
- HCV infection increases hepatic toxicity of ART: *see Hep B above & CID 38 (Suppl. 2):S90, 2004*.
- Liver decompensation can occur when treating HCV in HIV-HBV-HCV tri-infected patients who are not on specific anti-HBV Rx at time of treating HCV. **All HIV-HBV-HCV tri-infected patients MUST be on treatment for HBV at time of initiating HCV therapy** (typically a tenofovir based Rx regimen).

- Screen pts for past exposure to HAV & HBV. **If no evidence of past infection, give HAV & HBV vaccines.**
- Look for occult HBV—order antibody to HB core (IgG Anti-HBc). Co-infection with HB and HC increases risk of hepatocellular carcinoma *(AnIM 146:649, 2007)*.
- Assess degree of hepatic fibrosis by non-invasive marker of fibrosis: e.g., panels of common laboratory tests, liver stiffness by elastography (Fibroscan) or if neither of these tests are available, consider liver biopsy.
- For differential diagnosis of glomerular disease in pts with HCV/HIV co-infection, *see NEJM 362:636, 2010*.
- Emerging data: polymorphisms adjacent to IL28B gene determines degree of spontaneous clearance and response to interferon rx *(Nature 461:399, 2009; Nature 461:798, 2009)*.

Hepatitis D (delta agent): defective virus; requires chronic Hep B co-infection. Antibodies to delta agent in 25% of HIV+, HBV– individuals.

Do anti-HDV serology at baseline and/or with flares of hepatitis. Ref: *CID: 44:988, 2007*.

Hepatitis E (HEV): usually acute and self-limited. Can cause chronic infection & cirrhosis in AIDS pts *(NEJM 351:1025, 2009)*.

HEV antibodies by EIA found in 33/162 (20%) homosexual men (Italy), 60/198 (30%) (Spain) *(Ln 344:1433, 1994; Ln 345:127, 1995)*. In the U.S., HEV prevalence is <1%.

TABLE 11A (19)

CLINICAL SYNDROME, ETIOLOGY, EPIDEMIOLOGY	CLINICAL PRESENTATION, DIAGNOSTIC TESTS, COURSE
Hepatic Disease/Viral hepatitis *(continued)*	
Hepatitis G • Related to Hep C • Replication in lymphocytes; replicates poorly in hepatocytes • 2% of blood donors viremic & 13% have antibodies	So far, no association with any clinical illness. Transmitted sexually, by contaminated blood and mother to child. Infections (past or current) with **HGV were associated with ↑ CD4 counts & better AIDS-free survival rates** in hemophilia pts with HIV *(AnIM 132:959, 2000)*, & slower progression & ↓ mortality in others.
Hepatitis, viral, other	There are isolated reports of hepatitis associated with other viruses: EBV, CMV.
Lipomatosis/Lipodystrophy *(See Table 6C)*	
Lung Most common causes are PJP pneumonia, bacterial pneumonia, tuberculosis. Viral pneumonia dx increasingly common in older adults but not unique in HIV infected patients. Decreased incidence in ART era (0.8/100 pt yrs). Risk factors: ↑ age, IDU, smoking, non-adherence to ART.	
Pneumonia • Clinical syndrome ranges from abrupt onset of chills, fever and productive cough to weeks of cough, fever, night sweats and weight loss to months of gradually progressive dyspnea. • Clinical syndrome depends on pathogen, co-morbidities (other than HIV) and especially the patient's CD4 T lymphocyte count. • Need detailed epidemiologic history, e.g., TB exposure, influenza immunization, exposure to endemic area of deep fungi, compliance with ART • Pattern of illness varies with degree of immunocompromise.	• The lower the CD4 count, the broader the differential diagnosis, the more severe the illness and the more aggressive the diagnostic effort. • Clinical presentation can be acute or chronic. • Patterns of infection change as CD4 counts falls. Risk of ARV-induced IRIS increases as CD4 count falls. • Spectrum of potential pathogens broadens as AIDS patients are susceptible to opportunistic pathogens as well as neoplastic disease.
Any CD4 count (high or low):	
Pulmonary tuberculosis (Mycobacterium tuberculosis)	
Common: **ANY PT SUSPECTED OF TB SHOULD BE ISOLATED** [private room, negative pressure, health care workers (HCW) & visitors entering should wear high efficiency disposable masks]. Concomitant HIV and M. tuberculosis infections remain a major problem in the developing world where they are a significant cause of mortality, especially in patients with multi-drug resistant and extensively drug-resistant strains *(CID 48:829, 2009; CMR 24:351, 2011)*. Note that in certain areas such as CA & Mexico ~25% of HIV-associated TB is caused by M. bovis (esp. abd TB) rather than M. tuberculosis *(CID 51:1343, 2010)*.	**Clinical presentation varies with stage of HIV infection:** • **Early HIV infection** (CD4 >400/mm^3): Reactivation. Typical presentation **with upper lobe cavitary disease most common.** Extrapulmonary disease uncommon. PPD (5 TU) is + (≥5 mm induration) in 80%. Always consider in pts with chronic cough. • **Late HIV infection** (CD4 <400/mm^3): Either reactivation or progressive primary disease (30–50%). Clinical: Fever, cough (may be absent), shortness of breath, weight loss, night sweats but a small proportion of HIV+ patients (esp. in developing countries) have minimal or no symptoms of TB *(CID 50 (Suppl. 3): S223, 2010)*.
In resource-constrained countries TBc & HIV are closely linked: HIV and TBc coinfection as high as 50% *(CID 50:1377, 2010)*. Nearly 20% of patients starting ART in Durban, SA, had undiagnosed, culture positive TB in 2008 *(CID 51:823, 2010)*.	**X-ray: Mediastinal-hilar adenopathy most common with progression to diffuse, somewhat coarse interstitial densities or localized infiltrates,** especially in mid or lower lung fields. Pleural effusion in 10–20%. Disseminated (reticulonodular infiltrates, not classic "miliary" since "millets" are granulomata, usually not seen in HIV with low CD4) the most common with CD4 <200/mm^3. Hilar/peritracheal adenopathy is uncommon with PJP or bacterial pneumonia, common in TB. Sputum: Smears + for AFB in 40–50% pts with pulmonary TB, BAL + in 50–60%, culture + in 80–90%.
Tuberculosis often occurs before the pt has AIDS-defining illness, but ART sig. ↓ risk. Most cases due to reactivation but primary tuberculosis being recognized with increasing frequency. MDR and XDR TB emerging threats in sub-Saharan Africa *(Trop Med Int Health 15:1052, 2010)*.	In general, in patient with HIV and pulmonary TB, early ART improves outcomes but needs to balanced against risk of IRIS. Recommendations are if CD4 <50, start ART within 2 wks of starting TB treatment. If CD4 >50 start ART 8-12 weeks of starting TB. Rx: *Table 12, page 115.*

CLINICAL SYNDROME, ETIOLOGY, EPIDEMIOLOGY	CLINICAL PRESENTATION, DIAGNOSTIC TESTS, COURSE
Lung/Any CD4 count (high or low) *(continued)*	
Community-Acquired Pneumonia (CAP)	
• Bacterial pneumonia occurs at any CD4 count.	
CD4 Count ≤200 cells/mm³:	
Pneumocystis pneumonia (PJP)	
• Dry cough, fever and progressive dyspnea over period of several weeks. • With effective ART dramatic ↓ in incidence of PJP. Most cases now in pts. with previously undiagnosed HIV/AIDS or pts. who are non-compliant with ART. • Remember, may co-exist with TB. • Also, same organisms, i.e., S. pneumoniae, common in absence of HIV/AIDS also common in pts. with HIV/AIDS.	**S&S:** Dry cough, progressive dyspnea and fever. **Chest X-ray:** Most often—diffuse bilateral symmetrical fine reticular infiltrates. Less common—focal nodules without cavitation, thick wall cysts, pneumatoceles/pneumothorax. **Pulmonary physiology:** Low PaO_2, decreased vital capacity and diffusing capacity. **Diagnosis:** Presence of organism on induced sputum or BAL; PCR also sensitive. Beta-D-glucan sensitive for screening *(J Clin Microbiol 50:7-15, 2012).*

Comparison of clinical features of bacterial pneumonia (Bact Pn), PJP and M. tuberculosis (TBC) *(AIDS 16:85, 2002)*

Clinical Feature	Diagnosis ( ) = # of Pts					
	Bact Pn (94)		PJP (101)		TBC (37)	
(OR=Odds Ratio)	%	OR	%	OR	%	OR
Fever >7 days	11%	1.0	34%	4.3[†]	54%	9.9[†]
Cough >7 days	20%	1.0	50%	3.9[†]	51%	4.2[†]
Yellow-green sputum	54%	2.8[†]	30%	1.0	30%	1.0
DOE	43%	1.5	81%	9.0[†]	32%	1.0
Weight loss	23%	1.0	44%	2.2[†]	68%	6.8[†]
Night sweats	23%	1.0	46%	2.7[†]	54%	3.9[†]
Tachycardia	57%	2.8[†]	39%	1.3	32%	1.0
Abn auscultation	77%	3.5[†]	62%	1.8	49%	1.0
LDH >400	29%	1.0	62%	4.0[†]	43%	1.9
pO_2 <75	36%	1.8	66%	6.0[†]	24%	1.0
Interstitial infiltrate	17%	1.3	69%	14.5[†]	14%	1.0
Lobar infiltrate	54%	59[†]	22%	1.0	32%	24.8[†]

OR: 95% CI does not include 1.0 when indicated by †

TABLE 11A (21)

CLINICAL SYNDROME, ETIOLOGY, EPIDEMIOLOGY	CLINICAL PRESENTATION, DIAGNOSTIC TESTS, COURSE
Lung/CD4 Count ≤200 cells/mm³ *(continued)*	
Kaposi's sarcoma (KS) (in lung) Etiology is HHV-8 (KS-associated herpes virus)	**Clinical:** Usually but not always associated with cutaneous &/or mucosal KS. Present with cough (92%), dyspnea (82%) & fever (67%); less likely than pts with concurrent OI to have temp >38.3 & RR >20 breaths/min. Symptoms may be prolonged. X-ray: Findings are somewhat distinctive: **coarse, poorly defined nodular densities throughout the lungs with concomitant coarse linear densities in the perihilar regions.** Nodules increase slowly in size, rapid ↑ suggests hemorrhage. Pleural effusions common (up to 50%). Hilar adenopathy rare (<10%). Dx: Bronchoscopy will usually show typical violaceous endobronchial lesions. Rx: *Table 18.* May respond to antiretroviral rx or specific antiviral Rx *(Curr Top Microbiol Immunol 312:289, 2007).*
Lymphoma: HHV-8 also identified in body cavity lymphomas— *see above*	Lymphomas associated with advanced HIV infection are increasingly common, are usually non-Hodgkin B cell type, with extranodal involvement the rule. Thoracic involvement is uncommon (10%) but when it occurs it produces pleural effusion in 50%, hilar &/or mediastinal adenopathy in ¼ & either reticulonodular interstitial infiltrates or alveolar consolidation in 25%.
Lymphoid interstitial pneumonia (LIP) (children) *(Chest 112:2150, 2002)*	A disease of unknown etiology which may present with shortness of breath in children with HIV infection *(see Table 8E).* **X-ray: Resembles PJP with diffuse or focal, fine to medium reticular interstitial infiltrate. Findings gradually worsen over mos.** Dx: Lung biopsy is necessary for dx; shows an accumulation of lymphocytes & plasma cells in interstitial areas. Rx: Corticosteroids may be beneficial.
CD4 Count <100 cells/mm³	
Cryptococcosis (Cryptococcus neoformans) (common)	Site of entry is usually the lungs & pneumonia has been reported. X-ray: Variable pattern: single or multiple well-defined nodules with or without cavitation or diffuse reticular infiltrates &/or hilar/mediastinal adenopathy. Occasionally a reticulonodular pattern or isolated pleural effusion may occur. Dx: Isolation of C. neoformans from respiratory secretions or blood cultures. Serum CRAG may be positive. Rx: *Table 12, page 122.*
Coccidioidomycosis (Coccidioides immitis) (common—endemic areas) Risk factors include Afro-American race & ↑ level of immunosuppression. Reactivation or primary infection in patients from "cocci belt" (southwest U.S.) with CD4 <150/mm³.	**Presentation is similar to histoplasmosis—fever, chills, night sweats & weight loss; severe shortness of breath is common.** Cutaneous lesions common: generalized, erythema nodosum, granulomatous dermatitis and Sweet's syndrome. X-ray: Diffuse bilateral reticulonodular infiltrate (65%) similar to histoplasmosis or focal pulmonary infiltrate (14%) or normal (16%). Dx: While complement fixation antibody tests are frequently positive (68%), dx is established by identification of large spherules of C. immitis in sputum, BAL, biopsy or on culture. Rx: *Table 12, page 121.*
Histoplasmosis (Histoplasma capsulatum) (common—endemic areas) Reactivation infection common when CD4 <200/mm³ in pts with geographical history of having been in the "histo belts" (Ohio-Mississippi River Valley, southeastern U.S., St. Lawrence River Valley, Central America & northern South America).	Presents with nonspecific systemic complaints: fever, weight loss, night and dyspnea. Hepatosplenomegaly & focal cutaneous pustules or ulcers may be presenting findings. Pts may also present with "septic shock" including DIC. CD4 count <150. X-ray: Commonly shows diffuse, bilateral poorly defined small (1–2 mm) nodular infiltrates with or without hilar/mediastinal adenopathy. Diagnosis: 95% of pts. have detectable histo antigen in urine *(Mira Vista: Tel 866-647-2847).* Organism sometimes visible in PAS or silver stains of peripheral blood or bone marrow. Serologic tests also available.
Blastomycosis (uncommon)	Pulmonary, disseminated, and/or CNS disease.

CLINICAL SYNDROME, ETIOLOGY, EPIDEMIOLOGY	CLINICAL PRESENTATION, DIAGNOSTIC TESTS, COURSE
Lung/CD4 Count <100 cells/mm³ *(continued)*	
Paracoccidioidomycosis (South America)	Reported in Brazil. Lymphadenopathy, interstitial lung disease, with papule-nodular skin lesions with central ulceration, ulcerative lesions of the mouth *(Clin Dermatol 30:616, 2012)*.
Mycobacterium kansasii (may also occur at higher CD4 counts) Important to distinguish from M. tuberculosis, as all M. kansasii are resistant to PZA	Clinical: Fever, cough, weight loss, dyspnea, night sweats. X-ray: Infiltrates "atypical", alveolar, interstitial or diffuse parenchymal or pleural effusion. Upper lobe cavities. ½ have extrapulmonary dissemination. Cavitation more common at ↑ CD4 counts, hilar adenopathy with dissemination more common at ↓ CD4 counts.
Penicillium (Talaromyces) marneffei	Primarily presents as fever, anemia, weight loss & skin lesions (70%) with lymphadenopathy but ½ have cough & organism cultured from lung in 15%. Pulmonary infiltrates (densities, abscesses & cavities) have been seen. **Essentially all cases from SE Asia.** Dx by isolation from skin, blood or bone marrow. Rx: *Table 12, page 124*.
Rhodococcus equi (uncommon) Can be confused with TBC	Rhodococcus presentations vary: slowly progressive mass lesion which cavitates, consolidation with & without cavitation, ground glass opacities, peribronchial nodules and centrilobular nodules ("tree in bud" pattern). Rx: *Page 119*.
Toxoplasma gondii (uncommon, frequency reflects background population prevalence)	Rare in U.S., in France represents up to 5% of cases of suspected PJP. Febrile illness, minimal cough, ↑ dyspnea. Chest x-ray: Diffuse interstitial or diffuse coarse nodular infiltrates (resembles PJP). Pleural effusion occurs. Lab: ↑ transaminase, ↑ LDH. Sputum: BAL + for T. gondii. Rx: *Table 12, page 127*.
CD4 <50 cells/mm³	
Aspergillosis (uncommon) • Aspergillus sp. are commonly isolated but rarely invasive. AIDS & neutropenia increases risk.	Fever, cough, hemoptysis, fungus invades blood vessels and lung infiltrates and/or cavities. **Diagnosis:** serum or BAL galactomannan; airway culture; sometimes need biopsy.
Cytomegalovirus (CMV) • CMV pneumonia is rare.	Diagnosis of pneumonia more likely if CMV inclusions, with no other pathogens, seen on lung biopsy. Positive blood RT-PCR for CMV supports diagnosis.
Hilar adenopathy, mediastinal adenopathy M. tuberculosis, M. avium-intracellulare (MAI, MAC). Fungal: Histoplasmosis, coccid oidomycosis, cryptococcosis, blastomycosis Lymphoma, Kaposi's sarcoma.	Following ART & ↑ CD4, IRIS may manifest as hilar adenopathy with MAC, M. Tbc, crypto & other pathogens. Clinical predictors of etiology in 110 HIV+ pts: • Cough + necrosis of nodes = mycobacteria (51) • ≤7 days symptoms, dyspnea, airway disease = bacterial pneumonia (26) • >7 days symptoms, no cough or pulmonary nodules = lymphoma (2) *(J AIDS 31:291, 2002)*
Mass lesion ± necrosis (abscess) Histoplasmosis, coccidioidomycosis, cryptococcosis, anaerobes, S. aureus, M. kansasii, Rhodococcus equi Mycobacterium tuberculosis, Pneumocystis jirovecii (carinii), lymphoma, Kaposi's sarcoma, aspergillus, MAC, Nocardia asteroides, P. aeruginosa, CMV all possible etiologies.	Broad differential diagnosis. Frequent etiology: aspergillus, mycobacteria, bacteria (e.g., P. aeruginosa, R. equi). Less common etiology: crypto, cocci, histo among others.

TABLE 11A (23)

CLINICAL SYNDROME, ETIOLOGY, EPIDEMIOLOGY	CLINICAL PRESENTATION, DIAGNOSTIC TESTS, COURSE
Lung/CD4 <50 cells/mm³ *(continued)*	
Mycobacterium avium-intracellulare complex (MAI, MAC) • Usually presents as FUO in pts with fever, night sweats and weight loss.	**Diagnosis:** positive mycobacterial blood cultures. Following initiation of ART, pts with MAC at risk for IRIS. Manifests as: painful generalized lymphadenopathy, massive abdominal & thoracic adenopathy, pulmonary infiltrates, fever, leucocytosis & cutaneous nodules *(see Table 11B).*
Non-tuberculous mycobacteria, other than MAC: Mycobacterium genavense	Variety of presentations besides pulmonary, including cutaneous, or bone/joint, deep tissue, or disseminated disease.

Pleural effusion *(Sex Trans Infect 76:122, 2000)*
  Infections (66–70%):
  Bacterial pneumonia   31–57%
  Pneumocystis pneumonia   15%
  M. tuberculosis   8–16%
  Others (each <5%): Septic embolism, aspergillosis,
  C. neoformans, MAC, nocardia, all rare
  Non-infectious (31%): *(see Curr HIV Res 1:385, 2003)*
  KS   10–40%
  Hypoalbuminemia   19%
  Heart failure   5%
  Others: Kaposi's sarcoma (10% in 1 series), non-Hodgkins lymphoma (18% in 1 series), atelectasis, uremia, ARDS, pulmonary emboli (4%)
	Large effusions & bilateral effusions suggest Kaposi's sarcoma & lymphoma. Tuberculosis more likely when effusions suggest miliary nodules or mediastinal adenopathy. Dx usually requires pleural bx for histology & culture.

Pneumocystis pneumothorax • More common after aerosolized pentamidine	High mortality rate if associated with PJP.
Pulmonary eosinophilia (Loeffler's syndrome)	Can be caused by drugs commonly used in HIV+ pts: sulfonamides, dapsone, penicillin.
Pulmonary nodules (1 or more on CT scan)	Lengthy differential **diagnosis:** neoplasia, bacteria, mycobacteria and fungi all possible. Culture sputum and blood. May need tissue.
Selected Viral Etiologies	
Adenovirus (different serotypes with variable severity of viral pneumonia-- winter & spring)	Outbreaks of severe pneumonia due to adenovirus—14. No predilection for HIV pts.
Human herpesvirus 6 (HHV-6)	HHV-6 infected cells detected in tissues obtained at necropsy in 9/9 pts. In one pt, probably primary cause of fatal pneumonitis. Relevance is that HHV-6 infections treatable with ganciclovir & foscarnet *(Ln 343:577, 1994).*
Influenza A or B common in outbreaks; vaccine effective: incidence 6.1% in vaccinated vs. 21.2% in unvaccinated (p=0.001); Ab response ↑ when CD4 count >200 or on ART; immunization recommended	No evidence that influenza in general is more severe in HIV+ pts. **Diagnosis:** rapid nasal/oropharyngeal swabs only 50% sensitive. Need nasal RT-PCR to optimize sensitivity.
Varicella	Pneumonia common with typical diffuse reticulonodular infiltrates.

TABLE 11A (24)

CLINICAL SYNDROME, ETIOLOGY, EPIDEMIOLOGY	CLINICAL PRESENTATION, DIAGNOSTIC TESTS, COURSE
Lymph Nodes	
Generalized lymphadenopathy **(applies to lymphadenopathy without an obvious primary source)** Etiologies: acute HIV infection, TB, atypical mycobacteria, histoplasmosis, coccidioidomycosis, lymphoma, Kaposi's sarcoma, syphilis, Epstein-Barr virus, toxoplasma, tularemia, sarcoid, CMV, & Castlema's disease.	History & physical exam direct evaluation. If nodes fluctuant, aspirate & base rx on Gram & acid-fast stains. Pts receiving ART may demonstrate fever & generalized lymphadenopathy from MAC infection following robust ↑ CD4 cells; **immune reconstitution inflammatory syndrome (IRIS).**
Musculoskeletal System	
Pyomyositis Staphylococcal; aerobic Gm-neg. bacilli (uncommon).	May follow exercise, local trauma or injections. Swelling in muscular area, localized pain & fever. ESR usually ↑. Erythema often absent, can be indolent. ↑ bilateral in HIV. WBC may be normal & blood cultures usually negative Diagnosis: CT or MRI.
Osteonecrosis (avascular necrosis): osteoporosis, & osteopenia, assoc. with advanced HIV & traditional risk factors (↓ body mass, weight loss, steroid use, & smoking). Likely a complication of HIV itself, not ART. Can be complication of ongoing HIV replication. ARVs implicated: tenofovir, atazanavir, efavirenz.	Evaluate for osteonecrosis in pt with persistent groin & hip pain. Plain films not usually revealing; usually requires MRI for definitive diagnosis. Risk factors: ↑ lipids, alcoholism, pancreatitis, **corticosteroid rx**, hypercoagulable state. Multiple joints often involved. MRI best test for diagnosis. Hip replacement surgery usually required for optimal treatment outcomes. In a prospective multicenter randomized open-label study, alendronate 70 mg qw + Vit. D 500 intl units q24h & calcium 1000 mg q24h improved lumbar bone mineral density & minimized femoral bone mineral density decrease after 52 wks vs. Vit. D & calcium alone in 41 HIV+ persons on ART (*HIV Clin Trials 5:269, 2004*). Other studies also confirm use of bisphosphonates while hormonal therapies such as raloxifane, testosterone and growth hormone-releasing hormone promising but require more study (*see CID 42:108, 2006*).
Arthritis, polyarticular Reiter's syndrome; Reiter's arthritis: urethritis or cervicitis, conjunctivitis, arthritis, & mucocutaneous lesions (circinate balanitis, keratoderma blennorrhagica).	Typically, non-bacterial urethritis 7–14 days after sexual exposure. Asymmetric polyarticular arthritis involving large joints of legs, including toes, develops over several weeks. Typically resolves in 3–4 mos but ~50% have recurrences. HLA B27 uncommon in Africans but reactive spondyloarthropathies still common in HIV+ persons. Lab: Synovial fluid typically is translucent, 2000–100,000 cells/μl, >50% PMNs, culture negative, glucose <50 mg/dl lower than blood glucose. Rx: Since often assoc. with C. trachomatis, empirical rx for chlamydia is appropriate. In non-HIV+ patients, methotrexate or folic acid antagonists have been used; they should not be used in HIV+ pts.
Myopathy (progressive proximal muscle weakness)	
HIV-1 associated myopathy.	Proximal muscle weakness, ↑ creatinine kinase levels. Muscle biopsy: inflammatory infiltrates. Rule out statin toxicity; especially simvastatin with ritonavir (increased simvastatin levels).
Drug-associated: zidovudine (ZDV, ddI & ddC, may be assoc. with d4T, lactic acidosis & mitochondrial tox city.	Proximal muscle weakness & atrophy (legs >arms, "saggy butt" syndrome) with ZDV >6 months. Creatinine kinase ↑. Typically associated with high-dose zidovudine use in the past. Muscle biopsy: "Ragged red fibers" on histology, abnormal mitochondria on EM. Improves with discontinuation of ZDV, recurs with rechallenge. ddC other NRTIs can cause a selective loss of mitochondrial DNA in vitro. Rhabdomyolysis rarely associated with TMP-SMX.
Polymyositis—also reported from IRIS (*Clin Exp Rheumatol 22:651, 2004; Sex Trans Inf 80:315, 2004*).	A dermatomyositis-like disease has been described in AIDS.

TABLE 11A (25)

CLINICAL SYNDROME, ETIOLOGY, EPIDEMIOLOGY	CLINICAL PRESENTATION, DIAGNOSTIC TESTS, COURSE
Renal. Review of HIV-associated renal disease, *see Curr HIV/AIDS Rep 9:187, 2012.*	
HIV-associated nephropathy (glomerulosclerosis) (HIVAN) Incidence HIVAN 8/1000 person yrs for HIV+ but 26.4/1000 person yrs in those with AIDS. ART ↓ risk of HIVAN. Etiology likely due to direct infection of renal cells by HIV. HIV also shown to infect renal tubular epithelial cells with production of the various proinflammatory mediators.	**HIVAN is an indication for immediate initiation of ARV therapy.** Usually occurs in advanced HIV with ↑ viral load *(CID 43:377, 2006).* Massive proteinuria of sudden onset, hypoalbuminemia, renal insufficiency rapidly progressing to endstage renal disease. Peripheral edema & hypertension minimal or absent. Biopsy recommended to differentiate from other causes of GN. Renal bx: Focal glomerulosclerosis with mesangial deposits of C3 & IgM, tubular ectasia & tubulo-interstitial disease. Significance of antiglomerular basement membrane antibody uncertain *(Am J Kidney Dis 48:e55, 2006).* Treatment: **Antiretroviral therapy is imperative!** 60 mg prednisone for 1 mo. followed by 2 mos. taper ↓ serum creatinine, ↓ proteinuria, & preserved renal function at 6 mos. in 7/13 pts vs. 0/8 control *(Kidney Int 58:1253, 2000).* Angiotensin-converting enzyme (ACE) inhibitor has also had some limited success *(Pharmaco Therapy 25:1761, 2005).* ART rx improves outcome of HIV-assoc. nephropathy but not other renal diseases found in HIV+ pts *(Clin Nephrol 64:124, 2005).* **Renal Transplant:** Survival rates at 1 and 3 yrs were 95% and 88% among HIV+ transplant recipients; graft survival rates were 90% and 74%, respectively. Survival rates are similar to non-HIV+ individuals, rejection rates are a bit higher *(NEJM 2010; 363:2058-2059).* Transplants from HIV+ donors to HIV+ recipients now allowed and encouraged.
HIV-associated IgA nephropathy Rarer than HIV glomerulosclerosis. Majority of pts are white.	Microscopic hematuria, minimal proteinuria. ↑ serum IgA. Progression of disease is slow. Thought to be immune complex disease *(Kid International 81:833, 2012).*
Nephrotoxic drugs: pentamidine, foscarnet, aminoglycosides, amphotericin B; tenofovir (TAF much less nephrotoxic than TDF), cidofovir, adefovir.	Causes renal tubular damage. Cobicistat causes increase in serum creatinine of 0.1-0.4 mg/dl but NO concomitant decrease in GFR (as determined by Iohexol clearance). Cobi inhibits multidrug and toxin extrusion protein 1 (MATE1) in the proximal tubule and has no effect on kidney function. DTG and BIC inhibits a different proximal tubule extrusion molecule (OCT2) resulting in a mild increase in serum creatinine without any impact on glomerular filtration.
Immune reconstitution syndrome (IRIS) *(See Table 11B)*	Inflammatory response following 8 wks of ART. Pt with miliary TB with AFB urinary shedding, developed acute renal failure *(CID 38:e32, 2004).*
Sinuses, paranasal, sinusitis *(Otolaryngol Head Neck Surg 2015, 152(Suppl 2):51)* **Etiology (CD4 > 200):** S. pneumoniae, H. influenza, M. catarrhalis, S. aureus (rare). **Etiology (CD4 < 200):** As above, plus Aspergillus. sp., other fungi, Kaposi's sarcoma, lymphoma, other opportunistic pathogens (rare).	**Management (CD4 > 200):** Symptomatic x 10 days, e.g., saline irrigation; empiric antibiotics if symptoms >10 days, fever, focal pain, purulent discharge. **Management (CD4 < 200):** Image sinuses; consider culture/biopsy of sinus content; if febrile, empiric therapy pending culture results.
Skin/Hair *(See Dermatol Clin 24:473, 2006 for excellent review).* Selected skin conditions in HIV: *Topics Antiviral Med 22:680, 2014.*	
HIV-associated pruritus Etiology: Skin infections or infestations; papulosquamous disorders; photodermatitis; xerosis; drug reactions; rarely lymphoproliferative disorders.	One of the most common symptoms in pts with HIV. Workup with careful exam of skin, nails, hair & mucous membranes to establish primary dermatological diagnosis; biopsy skin if necessary. ART may improve idiopathic HIV pts but some may flare with immune reconstitution.
Eosinophilic folliculitis *(see J Am Acad Dermatol 55:215, 2006)* Low CD4 counts & marked pruritus, discrete, erythematous urticarial, follicular painless papules on trunk, head, neck, proximal extremities, 90% above nipple line. ↑ eos, ↑ IgE. CD4 usually <250. Metronidazole 250 mg po q8h for 3–4 wks works in some. May represent auto-immune reaction to sebum. Difficult to differentiate from infective folliculitis; bx is useful. ART may decrease folliculitis.	

CLINICAL SYNDROME, ETIOLOGY, EPIDEMIOLOGY	CLINICAL PRESENTATION, DIAGNOSTIC TESTS, COURSE
Skin/Hair (*continued*)	
Macular or papular lesions (*See papulo-squamous differential below*)	
Acute retroviral syndrome	Lesions 5–10 mm diam., symmetrical, esp. on face or trunk (may involve palms & soles), erythematous, non-pruritic. Constitutional "mono-like symptoms:" fever (87%), skin rash (68%). Average duration of symptoms/signs 21 days. *See page 84.*
Drugs: Common cause of rash (esp. TMP/SMX & nevirapine) HIV+ pts have ↑ frequency of skin reactions to most drugs	Drug-associated rashes occur in about 5% of those initiating ART. Overall, ART assoc. with ↓ of dermatological manifestations.
Molluscum contagiosum More common in young women (*CID 38:579, 2004*)	Occurs in 8–15% AIDS pts. 2–5 mm pearly flesh-colored papules, often with **central umbilication** on face, anogenital region. Disseminated cryptococcosis, P. marneffei, granuloma annulare may mimic. Rx: *see Table 12, page 132.*
Syphilis, secondary	*See above, Genital Tract.* Rx: *see Table 12, page 120.*
Candidiasis (47% of AIDS pts had mucocutaneous candidal infections in 1 series)	Children: diaper-rash type rash involving trunk & extremities. Adults: red, hemorrhagic macular or papular lesions. Rx: *see Table 12, page 120.*
Cryptococcosis	Common. Widespread skin-colored, dome-shaped translucent papules 1–4 mm in diameter. Resemble Molluscum contagiosum. Rx: *see Table 12, page 122.*
Emmonsia spp.	Disseminated infection in HIV, particularly southern Africa. with plaques, papules (possibly necrotic centers), macules (*Emerg Inf Dis 20:2164, 2014; ID Cases 2:35, 2015*).
Histoplasmosis	Slightly pink 2–6 mm cutaneous papules to larger reddish plaques & multiple shallow crusted ulcerations, usually in febrile patient. Rx: *see Table 12, page 123.*
Mycobacterial infections: M. tuberculosis, M. avium-intracellulare, M. kansasii, M. marinum, M. haemophilum, M. genavense	Vary from acneiform plaques, pustules or indurated verrucous plaques to ulcerative nodular lesions. *See page 102.* Lupus vulgaris from disseminating M. TBc or BCG.
Penicillium (Talaromyces) marneffei (*Curr Opin Infect Dis 21:31, 2008*)	Clinically present with fever, weight loss, small **umbilicated** macular or papular skin lesions (2/3 pts), hepato-splenomegaly, adenopathy. Almost all pts lived or traveled in Southeast Asia. Rx: *see Table 12, page 124.*
Human papillomavirus (warts, condyloma acuminatum)	Diffuse flat & filiform lesions, often in unusual sites. *See GI & Genital Tract, above.* Rx: *see Table 12, page 132.*
Kaposi's sarcoma (CD4: mean 87/mm³, median 37/mm³)	Early lesions are round or irregular pinkish-red to violaceous macules to papules, usually non-tender. Often symmetrical along skin tension lines. *See Table 18.*
Nodular, verrucous, &/or ulcerative lesions	
Mycobacterial infections	*See above.*
Bacillary angiomatosis (*Clin Dermatol 27:271, 2009*)	Friable vascular papules, cellulitis, plaques & subcutaneous nodules, usually tender. Pts may be febrile. May be confused with KS. Etiology: Bartonella henselae & B. quintana. May be isolated from blood (5–15 days incubation of lysis centrifugation cultures on blood agar, 5% CO₂) & identified with Warthin Starry stain. Serology available. Rx: *see Table 12, page 115.*
Cryptococcosis	*As above.*
Histoplasmosis	*As above.*
Furunculosis can be severe	Most due to MRSA. Contagious. Spread with households, partners.

TABLE 11A (27)

CLINICAL SYNDROME, ETIOLOGY, EPIDEMIOLOGY	CLINICAL PRESENTATION, DIAGNOSTIC TESTS, COURSE
Skin/Hair/Nodular, verrucous, &/or ulcerative lesions *(continued)*	
Kaposi's sarcoma: Kaposi-associated herpesvirus (KSHV) now called HHV 8 is found in biopsy samples & blood mononuclear cells of pts with AIDS-related or classical KS.	Skin usually 1st site of presentation. Lesions palpable, firm, non-tender nodules. Early lesions may resemble ecchymoses. Typically violaceous, hyperpigmented, involving head, neck. Later become confluent, form large tumor masses & occur throughout the body. Up to 40% GI involvement. Oral lesions may precede skin lesions. Responds to ART but often requires chemotherapy.
Non-Hodgkins lymphoma	Skin involved in 15% of pts with non-Hodgkin lymphoma. Lesions are usually papules or nodules.
Mycobacterium avium-intracellulare (MAI/MAC)	Fever & extensive cutaneous nodules (granulomas or focal necrosis) have been reported in pts infected with MAC who responded to ART **with immune reconstitution** (↑ CD4 counts & ↓ viral load). Steroids may be useful rx *(Table 11B)*.
Leishmania	May produce a wide spectrum of localized or disseminated cutaneous, mucosal or diffuse lesions. Most lesions are small, papular with ulceration but with HIV may widely disseminate with hundreds of lesions. Common in the Middle East/Iraq, other endemic regions.
Vesicular bullous or pustular lesions	
Herpes simplex virus	Grouped vesicles on erythematous base rapidly evolve into ulcerations or fissures. May persist as chronic large ulcerative lesions, esp. in perianal area. Rx: *see Table 12, page 131.*
Varicella zoster virus: Common in HIV+ pts & frequently precedes AIDS; 10–20%, frequency overall	Grouped vesicles on erythematous base. May be verrucous. In chronic form may persist as hyperkeratotic lesions. Dermatomal distribution. May be multidermatomal. Rx: *see Table 12, page 133.*
Cytomegalovirus	Rare. Small reddish-purple macules that ulcerate. May present with non-healing perianal ulceration. Rx: *see Table 12, page 129.*
Staphylococcal impetigo	Fragile bullae that rupture easily. No specific distribution.
"Typical scabies" *(see Crusted scabies below)*	Extremely pruritic, papular & vesicular lesions characterized by linear or serpentine burrows most commonly on hands, wrists, elbows, ankles. Average number of mites is 11.
Stevens-Johnson syndrome	Most often drug-related: TMP/SMX, fluconazole, ddI, anti-TBc drugs.
Porphyria cutanea tarda	Association with HIV described but the co-occurrence may reflect coexistence of risk factors, esp. alcohol use, Hep C, rather than causal association. Lesions especially over sun-exposed areas.
Papulosquamous lesions	
Seborrheic dermatitis	Occurs in 20–80% HIV+ individuals, dandruff to patches & plaques of erythema with indistinct margins & yellowish scale on "hairy" areas. Malassezia furfur may be causative agent.
Xerotic eczema (dry-skin syndrome). ↑ with ↓ CD4 counts	Occurs in 5–20% HIV+ individuals. Often severely pruritic & resistant to antihistamines.
Dermatophytosis (T. rubrum most common, then T. mentagrophytes & E. floccosum)	Occurs in 20–35% HIV+ individuals. Widespread, often severe with scaly red pruritic papules & plaques.
Crusted (Norwegian) scabies Occurs in 1.3–5% HIV+ individuals. Other: psoriasis, Lichen planus, secondary syphilis	**Highly contagious** to close contacts (health care workers). Usually occurs in patients with severe immunodeficiency. Characterized by erythema, hyperkeratosis & crusting. Pruritus is typically present but in hyperkeratotic, crusted form may be absent. Burrows usually not seen. Gross nail thickening & subungual debris common. Alopecia, hyperpigmentation, pyoderma & eosinophilia may occur. Dx is based on demonstration of heavy mite burden (1000s) on scraping vs. a few in typical scabies. Crusted scabies is resistant to therapy and treatment failure is common. Concomitant oral and topical treatment is most effective: permethrin 5% cream + oral ivermectin or topical benzyl benzoate emulsion with ivermectin.

CLINICAL SYNDROME, ETIOLOGY, EPIDEMIOLOGY	CLINICAL PRESENTATION, DIAGNOSTIC TESTS, COURSE
Skin/Hair *(continued)*	
Folliculitis	
Staphylococcal folliculitis	An uncommon presentation is violaceous plaques (up to 10 cm) in groin, axilla & scalp.
Eosinophilic folliculitis	*See above, Skin, eosinophilic folliculitis.*
Splenomegaly	23% of 70 consecutive HIV+ pts were found to have splenomegaly on physical exam & 66% by ultrasound. Pts with liver disease were more likely to have ↑ (RR=1.84, P<0.001). ↑ spleen was not predictive of any clinical event during a 1-yr follow-up or with developing AIDS in a 6-yr follow-up. **Massive splenomegaly: think leishmaniasis!**
Systemic, wasting syndromes "Slim" disease (enteropathic AIDS), rule out: Cryptosporidium & other causes of chronic diarrhea Mycobacterium avium-intracellu are complex (MAC) Mycobacterium tuberculosis Histoplasma capsulatum Kaposi's sarcoma Non-Hodgkin lymphoma	Weight loss is common (29% in one series). Causes: opportunistic infections, chronic diarrhea, psychosocial factors, drug associated, unexplained. Rapid weight loss (>4 kg in <4 mos.) accompanied by anorexia is usually a sign of secondary infection, slower weight loss (>4 kg in >4 mos.) is often due to GI disease with diarrhea, less marked weight loss may be due to ↓ caloric intake. Responds to ART. **Watch for 'refeeding syndrome'** in those with profound malnutrition and weight loss *(PLoS ONE 5(5): e10687, 2010).*

TABLE 11B: IMMUNE RECONSTITUTION INFLAMMATORY SYNDROME (IRIS)

Diagnostic criteria in patients with improving immune function due to ART.
- Either worsening of known pre-existing infection (paradoxical IRIS) or clinical appearance of an unrecognized pre-existing infection (unmasking IRIS)
- Usual features *(CID 49:1424, 2009)*
  - CD4 count usually <100; with treatment of TB, IRIS can occur with CD4 counts >200
  - Falling plasma HIV quantitation and rising CD4 count
  - Clinical findings consistent with active inflammatory response
  - No evidence of adverse reaction to ART
  - Onset between 30-100 days after starting ART *(AIDS 22:601, 2008)*
- Incidence of IRIS approximately 13% *(LnID 10:251, 2010)*.

Timing of treatment of known opportunistic infection (OI) and ART if new. OI diagnosis:
- Initiate OI therapy as soon as OI is recognized
- In general, start ART roughly 2 weeks after starting OI therapy *(JAMA 312:410, 2014)*.

Management of common IRIS syndromes: See also IRIS complicating specific opportunistic infections in Guidelines for the Prevention and Treatment of Opportunistic Infections in HIV-Infected Adults and Adolescents at *https://aidsinfo.nih.gov/guidelines/html/4/adult-and-adolescent-oi-prevention-and-treatment-guidelines/0*

Pathogen	Clinical Syndrome	Treatment Comments
Cytomegalovirus (CMV) *(HIV Clin Trials 6:136, 2005)*	4 wks – 4 yrs post start of ART. Progression of retinitis and/or uveitis. Rarely: pneumonia, colitis, pancreatitis cholangiopathy.	Continue ART. Start anti-CMV therapy. Start systemic corticosteroids (Prednisone 1 mg/kg/day with taper over 10-14 days). IF CMV eye disease occurs before ART, do not defer ART for >2 wks *(aidsinfo.nih.giv/guidelines)*.
Cryptococcus sp. *(JAIDS 45:595, 2007; JID 202:962, 2010)*	2-6 mos post start of ART. Meningitis, cavitary pneumonia.	For crypto meningitis, try to delay ART for >5 weeks after starting anti-fungal therapy *(NEJM 370:2487, 2014)*. IDSA guidelines range 2-10 weeks. Carefully manage ICP. Possible role of brief corticosteroid course.
Herpes simplex virus (HSV), **Varicella zoster virus** (VZV)	Perianal herpes, localized zoster.	Continue ART. Start Acyclovir or Famciclovir or Valacyclovir.
Hepatitis B virus (HBV)	Hepatitis B	Consider ART hepatotoxicity in differential. Use ART with activity against HBV in HBV/HIV co-infected patients.
JC Virus	Progressive multifocal leukoencephalopathy (PML) with evidence of inflammatory response on MRI with contrast.	Continue ART. Can try corticosteroid therapy. Most pts stabilize, rarely fatal *(CID 36:1047, 2003; Acta Neuropath 109:449, 2005)*.
Kaposi's sarcoma (KS) due to HHV-8	Clinical progression of KS with initiation of ART.	Corticosteroid use may exacerbate process *(Int J STD AIDS 27:1026, 2016)* and may be a risk factor for mortality *(AIDS 30: 909, 2016)*.
Mycobacterium tuberculosis (MTBc), **Mycobacterium avium complex** (MAC, MAI)	Can occur with and without HIV infection. Within 60 days post start of ART. Fever and weight loss. Enhanced inflammation at pulmonary or extrapulmonary sites of infection.	Studies support starting ART within 2 wks of starting antimycobacterial therapy to optimize survival if CD4 <50. Survival benefit exceeds risk of IRIS *(NEJM 365:1471, 1482 & 1492, 2011)*. Otherwise, start within 8 wks. In TB meningitis, very early ART may be more risky *(aidsinfo.nih.gov/guidelines)*.
Pneumocystis jirovecii (PJP pneumonia)	Pneumonia	Start ART within 2 wks of PJP diagnosis *(aidsinfo.nih.gov/guidelines)*.For moderate or severe disease, start course of corticosteroids concomitant with TMP/SMX for PJP pneumonia. Continue ART.

TABLE 11C: NOVEL SYNDROMES AFTER STARTING ART

Opportunistic Infection	Common Clinical Presentation	Presentation After Starting ART
Castleman's disease (HHV-8)	Fever, lymphadenopathy	Clinical resolution of lymphadenopathy in multicentric disease with ART and ganciclovir. Relapse after initial response less likely with rituximab therapy.
Cryptococcus neoformans	Meningitis usually indolent, cerebro-spinal fluid leukocytosis uncommon	Overt meningitis, marked cerebrospinal fluid leukocytosis. IRIS seen in 13% of patients with cryptococcal meningitis and was associated with elevated baseline serum cryptococcal antigen *(CID 49:931, 2009)*.
Cryptosporidiosis, microsporidiosis	Diarrhea	Clinical, microbiological resolution associated with significant reduction in viral load.
Cytomegalovirus	Retinitis, vitreitis, uveitis uncommon	Atypical (non-retinitis) manifestations of CMV, including pneumonitis, pseudotumoral colitis, adenitis & symptoms of viremia. Immune recovery uveitis.
Eosinophilic folliculitis	Inflammatory reaction involving new hair follicles—especially on face and trunk	One etiology is inflammatory reaction to Demodex mites. May respond to ivermectin *(Clin Exper Dermatol 34: e981, 2009)*.
Hepatitis B (chronic)	Asymptomatic or nonspecific symptoms	Acute flare of clinical hepatitis 5–12 wks after beginning ART. Usually resolves without change in therapy.
Hepatitis C (chronic)	Asymptomatic	Acute hepatitis, cirrhosis or HCV-associated disorder such as cryoglobulinemia within 1–9 months after initiation of ART.
Herpes simplex (ano-genital)	Painful ulcerated lesions	Recrudescence of recurrent episodes of ano-genital lesions.
Herpes zoster	May be severe accompanied by complications	Mild presentation, uncomplicated. May see increased incidence of zoster after initiation of ART, possibly due to ↑ CD8 cells.
Histoplasma capsulatum	Pulmonary infection	Disseminated cutaneous infection with laryngeal *(S Afr J HIV Med 18:693, 2017)*.
HIV-1 associated nephropathy	Impaired renal function	Reversal of pathology & recovery of function.
HIV-associated non-Hodgkin's lymphoma	Typical Stage I-IV lymphoma	Improved clinical outcome & survival.
Human papillomavirus (HPV) infection in women	Genital warts, squamous intraepithelial lesions (SILs) of cervix, cervical cancer.	Effective and adherent ART associated with reduced burden of HPV infection and SILs *(JID 201:681, 2010)*.
Kaposi's sarcoma (HHV-8)	Skin lesions, disseminated disease, oral lesions	Regression of lesions coincident with significant reduction in viral load. Laryngeal obstruction from mucosal edema is rare complication of ART. ↓ incidence in US after introduction of ART *(JAMA 305:1450, 2011)*.
Lymphoepithelial parotid cysts	Parotid cysts	Resolution on antiretroviral therapy.
Molluscum contagiosum	Disseminated skin lesions	Resolution of severe disease coincident with 10-fold increase in CD4 cells.
Mycobacterium avium complex	Disseminated disease, weight loss, diarrhea, mycobacteremia	Focal lymphadenitis, granulomatous masses, endobronchial proliferative lesions, abdominal lymphadenopathy & pain, chylous ascites, clearance of bacteremia without antimycobacterial therapy, development of cavitation in pulmonary nodules. Immune reconstitution lymphadenitis may occur despite azithromycin prophylaxis *(CID 42:418, 2006)*. Intraabdominal disease results in greater morbidity than peripheral lymphadenitis.
M. tuberculosis	Subclinical disease	Can develop "unmasked TB-IRIS syndrome" after initiation of ART *(JID 199:437, 2009)*. May also occur in patients with drug-resistant infections *(CID 48:667, 2009)*.
Oral candidiasis	White plaques on oral & pharyngeal mucosa (thrush)	May resolve on ART without anti-fungal. Early work attributed to PI effect other than CD4 recovery *(JID 185: 188, 2002)*; later evaluation did not confirm this association *(J Microbiol Immunol Infect 46: 129, 2013)*.
Oral warts	Relatively rare oral lesions	Oral warts reported to increase on ART; prospective study did not find increase in prevalence/incidence of warts, but showed increased oral HPV DNA after starting ART *(AIDS 30:1573, 2016)*.

TABLE 11C (2)

Opportunistic Infection	Common Clinical Presentation	Presentation After Starting ART
Chronic parvovirus B-19 infection	Anemia; AIDS wasting syndrome; encephalitis	Anecdotal case reports of response in patients with each syndrome receiving ART.
Progressive multifocal leuko-encephalopathy (JC virus)	Neurologic deficits, MRI demonstration of focal or multifocal lesions without contrast enhancement	Neurologic deficits; typically with subcortical white matter areas of $\downarrow$T1 and $\uparrow$T2 signals on MRI. IRIS in PML may show contrast enhancement on MRI. Long-term, see remission of neurologic symptoms & improvement of radiographic findings & increased survival in approx. 50% of cases. Steroids may be beneficial (aidsinfo.nih.gov/guidelines). Fatal, paradoxical worsening of PML (non-responsive to steroids) has also been described in pts shortly after initiation of ART.
Pulmonary tuberculosis	Pulmonary infiltrates	Fever, lymphadenopathy, worsening pulmonary infiltrates. Note: incidence of Tbc decreased with ART.
Sarcoidosis	Cutaneous lesions; diffuse pulmonary involvement; adenopathy	Flares of preexisting or new onset sarcoidosis described in patients on ART.
Systemic lupus erythematosus	Incidence of SLE decreased in immuno-suppressed AIDS pts	Anecdotal reports of new onset of SLE & flares of preexisting SLE following ART.
Tegumentary leishmaniasis	No lesions or few erythematous papules	Worsening of prior lesions or development of disseminated lesions.
Visceral leishmaniasis	Fever, hepatosplenomegaly	Long-term remission; development of post-kala-azar dermal leishmaniasis.

Effect on incidence of AIDS-related opportunistic infections. The immune reconstitution associated with ART has clearly led to a striking decline in the incidence of AIDS-related opportunistic infections, although the spectrum of these diseases, in general, has not been altered. The incidence is highest immediately after starting ART & declines progressively thereafter. There has been a significant decrease in AIDS-defining malignancies (KS, NHL) since introduction of ART *(JAMA 305:1450, 2011)*. ART may be a more common cause of diarrhea now than the formerly frequent opportunistic pathogens.

TABLE 12: TREATMENT OF SPECIFIC SELECTED COMMON OIs OR PROBLEMATIC INFECTIONS

CAUSATIVE AGENT/DISEASE	MODIFYING CIRCUMSTANCES	SUGGESTED REGIMENS		COMMENTS
		PRIMARY	ALTERNATIVE	
BACTERIAL INFECTIONS				
Bartonella				
Bacillary angiomatosis; Peliosis hepatis— patients with AIDS (*Guidelines at AAC 48: 1921, 2004 or https://aidsinfo.nih.gov/ contentfiles/lvguidelines/ glchunk/glchunk_329.pdf*)	Etiology: B. henselae, B. quintana	**Doxy** 100 mg po/IV q12h or **Erythro** 500 mg po/IV q6h	**Azithro** 500 mg po once daily or **Clarithro** 500 mg po bid (neither should be used for CNS disease or endocarditis)	For documented endocarditis, doxy +gent 1 mg/kg IV q8h for 2 weeks, then doxy as a single agent; for CNS disease, other severe infections doxy + rifampin 300 mg po bid (may also be used for endocarditis). Duration of therapy for 3 months. Suppression with macrolide or doxycycline as long as the CD4 count remains <200 cells/mm. May discontinue long-term suppression if at least 3 months of treatment and CD4 count >200 cells/mm for at least 6 months
For chronic suppression in AIDS patients	With CD4 count <200			

Treatment, active Mycobacterium tuberculosis

Overlapping TB (especially MDR TB) and HIV remains a major problem in developing countries.

Isolation essential

See https://aidsinfo.nih.gov/contentfiles/lvguidelines/ adult_oi.pdf

General principles TB therapy in pts co-infected with HIV *(See 2012 DHHS Guidelines cited under general references):*
- Rx of TBc in pts with HIV infection should follow same principles as for persons without HIV.
- Presence of active TBc requires immediate initiation of rx. All HIV-infected pts with active TB should receive ART.
- In antiretroviral-naïve pts, delay of ART for 2-4 wks after initiation of TBc rx permits better definition of causes of adverse reactions & paradoxical reactions, but data shows that initiation of ART with TB rx significantly improves survival despite risk of IRIS (paradoxical reactions) *(NEJM 365:1471, 1482 & 1492, 2011).*
- Specific recommendations on timing of ART.
  - In pts with CD4 <50, start ART within 2 wks of starting TB treatment.
  - In pts with CD4 >50 and clinical disease of major severity, start ART within 2-4 wks after starting TB treatment.
  - In pts with CD4 >50 but without severe clinical disease, ART can be delayed beyond 2-4 wks of starting TB treatment, but not beyond 8-12 wks.
  - All HIV-infected pregnant women with active TB should receive ART as early as feasible.
  - In HIV infected pts with documented MDR-TB or XDR-TB, start ART within 2-4 wks of confirmation of TB drug resistance & initiation of 2nd-line TB therapy.
- Directly observed therapy strongly recommended for HIV/TB co-infected.
- Rifampin/rifabutin-based regimens should be given at least 3x weekly in pts with CD4 <100/mm^3. Rifabutin is preferred rifamycin for pts on PIs.
- Rifapentine is not recommended in HIV-infected pts unless in the context of a clinical trial.
- Despite drug interactions, a rifamycin should be included in pts receiving ART, with dosage adjustment as necessary.
- Paradoxical reaction should be treated with continuation of rx for TBc & HIV, along with use of NSAIDs.
- In severe cases of paradoxical reaction, some suggest use of high-dose prednisone.

Multiresistant (MDR) TB: *defined as resistant to both INH and RIF.*

Extensively Drug-Resistant TB (XDR-TB): defined as resistant to INH & RIF plus any FQ and at least one of 3 second-line drugs: capreomycin, kanamycin or amikacin.

TABLE 12 (2)

BACTERIAL INFECTIONS/Treatment, active Mycobacterium tuberculosis *(continued)*

NOTES:

1. Clinical & microbiologic response same as in HIV-neg patient.
2. Post-treatment long-term suppression not necessary for drug-susceptible strains.
3. Twice weekly regimens not recommended for HIV-infected patients.

	INITIAL PHASE			CONTINUATION PHASE OF THERAPY (in vitro susceptibility known)			
	SEE COMMENTS FOR DOSAGE						
	Regimens	Drugs	Interval/Doses (min. duration)	Regimen	Drugs	Interval/Doses (min. duration)	Range of Total Doses (min. duration)
Rate of INH resistance known to be <4% (drug-susceptible organisms)	1	INH RIF or RFB* PZA EMB	7 d/wk x 56 doses (8 wk) or 5 d/wk x 40 doses (8 wk).	1a	INH RIF or RFB	7 d/wk x 126 doses (18 wk) or 5 d/wk x 90 doses (18 wk)	182–130 (26 wk)
				1b	INH RIF or RFB	3x/wk x 54 doses (18 wk)	92–76 (26 wk)
	2	INH RIF* PZA EMB	7 d/wk x 14 doses (2 wk), then 2x/wk x 12 doses (6 wk) or 5 d/wk x 10 doses (2 wk) then 2x/wk x 12 doses (6 wk)	2	INH RIF or RFB	3x/wk x 54 doses (18 wk)	62–58 (26 wk)

** See end of Section for options regarding concomitant use of protease inhibitors & **RIF** or **RFB**.*

COMMENTS

Dose in mg/kg (max. daily dose)

Regimen	INH	RIF*	PZA	EMB	SM	RFB*
Daily:						
Child	10–20 (300)	10–20 (600)	15–30 (2000)	15–25 (1600)	20–40 (1000)	10–20 (300)
Adult	5 (300)	10 (600)	15–30 (2000)	15–25 (1600)	15 (1000)	5 (300)
3x/wk (DOT):						
Child	20–40 (900)	10–20 (600)	50–70 (3000)	25–30 (2000)	25–30 (1500)	NA
Adult	15 (900)	10 (600)	50–70 (3000)	25–30 (2000)	25–30 (1500)	NA

Include pyridoxine in all INH regimens.

Preferred regimens are 1 and 1a which because of more intensive dosing are less likely to have treatment failure.

Extend duration of therapy with INH + RIF or RFB to 9 months for pulmonary TB if cultures are positive at 2 months on therapy or for bone/joint disease and to 12 months for CNS disease.

TABLE 12 (3)

MODIFYING CIRCUMSTANCES	SUGGESTED REGIMENS	DUR. OF TREATMENT (MO.)	SPECIFIC COMMENTS	COMMENTS
INH (± SM) resistance	(**RIF** or **RFB**) + **PZA** + **EMB** + (**Moxifloxacin** or **Levofloxacin**) for 2 months then (**RIF** or **RFB**) + **EMB** + (**Moxifloxacin** or **Levofloxacin**) x 7 months	9	No need to continue INH once resistance is confirmed.	**NOTE:** FQ resistance may be seen in pts previously treated with FQ. Linezolid has excellent in vitro activity, including MDR strains.
MDR TB (INH + RIF resistance): Expert consultation strongly advised. *See WHO Treatment Guidelines for Drug-Resistant Tuberculosis, revised October 2016.*	At least 5 effective drugs should be used: **PZA** + **FQ** + an injectable agent + two core second-line agents (WHO also recommends addition of high dose **EMB** unless there is confirmed resistance)	18–24	**Injectables:** amikacin, capreomycin, kanamycin, streptomycin (if confirmed susceptible). **Core second-line agents:** ethionamide or prothionamide, cycloserine or terizidone, linezolid, clofazimine. **In patients not previously treated with second-line drugs** and in whom resistance to FQ and second-line injectable agents is excluded or is considered highly unlikely, a shorter MDR-TB regimen of 9–12 months may be used instead of the longer regimens.	
Resistance to RIF	Mono-rifampin resistance is rare and RIF resistance usually indicates MDR (resistance to both INH and RIF). Same as for **MDR TB** + **INH** + **EMB** unless there is confirmed resistance.	12–18	*See comments for MDR TB.*	
XDR TB (extensively drug resistant, MDR + resistance to any FQ plus least one of following: capreomycin, kanamycin or amikacin)	*See comments - need expert consultation*	18–24	Therapy with 5 drugs to which the isolate is susceptible including bedaquiline or delamanid if needed.	

* Alternative agents = ethionamide, cycloserine, p-aminosalicylic acid, clarithromycin, AM/CL, linezolid.

INITIAL & CONTINUATION THERAPY		ALT. REGIMEN	COMMENTS
Concomitant protease inhibitor (PI) therapy requires dose modification	**INH** 300 mg + **Rifabutin** 150 mg po q24h+ **PZA** 25 mg/kg + **EMB** 15 mg/kg q24h x 2 mos.; then **INH** + **RFB** x 4 mos. (7 months for patients with cavitary disease who are culture positive at 2 months)	Consider switching from protease regimen to a reverse-transcriptase integrase inhibitor combination regimen (e.g., tenofovir + emtricitabine + dolutegravir)	Rifamycins induce cytochrome CYP450 enzymes (RIF > rifapentine > RFB) & reduce serum levels of concomitantly administered PIs including 1st line drugs, e.g., Darunavir, Atazanavir. Conversely, PIs inhibit CYP450 & cause ↑ in serum levels of RIF & RFB. If dose of RFB is not reduced, toxicity ↑. RFB/PI combinations are therapeutically effective. Based on new data, RIF can be used for rx of active TB in pts on regimens containing efavirenz or ritonavir. **RIF should not be administered to pts on ritonavir + saquinavir because drug-induced hepatitis with marked transaminase elevations has been observed in healthy volunteers receiving this regimen** *(www.fda.gov).* RFB can also be used with efavirenz or ritonavir but dose should be 450–600 mg/day with efavirenz & 150 mg qod or 300 mg 2x weekly with Ritonavir. Monitor plasma levels of RFB when given with Lopinavir/Ritonavir. RIF preferred rifamycin with efavirenz-based ART regimen.

TABLE 12 (4)

CAUSATIVE AGENT/DISEASE	MODIFYING CIRCUMSTANCES	SUGGESTED REGIMENS		COMMENTS
		PRIMARY	ALTERNATIVE	
BACTERIAL INFECTIONS *(continued)*				
Mycobacterium avium-intracellulare complex (MAC or MAI)	**Primary prophylaxis:** Pt's CD4 count <50–100/mm³ NOTE: Prophylaxis may be discontinued in pts with sustained ↑ in CD4 cells of ≥100/mm³ on ART.	**Azithro** 1200 mg po weekly OR **Clarithro** 500 mg po q12h	**Rifabutin** 300 mg po q24h	If disseminated MAC is a consideration, obtain blood cultures and treat empirically and de-escalate once active infection is ruled out.
	Treatment: Either presumptive dx or after positive culture of blood, bone marrow, or other usually sterile body fluids, e.g., liver.	[**Clarithro** 500 mg po q12h or **azithro** 600 mg po q24h] + **EMB** 15–25 mg/kg/day +/- **Rifabutin** 300 mg po q24h	Clarithro or Azithro + EMB + third or fourth drug for patients with advanced immunosuppression (CD4 counts <50 cells/µL), high mycobacterial loads (>2 log CFU/mL of blood), or in the absence of effective ART. Options include: RFB 300 mg PO, Amikacin 10–15 mg/kg IV daily, Moxifloxacin 400 mg po daily, Levofloxacin 500 mg po daily.	
	Chronic post-treatment suppression—secondary prophylaxis (until CD4 >100 x several mos)	[**Clarithro** or **azithro**] + **EMB** (lower dose to 15 mg/kg/day) *(Dosage above)*	**Clarithro** or **azithro** or **Rifabutin** *(dosage above)*	
Neisseria gonorrhoeae (gonococcus) Ref: *MMWR 64 (RR-3) 1, 2015; CID 61:5785, 2015.* Cephalosporin resistance *(JAMA 309:163 & 185, 2013)*	Gonorrhea; urethritis, conjunctivitis, proctitis; mucopurulent cervicitis; epididymoorchitis (sexually acquired); for disseminated disease, *see Sanford Guide to Antimicrobial Therapy*	[(**Ceftriaxone** 250 mg IM x 1) (**Azithro** 1 gm po x 1)] **Evaluate & rx sex partner.** **Note:** Due to increasing resistance, **fluoroquinolones** no longer recommended.	**Treat for both GC & C. trachomatis even if NAAT indicates single pathogen. Screen for syphilis.** Other alternatives for **GC (Test of cure recommended):** • Spectinomycin[NUS] 2 gm IM x 1. No efficacy for pharyngeal infection. Mono-therapy no longer recommended. • Azithro 1 gm po x 1 effective for chlamydia but need 2 gm po x 1 for GC; not recommended for GC due to GI side effects & expense. • For severe Penicillin allergy, replace penicillin with cephalosporin or, (Azithromycin 2 gm po x 1 + Gent 250 mg IM) or (Azithro 2 gm + Gemi 320 mg). Due to ↑ resistance, Cefixime not recommended for primary therapy. If Ceftriaxone not available, can try Ceftizoxime 500 mg IM, Cefotaxime 500 mg IM, (Cefoxitin 2 gm IM + Probenecid 1 gm po). Due to increasing resistance, double coverage of GC recommended. Therefore Doxy no longer a primary rec though still effective for Chlamydia.

TABLE 12 (5)

CAUSATIVE AGENT/DISEASE	MODIFYING CIRCUMSTANCES	SUGGESTED REGIMENS		COMMENTS
		PRIMARY	ALTERNATIVE	
BACTERIAL INFECTIONS (continued)				
Pelvic inflammatory disease (PID), salpingitis, tubo ovarian abscess. Etiology polymicrobic: *gonococcus, C. trachomatis, bacteroides, enterobacteriaceae, strepto-cocci, mycoplasma.* Ref: *MMWR 64 (RR-3):1, 2015; NEJM 372:3029, 2015*	Outpatient (limit to pts with temp <38 °C, WBC <11,000/mm³, minimal evidence of peritonitis, active bowel sounds & able to tolerate oral nourishment *See www.cdc.gov/std/ treatment*	**Outpatient rx: (ceftriaxone** 250 mg IM x 1 + **doxy** 100 mg po q12h ± **metro** 500 mg po q12h) OR (**cefoxitin** 2 gm IM with **probenecid** 1 gm po—both as single dose)+ (**doxy** 100 mg po bid with **metro** 500 mg po bid). Treat for 14 days.	**Inpatient regimens:** [(**Cefotetan** 2 gm IV q12h or **cefoxitin** 2 gm IV q6h) + (**doxy** 100 mg IV/po q12h)] (**Clinda** 900 mg IV q8h) + (**gentamicin** 2 mg/kg loading dose, then 1.5 mg/kg q8h or single daily dosing), then **doxy** 100 mg po q12h x 14 d	Alternative parenteral regimen: • **AM-SB** 3 gm IV q6h + **doxy** 100 mg IV/po q12h • **FQs** not recommended due to resistance. **Remember: Evaluate & treat sex partner.** Current recommended treatments don't cover M. genitalium, so if no response after 7-10 d consider M. genitalium NAAT and treat with Moxi 400 mg/d x 14d
Prostatitis—Review: *CID 50:164, 2010*				
Acute			**In AIDS pts, prostate may be focus of Cryptococcus neoformans. FQs** no longer recommended for gonococcal infections *(MMWR 65: RR-3, 2015 – STD Guidelines).*	
≤35 years of age	N. gonorrhoeae C. trachomatis *See Comments*	(**ceftriaxone** 250 mg IM x 1, then **doxy** 100 mg po q12h x 10 d)		
>35 years of age	Enterobacteriaceae (coliforms)	**FQ: CIP-ER** 500 mg po 1x/day or **CIP** 400 mg IV bid or **levo** 750 mg IV/po 1x/day for 10-14 d. *See comment.*	**TMP/SMX-DS** 1 tab po bid x 10-14 d. *See comment.*	Treat as acute urinary infection, 10-14 d (not single dose regimen). **Some authorities recommend 3–4 wk therapy.** If uncertain, do urine NAAT for C. trachomatis & N. gonorrhoeae.
Chronic bacterial	Enterobacteriaceae (80%), enterococci (15%), P. aeruginosa	**FQ (CIP** 500 mg po q12h x 4 wks, OR **levo** 750 mg po q24h x 4 wks)—*see Comment*	**TMP/SMX-DS** 1 tab po q12h x 1–3 mos. Case reports of Fosfomycin for resistant organisms	With rx failures, consider infected prostatic calculi. FDA-approved dose of levo is 500 mg; editors prefer higher 750 mg dose. If enterococci & susceptible isolate: Amoxicillin 500 mg po q8h. If XDR gram neg: ERTA 1 g qd; IMP 500 q6 or MERO 500 q8.
Chronic prostatitis/chronic pain syndrome *(NIH classification, JAMA 282: 236, 1999; World J Urol 21:54, 2003)*	The most common prostatitis syndrome, etiology is unknown; molecular probe data suggest infectious etiology *(Clin Micro Rev 11:604, 1998)*	**α-adrenergic blocking agents are controversial** *(AnIM 133:367, 2000).*		Definition of chronic prostatitis: pt. has sx of prostatitis, cells in prostatic secretions, but routine cultures negative. Chlamydia, ureaplasma suspected. Definition of chronic pair: pt. has sx of prostatitis but negative cultures & no cells in prostatic secretions. Review: *JAC 46:157, 2000.* In randomized double-blind study, CIP and alpha blocker were of no benefit *(AnIM 141:581 & 639, 2004).*
Rhodococcus equi (Corynebacterium equi) *CID 44:460, 2007*	Pulmonary infection (most common), CNS, skin, joint, IV line, others	2 drug combination: macrolide (**Azithro**) + FQ	2 drug combination: (FQ or macrolide) + **Rifabutin** (adjust dose if concomitant PI)	Secondary prevention with FQ until CD4 count >200. Macrolide resistance reported in animal infections; resistance mediated by novel erm gene product. *J. Antimicrob. Chemother. (2015)70 (12): 3784-3790.*

TABLE 12 (6)

CAUSATIVE AGENT/DISEASE	MODIFYING CIRCUMSTANCES	SUGGESTED REGIMENS		COMMENTS
		PRIMARY	ALTERNATIVE	
BACTERIAL INFECTIONS (*continued*)				
Syphilis **(Treponema pallidum)** Recommendations are for pts with normal CD4 T-lymphocyte counts. In AIDS pts, clinical course may be atypical. Higher doses/longer periods of rx may be required— *MMWR 64 (RR-3) 1, 2015; Diagnosis JAMA 312:1922, 2014; Treatment JAMA 312:1905, 2014*	Primary (chancre), secondary (rash, mucositis, lymphadenopathy), & early latent (<1 year)	**Benzathine penicillin G (Bicillin L-A)** 2.4 m units IM x 1. Dose for children: 50,000 units/kg IM up to max. of 2.4 m units	**Doxycycline** 100 mg po q12h x 14 d **or** **Tetracycline** 500 mg po q6h x 14 d **or** **Ceftriaxone** 1 gm IM/IV q24h x 8–10 d For failures of initial rx, re-treat with benzathine penicillin G 2.4 m units IM weekly x 3.	For all stages, penicillin best drug. If penicillin allergy, skin test if available or desensitize & treat with penicillin. Erythro not acceptable alternative agent; use doxycycline if unable to desensitize. Limited data on efficacy of alternative regimens. Need baseline titered VDRL (RPR) & repeat titered serology at 3, 6, 12, 24 mos. Repeat rx if (1) persistent clinical signs, (2) titer of VDRL increases 4-fold or fails to decrease 4-fold after 3–6 mos. Even with recommended rx, serologic relapse frequent. **CSF examination indicated if neurologic signs or symptoms are present.**
Azithro resistance in California, Ireland, & elsewhere (*CID 44:5130, 2007; AAC 54:583, 2010*)	Late latent: >1 year duration & neg. CSF exam	**Benzathine penicillin G (Bicillin L-A)** 2.4 m units qwk x 3 wks	**Doxycycline** 100 mg po q12h x 28 d or **Tetracycline** 500 mg po q6h x 28 d	**Azithromycin resistance in California, Ireland, & elsewhere: Do not use in pregnancy or MSM** *(MMWR 64 (RR-3):1, 2015; CID 61:S818, 2015).* **Azithro:** single 2 gm po dose effective for early syphilis in pts with severe pen allergy.
	Neurosyphilis or optic neuritis	**Pen G** 3–4 m units q4h IV x 10–14 d	**(Procaine pen G** 2.4 mUnits IM q24h + **probenecid** 0.5 gm po q6h) both x 10–14 d—*See Comment*	**Ceftriaxone** 2 gm q24h (IV or IM) x 14 d. Failure rate may be higher than with penicillin. For penicillin allergy: either desensitize to penicillin or obtain infectious diseases consultation. **Serologic criteria for response to rx: 4-fold or greater ↓ in VDRL titer over 6–12 mos.** (*CID 61:S818, 2015*).

TYPE OF INFECTION/ORGANISM/ SITE OF INFECTION	SUGGESTED REGIMENS		COMMENTS
	PRIMARY	ALTERNATIVE	
FUNGAL INFECTIONS			
Blastomycosis (*IDSA Treatment Guidelines: Clin Infect Dis 46:1801, 2008*) (*J Clin Micro 7:196, 2015*).	(**Liposomal Ampho B** 3-5 mg/kg/day or **Ampho B** 0.7 mg/kg/day) x 1-2 weeks or until clinical response, then **Itra** 200 mg tid x 3 days followed by **Itra** 200 mg bid.	Mild or moderate disease: **Itra** 200 200 mg tid x 3 days, then 200 mg bid or **Fluconazole** 400-800 mg/day	Itraconazole is drug of choice. In HIV+ pts, because of potential for drug-drug interactions, fluconazole 400-800 mg/day may be used instead of itraconazole. Duration of therapy: 6-12 months in non-HIV but consider chronic suppressive therapy for patients not on ART and with low CD4 count.

Candidiasis: Oral, esophageal, or vaginal candidiasis is a major manifestation of advanced HIV & represents one of the most common AIDS-defining diagnoses. Candida is also a common cause of nosocomial bloodstream infection. A decrease in *C. albicans* & increase in non-albicans species show ↓ susceptibility among candida species to antifungal agents (esp. fluconazole). These changes have predominantly affected immunocompromised pts in environments where antifungal prophylaxis (esp. fluconazole) is widely used. *See CID 48:503, 2009* for updated IDSA Guidelines and *MMWR 58 (RR-1):1, 2009* for recommendations in HIV.

TABLE 12 (7)

TYPE OF INFECTION/ORGANISM/ SITE OF INFECTION	SUGGESTED REGIMENS		COMMENTS
	PRIMARY	ALTERNATIVE	
FUNGAL INFECTIONS/Candidiasis *(continued)*			
Oropharyngeal candidiasis	**Fluconazole** 100-200 mg daily for 7-14 days	Itraconazole solution 200 mg daily **OR** Posaconazole suspension 400 mg bid for 3 days then 400 mg daily **OR** **Voriconazole** 200 mg bid	ART recommended to prevent recurrent disease. Suppressive therapy not necessary, especially with ART and CD4 >200/mm^3, but if required to prevent recurrences Fluconazole 200 mg once daily recommended. Itra, posa, or vori for 28 days for fluconazole-refractory disease. IV echinccardin also an option. Dysphagia or odynophagia predictive of esophageal candidiasis.
Candida esophagitis	**Fluconazole** 200-400 mg daily	**An azole** (itraconazole solution 200 mg daily; or posaconazole suspension 400 mg bid for 3 days then 400 mg daily or voriconazole 200 mg bid) **OR** **An echinocandin** (caspofungin 50 mg IV daily; or micafungin 150 mg IV daily; or anidulafungin 200 mg IV loading dose then 100 mg IV daily) **OR** **Ampho B** 0.3-0.7 mg/kg daily	**Duration of therapy** 14-21 days. IV echinocandin or ampho B for patients unable to tolerate oral therapy. For fluconazole refractory disease, itra (80% will respond), posa, vori, an echinocandin, or ampho B. Echinocandins associated with higher relapse rate than fluconazole. ART recommended. Suppressive therapy with fluconazole 200 mg once daily for recurrent infections. Suppressive therapy may be discontinued once CD4 >200/mm^3.
Vulvovaginitis, Candida Common among healthy young females & unrelated to HIV status.	Topical **azoles** (clotrimazole, buto, mico, tico, or tercon) x 3–7 days; **OR** Topical **nystatin** 100,000 units/day as vaginal tablet x 14 days; **OR** Oral **flu** 150 mg x 1 dose		For recurrent disease 10-14 days of topical azole or oral fluconazole 150 mg, then fluc 150 mg weekly for 6 mo.
Coccidioidomycosis*(CID 63:e112, 2016)*	**Primary prophylaxis:** Not recommended.		
Pulmonary & extrapulmonary (not meningitis). Usually seen in pts with <250 CD4/mm^3. Usually involves generalized lymphadenopathy, skin nodules or ulcers, peritonitis, liver abnormalities, & bone/joint involvement.	**Acute phase (milder disease):** • **Flu** 400–800 mg po q24h; or **itra** 200 mg po q12h **Acute phase (diffuse pulmonary disease):** • **Ampho B** 0.5–1 mg/kg IV q24h, continue until clinical improvement, usually 500–1000 mg total dose **Disseminated disease:** • **Ampho B** 0.5–1 mg/kg IV q24h, continue until clinical improvement, usually 500–1000 mg total dose • **Flu** 400 mg/d (up to 2 g/d recommended by some) • **Itra** up to 800 mg/d as 200 mg doses **Suppression:** • **Flu** 400 mg/d (preferred) • **Itra** 200 mg po q12h	Acute phase (diffuse pulmonary or disseminated disease): Some specialists add azole to ampho B therapy.	Lung infection in approx. 80% of pts. Despite rx with ampho B ± subsequent po azole, mortality reported as 60%. Posaconazole 400 mg twice daily may be effective in cases of fluconazole failure.

TABLE 12 (8)

TYPE OF INFECTION/ORGANISM/ SITE OF INFECTION	SUGGESTED REGIMENS		COMMENTS
	PRIMARY	ALTERNATIVE	
Fungal Infections/Coccidioidomycosis *(continued)*			
Meningitis **Occurs in 1/10 to 1/3 of pts with disseminated cocci** CSF demonstrates lymphocytic pleo-cytosis. CSF glucose <50 mg/day & normal to mildly ↑ protein.	**Treatment: Fluconazole** 200–400 mg po q24h *(CID 63:e112, 2016)*	IV amphotericin B as for pulmonary + 0.2–0.5 mg intrathecal (intraventricular via reservoir device) 2–3x/wk	Flu effective in up to 80% of cases. Vori successful in high doses (6 mg/kg IV q12h) followed by oral suppression (400 mg po q12h). Itra should not be used for treatment or suppression of meningitis, as it does not penetrate into CSF.
	Suppression: Do not dc for patients with meningitis even with robust response to ART. **Fluconazole** 400 mg/day po as single dose or 200 mg po q12h	**Amphotericin B** 1 mg/kg IV once	Relapses are common in both HIV+ & HIV– pts. Lifelong suppression indicated for patients with meningitis.
Cryptococcosis IDSA Treatment Guidelines: *Clin Infect Dis 50:291, 2010.*	**Primary prophylaxis:** Not recommended. *See MMWR 58 (RR-1):1, 2009.*		
Cryptococcemia &/or Meningitis *(MMWR 58 (RR-1):1, 2009)*			
Treatment *(also see Table 11A)* ↓ in era of ART but still common presenting OI in newly diagnosed AIDS pts. Cryptococcal infection may be manifested by positive blood culture or positive test of serum for cryptococcal antigen (CRAG: >95% sens). CRAG no help in monitoring response to therapy.	**Ampho B** 0.7 mg/kg IV q24h + **flucytosine**[1] 25 mg/kg po q6h x 2 wks **OR** **Liposomal amphotericin B** 4 mg/kg IV q24h + **flucytosine** 25 mg/kg po q6h x 2 wks **OR** (Ampho B or Liposomal Ampho B) + Fluconazole 800–1200 mg/day	(**Liposomal Ampho B** 4 mg/kg IV or **Ampho B** 0.7 mg/kg IV) x 2 weeks if Flucytosine not tolerated **OR** **Fluconazole** 400–800 mg/day po or IV + **flucytosine** 25 mg/kg po q6h x 4–6 wks (only if Amphotericin-based therapy not tolerated). Note: Fluconazole 400–800 mg/day only for less severe disease and when Ampho B not tolerated.	**Outcome of treatment:** failure associated with dissemination of infection & high serum antigen titer, indicative of ↑ burden of organisms and lack of 5FC use during inductive Rx, abnormal neurological evaluation & underlying hematological malignancy. Mortality rates still 12% at 3 mos. Early Dx essential for improved outcome *(PLOS Medicine 4:e47, 2007).* **Ampho B + 5FC treatment** ↓ crypto CFUs more rapidly than ampho + flu or ampho + 5FC + flu. Ampho B 1 mg/kg/d alone much more rapidly fungical in vivo than flu 400 mg/d *(CID 45:76&81, 2007).* Ampho B + 5FC and Ampho B + Fluconazole 800–1200 mg/day had similar rates of clearance of crypto from CSF *(CID 54:121, 2012);* Fluconazole may be an acceptable alternative to 5FC in combo with Ampho B.
With ART, symptoms of acute meningitis may return: immune reconstitution inflammatory syndrome (IRIS) ↑ **CSF pressure associated with high mortality: lower with CSF removal.** If frequent LPs not possible, ventriculoperitoneal shunts an option. *(NEJM 370:2487, 2014)*	**Consolidation therapy:** CSF should be sterile before initiation of consolidation therapy, then **Fluconazole** 400 mg po q24h to complete a 10-wk course, then suppression *(see % below).* **Start ART if possible: generally after 5 weeks of antifungal therapy.**	**Then**	Monitor 5-FC levels: peak 70–80 mg/L, trough 30–40 mg/L. Higher levels assoc. with bone marrow toxicity. No difference in outcome if given IV or po.

[1] Flucytosine = 5-FC

TYPE OF INFECTION/ORGANISM/ SITE OF INFECTION	SUGGESTED REGIMENS		COMMENTS
	PRIMARY	ALTERNATIVE	
FUNGAL INFECTIONS/Cryptococcosis/Cryptococcemia &/or Meningitis (*continued*)			
Suppression (chronic maintenance therapy). Discontinuation of antifungal Rx can be considered among pts who remain asymptomatic with CD4 ≥200 for at least 6 months; completed ≥6 months of ART; resolution of signs and symptoms.	**Fluconazole** 200 mg/day po. If CD4 count rises to >100/mm³ with ART and is sustained for 6 mo, suppressive rx can be discontinued. Some perform a lumbar puncture before discontinuation of maintenance rx.	**Itraconazole** 200 mg po q12h if flu intolerant or failure.	Itraconazole less effective than fluconazole & not recommended because of higher relapse rate (23% vs. 4%). Recurrence rate (95% CI) of 0.4 to 3.9 per 100 patient-years with discontinuation of suppressive therapy in 100 patients on ART with CD4 >100 cells/mm³.
Histoplasmosis (IDSA treatment guidelines in *CID 45:807, 2007*) In a Colombian study comparing 30 pts with AIDS with 20 pts without HIV infection with disseminated histo, the AIDS pts had ↑ numbers of skin lesions, ↑ sed rate, anemia, leucopenia, fungal isolated from multiple sites, had ↓ response to itra which ↑ with ART to non-AIDS levels. Best diagnostic test is urinary histoplasma antigen (90% sensitivity) (*Curr Opin Infect Dis 21:421, 2008*): MiraVista Diagnostics (1-866-647-2847). Risk factors for death: dyspnea, platelet count <100,000/mm³, & LDH >2x upper limit normal. In 1 study suppression was safely dc after 12 mos. of antifungal rx & 6 mos. of ART with CD4 >150: 0 relapses after 2 yrs follow-up in 32 pts (*Medicine 93:11, 20'4*).	**Primary prophylaxis: itraconazole** (200 mg daily) for patients with CD4 cell counts <150 cells/mm³ in endemic areas where the incidence of histoplasmosis is >10 cases per 100 patient-years. **Severe disseminated: Acute phase** (1-2 wks): • **Liposomal ampho B** 3 mg/kg/d IV; or • **ABLC** 5 mg/kg/d IV **Continuation phase** (12 mos): **Itra** 200 mg po q12h **Less severe disseminated: Itra** 200 mg po twice daily for 12 mos **Meningitis: Liposomal ampho B** 5 mg/kg/d IV for 4-6 wks; **itra** 200 mg 2-3 times a day for 12 mos	**Fluconazole** 800-1200 mg/day for 12 mos	Institute ART as early as possible. ART improves outcome and although immune response inflammatory syndrome occurs, it is rare, usually not severe and easily managed. L-AMB less toxic and more effective than ampho B: higher response rate, lower mortality. Itra is the preferred azole: flu less effective; keto less expensive but has more adverse effects; vori and posa anecdotally effective, but too few patients to recommend. All are second-line agents and if any of these instead of itra is used, reasons for doing so should be documented in the medical record. Blood levels should be documented during the first month of itra Rx. **Itra is a potent CYP3A4 inhibitor: contraindicated drugs include efavirenz, statins, rifamycins, midazolam, triazolam, cisapride, pimozide, quinidine, dofetilide, or levacetylmethadol. Important drug interactions with antiretroviral agents, PIs in particular.**
	Suppression: Itra 200 mg po q24h. Suppressive therapy may be discontinued in pts who have completed 1 yr of therapy, neg. blood cultures, a serum and urinary hosto antigen <2 ng/mL, CD4 >150 cells/mm³, and who are on ART for ≥6 mos.	**Fluconazole** 200 mg daily or **Amphotericin B** 1 mg/kg IV weekly or biweekly	Itraconazole relapse rate is approx. 5%; 5% relapse rate; 10–20% relapses with ampho B.

TABLE 12 (10)

TYPE OF INFECTION/ORGANISM/ SITE OF INFECTION		SUGGESTED REGIMENS		COMMENTS
		PRIMARY	ALTERNATIVE	
FUNGAL INFECTIONS (*continued*)				
Penicilliosis [Penicillium (Talaromyces) marneffei Common disseminated fungal infection in AIDS pts in SE Asia (esp. Thailand & Vietnam). Most occur when CD4 <50/mm³		**Ampho B** 0.5-1 mg/kg/day x 2 wks followed by **itraconazole** 400 mg/day for 10 wks Then **suppressive therapy** 200 mg/day po **for HIV-infected pts.**	For less sick pts: **Itra** 200 mg po q8h x 3 days, then 200 mg q12h po x 12 wks, then 200 mg po q24h (IV if unable to take po); continue as suppressive therapy for HIV-infected pts.	3rd most common OI in AIDS pts in SE Asia following TB & cryptococcal meningitis. May resemble histoplasmosis or TB. Skin nodules are umbilicated (mimic cryptococcal infection or molluscum contagiosum). In AIDS pts, suppression with itra effective in **preventing relapses.** One retrospective study of 33 patients on ART and >6 mos of CD4 > 100 cells/mm³ in whom suppressive therapy was stopped found zero cases of recurrence per 641 person-months (95% confidence interval 0–0.6 cases per person-month) after a median follow-up of 18 months (range 6–45) (*AIDS 21:365, 2007*).
Pneumocystis pneumonia (PJP) Etiology: Pneumocystis jirovecii Beta-D-glucan with a sensitivity of 96% is an excellent screening tool for PJP (*J Clin Micro 50:7, 2012*)	**Not acutely ill,** able to take po meds. PaO₂ >70 mmHg on room air.	(**TMP/SMX-DS**, 2 tabs po q8h x 21 d) OR (**Dapsone** 100 mg po q24h + **TMP** 5 mg/kg po q8h x 21 d)	[**Clinda** (600 mg IV or 300–450 mg po) q6h + **primaquine** 15 mg to 30 mg base po q24h] x 21 d OR **atovaquone suspension** 750 mg po bid with food x 21 d or (Dapsone 100 mg po + TMP 15 mg/kg/day po in 3 divided doses)	**After 21 days of therapy, then chronic suppression in AIDS pts**
	NOTE: Concomitant use of corticosteroids usually reserved for sicker pts with PaO₂ <70			
	Acutely ill, po therapy not possible. PaO₂ <70 mmHg. Unclear whether anti-HIV therapy should start during or after treatment of PJP (*CID 46:625 & 635, 2008*).	[**Prednisone** 15–30 min. before TMP/ SMX— start with 40 mg po q12h x 5 d, then 40 mg po q24h x 5 d, then 20 mg po q24h x 11 d] + [**TMP/SMX** (15-20 mg of TMP component/ kg/day) IV div. q6–8h x 21 d]		After 21 days of therapy, then chronic suppression. Clinical failure defined as absence of clinical response after 7 days; then switch to **Clinda + primaquine** or **pentamidine** (*JAIDS 48:63, 2008*).
		Can substitute IV prednisolone (reduce dose 25%) for po prednisone		
	Primary prophylaxis & post-treatment suppression	(**TMP/SMX-DS**, 1 tab po q24h or 3x/wk) OR (**dapsone** 100 mg po q24h) OR (**TMP/SMX-SS**, 1 tab po q24h). DC when CD4 >200 x 3 mos.	(**Pentamidine** 300 mg in 6 mL sterile water by aerosol q4 wks) OR (**dapsone** 200 mg po + **pyrimethamine** 75 mg po + **folinic acid** 25 mg po— all once a week); OR **atovaquone** 1500 mg po q24h with food.	TMP/SMX-DS regimen also provides cross-protection vs. toxo & other bacterial infections. Dapsone + pyrimethamine protects vs. toxo.

TYPE OF INFECTION/ORGANISM, SITE OF INFECTION	SUGGESTED REGIMENS		COMMENTS
	PRIMARY	ALTERNATIVE	
FUNGAL INFECTIONS (continued)			
Sporotrichosis (See IDSA treatment guidelines: CID 45:1255, 2007; Am J Respir Crit Care Med 183:96, 2011)			
Cutaneous/Lymphonodular Dissemination is uncommon in immunocompetent pts, but tends to occur in AIDS.	**Itraconazole** 200 mg/day po x 3-6 mos. For non-responders, use itra 200 mg twice daily; or terbinafine 500 mg twice daily, or saturated solution of potassium iodide (SSKI) 5 drops 3x a day, increasing to 40-50 drops 3x a day as tolerated	**Fluconazole** 400-800 mg po q24h Only in those unable to tolerate other agents.	SSKI side effects: nausea, rash, fever, metallic taste, salivary gland swelling. Duration of itra suppressive therapy is indefinite. Based on experience w th other fungal infections, it seems reasonable to discontinue suppressive therapy in those treated with itra for at least 1 year and whose CD4+ cell counts have remained >200 cells/mm^3 for >1 year.
Osteoarticular	**Itraconazole** 200 mg po q12h for 12 mos. (IV if unable to take po)	**Lipid-based ampho B** 3-5 mg/kg/d or ampho B 0.7-1.0 mg/kg/d for initial therapy; then after a favorable response **itra** 200 mg q12h to complete 12 mos of therapy.	Determine itra serum concentrations at two weeks of therapy to document adequate levels.
Pulmonary	**For more severe disease:** **Lipid-based ampho B** 3-5 mg/kg/d **OR Ampho B** 0.7-1.0 mg/kg/d for initial therapy then after a favorable response itra 200 mg q12h to complete 12 mos of therapy	**For less severe disease itra** 200 mg po q12h for 12 mos. (IV if unable to take po).	Determine itra serum concentrations at two weeks of therapy to document adequate levels. Surgery is recommended for resection of localized disease.
Disseminated	**Lipid-based ampho B** 3-5 mg/kg/d for initial therapy then after a favorable response **itra** 200 mg q12h to complete 12 mos of therapy		Determine itra serum concentrations at two weeks of therapy.
Meningeal	**Lipid-based ampho B** 5 mg/kg/d for 4-6 weeks then **itra** 200 mg q12h to complete 12 mos of therapy		Determine itra serum concentrations at two weeks of therapy.
Suppressive therapy	**Itra** 200 mg once daily		Suppressive therapy is recommended for AIDS and other immunocompromised pts to prevent relapse of meningeal and disseminated disease and, because of propensity for dissemination in AIDS, should be considered for cutaneous, osteoarticular, and pulmonary disease. Duration of suppression is not defined, but may be lifelong in meningeal disease. In disseminated and localized disease discontinuation of itra may be reasonable in the patient treated with itra for at least 1 yr and whose CD4 counts are >100 cells/mm^3 for ≥1 yr.

TABLE 12 (12)

TYPE OF INFECTION/ORGANISM/ SITE OF INFECTION	SUGGESTED REGIMENS		COMMENTS
	PRIMARY	ALTERNATIVE	
PARASITIC INFECTIONS. Reference with pediatric dosages: Medical Letter online version: *Drugs for Parasitic Infections (Suppl.), 2007*			
Protozoan—Intestinal			
Cryptosporidium parvum & C. hominis Treatment unsatisfactory.	Effective ART best therapy	**Immunocompetent —no HIV: Nitazoxanide** 500 mg po q12h x 3 days (expensive)	**HIV with immunodeficiency--ART best treatment. Nitazoxanide** is not licensed for immunocompromised pts: no clinical or parasite response compared to placebo.	**Nitazoxanide:** Approved for immunocompetent pts: liquid formulation for rx of children & 500 mg tabs for adults. Ref: *CID 40:1173, 2005.* In AIDS pts, infection of respiratory and biliary tracts recognized. Post **C. hominis** syndrome: eye/joint pain, headache, dizziness *(CID 39:504, 2004).*
Entamoeba histolytica (Amebiasis) Refs: *Ln 361:1025, 2003; NEJM 348:1563, 2003*	Asymptomatic cyst passer	**Paromomycin**[NUS] (aminosidine in U.K.) 500 mg po q8h x 7 d OR **iodoquinol** (Yodoxin) 650 mg po q8h x 20 days	**Diloxanide furoate**[NUS] (Furamide) 500 mg po q8h x 10 days *(Source: Panorama Compound Pharm., 800-247-9767)*	Metronidazole not effective vs. cysts.
	Patient with diarrhea/ dysentery; mild/moderate disease. Oral therapy possible	**Metronidazole** 500–750 mg po q8h x 10 d or **tinidazole** 2 gm po q24h x 3 days, followed by: either [**iodoquinol** (was diiodohydroxyquin) 650 mg po q8h x 20 d] or [**paromomycin**[NUS] 500 mg po q8h x 7 d] to clear intestinal cysts.	**Ornidazole**[NUS] 500 mg po q12h x 5 days followed by:	Colitis can mimic ulcerative colitis; ameboma can mimic adenocarcinoma of colon. **Dx:** Antigen detection and PCR better than O&P. Watch out for non-pathogenic but morphologically identical *E. dispar (CID 29:1117, 1999). Another* alternative: **nitazoxanide** 500 mg po bid x 3 days *(Trans R Soc Trop Med & Hyg 101:1025, 2007).*
	Extraintestinal infection, e.g., hepatic abscess	(**Metronidazole** 750 mg IV/po q8h x 10 d **OR tinidazole** 800 mg po q8h x 20 d) followed by **paromomycin** 500 mg po q8h x 7 days **OR Iodoquinol** 650 mg po tid x 20 days		**Serology positive with extraintestinal disease.**
Isosporiasis: Cystoisospora belli (formerly Isospora belli) *(MMWR 58 (RR-4): 1, 2009)*	Hard to eradicate after ART *(PLoS One 7:e42884, 2012)*	Immunocompetent: **TMP/SMX-DS** tab 1 po bid x 7-10 d; if AIDS pt, then **TMP-SMX-DS** 1 tab qid for up to 4 weeks	**CIP** 500 mg po q12h x 7 d *(AnIM 132:885, 2000)* or Pyrimethamine 50-75 mg/day po + folinic acid 10-25 mg/day po	Chronic suppression in AIDS pts; either **TMP/SMX-DS** 1 tab daily or 3x/wk OR daily (**pyrimethamine** 25 mg/day po + **folinic acid** 5 mg/day po). 2nd line alternative: **CIP** 500 mg po 3x/week.
Microsporidiosis (Ref: *Curr Opin Infect Dis 19:485, 2006, Clin Micro Rev 23:795, 2010). **Effective ART is main therapy.**			
Ocular (Keratoconjunctivitis): Encephalitozoon hellum or cuniculi, Vittaforma (Nosema) corneae or Nosema ocularum.		If corneal infection and disseminated disease, use Fumagillin eyedrops + **Albendazole** 400 mg po bid x 3 weeks	If no disseminated infection: **fumagillin** eyedrops. For V. corneae, may need keratoplasty.	**To obtain fumagillin (Fumidil B):** 1-800-292-6773 or *www.leiterrx.com.* Neutropenia/thrombocytopenia serious side effects. Dx: Most labs use modified trichrome stain. Need electron micrographs for species identification. FA & PCR methods in development. Peds does ref: *PIDJ 23:915, 2004.*
Intestinal (diarrhea): Enterocytozoon bieneusi, Encephalitozoon (Septata) intestinalis		**Albendazole** 400 mg po bid x 3-4 wks. Peds dose: 15 mg/kg per day divided bid x 7 d *(PIDJ 23:915, 2004)* for E. intestinales.	**Fumagillin** 20 mg po tid reported effective for E. bieneusi *(NEJM 346:1963, 2002).* Oral prep is available internationally, but not in the U.S	Oral fumagillin causes Neutropenia/thrombocytopenia.
Disseminated: E. hellum, cuniculi or intestinalis; Pleistophora sp.		**Albendazole** 400 mg po q12h x 2-4 wks		

TABLE 12 (13)

TYPE OF INFECTION/ORGANISM/ SITE OF INFECTION		SUGGESTED REGIMENS		COMMENTS
		PRIMARY	ALTERNATIVE	
PARASITIC INFECTIONS (continued)				
Protozoan—Extraintestinal				
Toxoplasma gondii (AIDS)				
Cerebral toxoplasmosis (Toxoplasma encephalitis) Ref: *MMWR 58(RR-4):1, 2009; Acta Tropica 127:236, 2013* IgG toxo antibody positive in approx. 84% of pts with cerebral toxoplasmosis. **Note: Leucovorin = folinic acid**		**Pyrimethamine** (pyri) 200 mg po x 1 dose then 75 mg/day po] + (**sulfadiazine** [wt-based dose: 1 gm if <60 kg; 1.5 gm if ≥60 kg] po q6h) + (**folinic acid** 10–25 mg/day po) x 6 wks after resolution of signs/symptoms, & then suppressive rx *(see below)* **OR** **TMP/SMX** 10/50 mg/kg/day po or IV div. q12h x 6 wks)	[**Pyri + folinic acid** (as in primary regimen)] plus: (1) **Clinda** 600 mg po/IV q6h or (2) **Atovaquone** 750 mg po q6h **or** (3) **Azithro** 900-1200 mg po once daily All above for 4-6 weeks after resolution of signs & symptoms, then suppression.	Use alternative regimen for pts with severe sulfa allergy. If multiple ring-enhancing brain lesions (CT or MRI), >85% of pts respond to 7–10 days of empiric rx; if no response, suggest brain biopsy. **Dexamethasone:** 4 mg po/IV q6h if evidence of increased cranial pressure.
Primary prophylaxis, AIDS pts—IgG toxo antibody present + CD4 count <100/µl		(**TMP/SMX-DS**, 1 tab po q24h) or (**TMP/SMX-DS**, 1 tab po 3x weekly)	[(**Dapsone** 50 mg po q24h) + (**pyri** 50 mg po q week) + (**folinic acid** 25 mg po q week)] **or** [atovaquone 1500 mg po q24h].	Prophylaxis for pneumocystis with TMP/SMX also effective vs. toxo. Ref: *MMWR 58(RR-4):1, 2009*. Another alternative: (**Dapsone** 200 mg po + **Pyri** 75 mg po + **Folinic acid** 25 mg po) once weekly.
Suppression Secondary prophylaxis after treatment of cerebral toxo Ref: *CID 40 (Suppl. 3), 2005*		(**Sulfadiazine** 500–1000 mg po 4x/day) + (**pyri** 25–50 mg po q24h) + (**folinic acid** 10–25 mg po q24h)	(**Clinda** 300–450 mg po q6-8h) + (**pyri** 25–50 mg po q24h) + (**folinic acid** 10–25 mg po q24h) **or** [atovaquone 750 mg po q6-12h].	(**Pyri + sulfa**) prevents PJP & toxo; (**clinda + pyri**) prevents toxo only. Discontinue suppression when CD4 >200 for 3 months.
Vaginitis— *MMWR 64 (RR-3):1, 2015*				
Bacterial vaginosis Malodorous vaginal discharge, pH >4.5 Ref: *JID 193:1475, 2006*	Polymicrobic: associated with Gardnerella vaginalis, Mobiluncus, Mycoplasma hominis, Prevotella sp., Atopobium sp., et al. Etiology unclear.	**Metronidazole** (0.5 gm po bid x 7 d) **OR** **metronidazole vaginal gel**[1] (1 applicator intravaginally) once daily x 5 d (avoid in 1st trimester pregnancy) **OR** **tinidazole** (2 gm po once daily x 2 days) **OR** (1 gm po once daily x 5 days).	**Clinda** (0.3 gm bid po x 7 d) or 2% **clinda vaginal cream** 5 gm intravaginally at bedtime x 7 d OR **clinda ovules** 100 mg intravaginally at bedtime x 3 d	50% increase in cure rate with condoms or if abstain from sex (*CID:44:213 & 20, 2007*). **Rx of male sex partner not indicated unless balanitis present. Metro-ER** 750 mg po once daily available, efficacy unclear. **In pregnancy:** Rx same as non-pregnancy, except avoid clindamycin cream (↑ risk premature birth). Atopobium resistant to **metro** in vitro; susceptible to **clinda** (*BMC Inf Dis 6:51, 2006*).
Candidiasis vulvovaginal Pruritus, thick cheesy discharge, pH <4.5	Candida albicans 80–90%. C. glabrata, C. tropicalis may be increasing—less suscept. to azoles.	**Fluconazole** 150 mg single dose po or **itraconazole** 200 mg po q12h x 1 d	**Intravaginal azoles:** Variety of strengths. Regimens vary from 1 dose to 7–14 d. Examples (all end in –azole): butocon, clotrim, micon, tiocon, tercon	**Intravaginal azoles available both OTC & by prescription.** Nystatin vaginal tabs x 14 days less effective than azoles. Other therapies for azole-resistant strains: gentian violet, boric acid. With normal CD4 lymphocyte count, usual duration of rx; if AIDS pt, treat for 10–14 d. If 4 or more episodes/year: 6 mos suppression with fluconazole 150 mg po once weekly.

[1] 1 applicator contains 5 gm of gel with 37.5 mg metronidazole

TABLE 12 (14)

TYPE OF INFECTION/ORGANISM/ SITE OF INFECTION		SUGGESTED REGIMENS		COMMENTS
		PRIMARY	ALTERNATIVE	
PARASITIC INFECTIONS/Protozoan—Extraintestinal/Vaginitis *(continued)*				
Trichomoniasis Copious foamy discharge, pH >4.5 *(CID 61:S842, 2015)*	Trichomonas vaginalis	**Metronidazole** (2 gm as single dose) (contraindicated in 1st trimester of pregnancy) **OR** **Tinidazole** 2 gm po x 1 dose **Pregnancy:** *See Comment*	**For rx failure:** Re-treat with **metro** 500 mg po q12h x 7 d; if 2nd failure: **metro** 2 gm po q24h x 3–5 d or **Tinidazole** 2 gm po q24 x 5d. If still failure, suggest ID consultation &/or contact CDC: 770-488-4115 or *www.cdc.gov/std.*	**Treat male sexual partners (2 gm metronidazole po as single dose).** Nearly 20% of men with NGU infected with trichomonas *(JID 188:465, 2003).* **Pregnancy: Metro is not mutagenic or teratogenic. Less data for tinidazole.** Ref: *CID: S842, 2015.*
Nematode infections				
Strongyloides stercoralis (strongyloidiasis)	Risk of hyperinfection in AIDS pts	**Ivermectin** 200 mcg/kg po q24h x 2 d	**Albendazole** 400 mg po bid x 7 days	**For hyperinfection:** repeat rx at 15 days; can use veterinary ivermectin (IV or rectally) *(CID 49:1411, 2009).*
Ectoparasites. NOTE: Due to potential neurotoxicity and risk of aplastic anemia, use lindane products only as last resort.				
Pediculus humanus corporis **(body lice)** For use of ivermectin in outbreak *see JID 193:474, 2006.*		For clothing: either hot wash (149 °F), dry clean or discard. If washed, use hot iron, especially on seams. If nits on body hair (rare) 5% permethrin cream to entire skin x 1. Leave cream on for 6-8 hrs.		Organism lives, and deposits eggs, in clothing seams. Body louse leaves clothing only for blood meal. Nits in clothing viable for 1 month. *See Cutis 80:397, 2007.*
P. humanus var. capitis **(head louse,** nits) Refs: *NEJM 367:1687 & 1750, 2012*		**Permethrin**, 1% generic lotion or cream rinse (RID, Pronto, others): Apply to shampooed dry hair for 10 min; repeat in one week **OR** **Ivermectin** 200-400 mcg/kg po once (report that 3 doses at 7 day intervals works *(JID 193:474, 2006))*; does not affect nits **OR** **Malathion 0.5% lotion** (Ovide). Apply to dry hair for 8–12 hrs, then shampoo. Repeat in 7 days.		**Permethrin:** Success in 78%. Extra nit combing of no benefit. Resistance increasing. No advantage to 5% permethrin. **Malathion:** 98% effective. In alcohol—potentially flammable. Ref: *Ped Dermatol 24:405, 2007; NEJM 362:896, 2010; Ped Infect Dis J 29:991, 2010.*
Phthirus pubis (Crab louse) Eyelash infection: *see Comment*		**Topical: Permethrin** 1% cream to pubic & perianal skin, thighs, trunk & axillae, Wash off after 10 minutes. May need retreatment in 7 days OR **Malathion** 0.5% lotion. Apply as above; leave on for 8-12 hrs before washing off.	Oral therapy (if refractory to topical): **Ivermectin** 250 mcg/kg po x 1 dose; repeat in one week. DO not use in pregnancy or in children if wt <15 kg.	Pediculosis ciliaris (eyelash involvement) treatment: Occlusive petroleum jelly or yellow oxide of mercury to lid margin bid x 8-10 days then mechanical removal of lice and nits. For failures: oral **Ivermectin.** Ref: *MMWR 59 (RR-12):88, 2010.*
Sarcoptes scabiei **(scabies)** (mites) Ref: *NEJM 362:717, 2010*				
Immunocompetent patients		**Primary: Permethrin** 5% cream (ELIMITE). Apply entire skin except around eyes. Leave on 8-10 hrs. Repeat in 1 wk. Safe for children >2 mos. old. **Alternatives: Ivermectin** 200 mcg/kg po, repeat in 14 days OR **crotamiton** 10% cream topically q24h x 2 d (less effective).		Trim fingernails. Reapply cream to hands after handwashing. Pruritus may persist x 2 wks after mites gone. **Do not use lindane in pregnancy or in young children**—absorbed through skin; can use 6–10% precipitated sulfur in petrolatum q24h x 3 d.
AIDS patients, CD4 <150/mm³; lymphoma **(Norwegian scabies—"Crusted" scabies)**		For Norwegian scabies: (**Permethrin** 5 daily x 7 days, then 2x/week until cured + **Ivermectin** 200 mcg/kg po with food on days 1, 2, 8, 9 15 (and maybe 22 & 29)).		Norwegian scabies in AIDS pts: Extensive, crusted. Can mimic psoriasis. Not pruritic. **Highly contagious—isolate!**

TYPE OF INFECTION/ORGANISM/ SITE OF INFECTION	SUGGESTED REGIMENS		COMMENTS
	PRIMARY	ALTERNATIVE	
VIRAL INFECTIONS **Cytomegalovirus (CMV)** Marked ↓ in CMV infections & death from CMV with ART Rx: Progressive ↓ in CMV DNA & most pts become neg. after a median time of 3 mos *(JAC 54:582, 2004; EJCMID 23:550, 2004).*	**Primary prophylaxis** not generally recommended; preemptive rx in pts with ↑ CMV DNA titers in plasma & CD4 <100/mm³. If used: **valganciclovir** 900 mg po q24h. Discontinue primary prophylaxis after ↑ CD4 >100 for 6 mos and viral load suppressed on ART *(MMWR 53:98, 2004).*		Risk for developing CMV disease correlates with quantity of CMV DNA in plasma: each $\log_{10}$ ↑ associated with 3.1-fold ↑ in disease *(CID 28:758, 1999).*
Colitis, esophagitis Dx best by biopsy of ulcer base/edge *(Clin Gastro Hepatol 2:564, 2004).* Multiple biopsies (6 -10) required.	**Ganciclovir** as with retinitis except induction period extended for 3–6 wks. No agreement on use of maintenance; may not be necessary except after relapse. Responses less predictable than for retinitis. **Foscarnet** 90 mg/kg q12h effective. **Valganciclovir also likely effective.** Switch to oral **valganciclovir** 900 mg po q12h when po tolerated & when symptoms not severe enough to interfere with absorption.		
CMV of the nervous system: Encephalitis & ventriculitis, lesions usually periventricular. Molecular diagnostics *(CID 58:1771, 2014).* Treatment not defined, but should be considered the same as retinitis. Disease may develop while taking ganciclovir as suppressive therapy. *[See Herpes 11(Suppl.12):95A, 2004].* **Optimize ART!** *Most would use combination of ganciclovir & foscarnet, but high dose valganciclovir (900 mg po bid) successful in single case (AIDS Reader 17:133, 2007).*			
Lumbosacral polyradiculopathy	**Ganciclovir**, *as with retinitis*. Consider combination of ganciclovir & foscarnet, esp. if prior CMV rx used. Switch to **valganciclovir** when possible. Suppression continued until CD4 remains >100/mm³ for 6 mos.	**Cidofovir** 5 mg/kg IV, once weekly for 2 weeks followed by administration q2 weeks; MUST be administered with probenecid 2 gm po 3 hrs before each dose and further 1 gm doses 2 hours and 8 hours after completion of the cidofovir infusion. IV saline hydration is essential.	
Mononeuritis multiplex	Not defined		Due to vasculitis & may not be responsive to antiviral rx
CMV pneumonia—seen predominantly in transplants (esp. bone marrow), **rare in HIV** Rx only when histological evidence present in AIDS pts & other pathogens not identified. High rate of CMV reactivation in immunocompetent ICU patients; prolonged hospitalizations and increased mortality *(JAMA 300:413, 2008).*	**Ganciclovir/valganciclovir**, as with retinitis. Many transplant units also use IVIG or CMV specific immune globulin as adjunctive Rx (no studies).		In infants treated for pneumocystis, dual infection with CMV documented in 1/3 *(Ped Pulmon 45:650, 2010).*

TABLE 12 (16)

TYPE OF INFECTION/ORGANISM/ SITE OF INFECTION	SUGGESTED REGIMENS		COMMENTS
	PRIMARY	ALTERNATIVE	
VIRAL INFECTIONS/Cytomegalovirus (CMV) *(continued)*			

CMV Retinitis (most common in AIDS) Still the most common cause of blindness in AIDS patients with <50/mm³ CD4 counts.
 	
Differential dx: HIV retinopathy, herpes simplex retinitis, varicella zoster retinitis *(Am J Ophthal 145:397, 2008).*
 	
11.6% of 374 pts followed with CMV retinitis who responded to ART (↑ of ≥50 CD4 cells/ mL) developed immune recovery vitreitis (vision ↓ & floaters with posterior segment inflammation — vitreitis, papillitis & macular changes) *(Ophthal 113:684, 2006).*
 	
Corticosteroid rx ↓ inflammatory reaction of immune recovery vitreitis without reactivation of CMV retinitis, either periocular corticosteroids or short course of systemic steroid.
 	
Review: *Curr ID Reports 14:435, 2012.*
	Treatment:
	• **For immediate sight-threatening lesions:**
	Intravitreal injections of **ganciclovir** (2 mg/ infection) or **foscarnet** (2.4 mg/ injection) for 1-4 doses over a period of 7-10 days PLUS **valganciclovir** 900 mg orally BID for 14-21 days; then 900 mg orally once daily. (NB: GCV implants no longer manufactured).
	
	• **For peripheral lesions:**
	  Valganciclovir 900 mg po q12h x 14–21 d, then 900 mg po q24h
	  (Clin Ophthal 4:111, 2010)
	
	Suppression:
	• **Chronic maintenance Rx or secondary prophylaxis:**
	  Valganciclovir 900 mg po q24h
	  OR
	  Foscarnet 90 mg/kg IV q24h
	
	Dc with CD4 >100 x 6 mos.
		Ganciclovir 200 to 400 µgm/0.1 mL (of 4 mgm/mL solution) by intravitreal injection every other week until retinitis inactive: ↓ cost and useful in resource restricted regions *(J Med Assoc Thai 88: Suppl. 9:S63, 2005).*
		OR
		Ganciclovir 5 mg/kg IV q12h x 14–21 d, then **valganciclovir** 900 mg po q24h
		OR
		Foscarnet 60 mg/kg IV q8h or 90 mg/kg IV q12h x 14–21 d, then 90–120 mg/kg IV q24h
		OR
		Cidofovir 5 mg/kg IV x 2 wks, then 5 mg/kg every other wk; each dose should be administered with IV saline hydration & oral probenecid
		
		Suppression, 2°: Chronic maintenance therapy: **Cidofovir** 5 mg/kg IV every other week with **probenecid** 2 gm po 3 hrs before the dose followed by 1 gm po 2 hrs after the dose, & 1 gm by mouth 8 hrs after the dose (total of 4 gm)
			Valganciclovir po equal to GCV IV in induction of remission. Intravitreal ganciclovir qow effective in 827 pts with active retinitis also receiving ART in Thailand. A mean of 5 cc injections necessary and no relapses but follow up only 5 mos.
			
			Complications in 7 of 51 eyes (14%) included vitreous haze, retinal detachment, endophthalmitis & immune recovery vitreitis *(J Med Assoc Thai 88: Suppl. 9:S63, 2005).*
			
			Retinal detachments 50–60% within 1 yr of dx of retinitis. In 271 AIDS pts with CMV retinitis, both 2ⁿᵈ eye involvement & retinal detachment markedly ↓ with ART but only if good CD4 cell response *(Ophthal 111:2232, 2004).*

Maintenance can be discontinued if CD4 >100/mm³ x 6 mos. Pts who discontinue maintenance rx should undergo regular eye examination for early detection of relapses! Risk for reactivation very low 0.016 per person yr of follow up *(HIV Clin Trials 7:1, 2006).*			Potential emergence of resistant CMV. 27.5% pts treated 9 mos developed CMV isolates resistant to GCV *(JID 177:770, 1998),* hence may be reason for clinical failure.

TABLE 12 (17)

TYPE OF INFECTION/ORGANISM/ SITE OF INFECTION	SUGGESTED REGIMENS		COMMENTS
	PRIMARY	ALTERNATIVE	
VIRAL INFECTIONS (continued)			
Hairy leukoplakia (Epstein Barr virus, EBV)	Usually asymptomatic & no treatment indicated	**Acyclovir** (800 mg po 5x/day) or topical podophyllin resin (one application) (not currently FDA-approved for this indication)	Patients usually asymptomatic, lesions respond to rx but recur.
Hepatitis A *(Ln 351:1643, 1998)*	No therapy recommended. If within 2 wks of exposure, gamma globulin 0.02 mL/kg IM injection x 1 is protective. Hep A vaccine equally effective as IVIG in randomized trial and is emerging as preferred Rx *(NEJM 357:1685, 2007)*.		For vaccine recommendations, *see Table 19 (MMWR 48:RR-12, 1999)*. Based on increased severity of acute hepatitis A super-imposed on chronic liver disease, **HAV vaccine recommended for all patients with chronic liver disease** *(Am J Med 118:21S, 2005)*. Up to 20% of pts require hospitalization *(NEJM 353: 890, 2005)*.
Hepatitis B	**Truvada** (**TDF** 300 mg + **Emtricitabine** 200 mg) OR **Descovy** (**TAF** 25 mg + **Emtricitabine** 200 mg) po once daily + another anti-HIV drug. Use **Entecavir** 0.5 mg once daily if unable to use tenofovir-based therapy.		ALL patients should use tenofovir-based regimen as part of a fully suppressive anti-HIV/anti-HBV regimen. Continue therapy indefinitely. TAF effective vs HBV infection.
Hepatitis C	HCV treatment recommendations are changing rapidly with the advent of new direct-acting agents (DAAs). For current treatment options, see *The Sanford Guide to Hepatitis Therapy; webedition.sanfordguide.com* or *www.hcvguidelines.org*		

Herpes simplex virus (HSV)
Genital herpes ↑ transmission and acquisition of HIV *(See http://www.cdc.gov/std/tg2015/default.htm; MMWR Vol. 64 / No. 3, June 5, 2015)*

	PRIMARY	ALTERNATIVE	COMMENTS
Mucocutaneous (oral, anal, genital, skin) **Treatment** Mild	**Acyclovir** 400 mg po q8h x 7-10 d **OR** **Famciclovir** 500 mg po q12h x 7-10 d **OR** **Valacyclovir** 1000 mg po q12h x 7-10 d[NFDA]	Chronic suppression indicated if frequent recurrences &/or extensive disease. 1% foscarnet cream applied 5x/day in acyclovir-unresponsive ulcers had 65–90% partial to complete response *(J AIDS 21:301, 1999)*. Famcyclovir approved for "fever blister" at 1500 mg po x 1 dose and for acute exacerbations of genital lesions at 1000 mg po bid x one day for normal hosts. Not yet approved for HIV-infected persons at these doses.	
Severe—extensive disease, systemic toxicity	**Acyclovir** 5 mg/kg q8h IV x 5–10 d [For encephalitis, ↑ to 10-12 mg/kg IV q8h x 10 d] After lesions begin to heal, switch to **famciclovir** 500 mg po q12h or **valacyclovir** 1000 mg po q12h, or **acyclovir** 400 mg po q8h. Continue rx until lesions have completely healed.	If acyclovir-resistant: **Foscarnet** 80-120 mg/kg/day in 2-3 divided doses **OR** **Cidofovir** 5 mg/kg IV q wk until clinical response	Severe disease not responding to acyclovir may represent resist-ant virus. Acyclovir-resistant HSV occurs, esp. in large ulcers. Most will respond to IV foscarnet or cidofovir, but recur after drug discontinued [median 6 wks *(NEJM 325:551, 1991)*]. HSV that becomes resistant to both acyclovir & foscarnet will usually remain sensitive to cidofovir *(JID 180:487, 1999)*.
Suppression, post-treatment, only if recurrences are frequent or severe *See CID 39 (Suppl. 5):S237, 2004*	**Valacyclovir** 500 mg (or 1000 mg for those with very frequent recurrences) po q24h; Valacyclovir more effective overall than other agents *(Meta-analysis in J Oral Path Med 46:561, 2017)* **OR** **Acyclovir** 400 mg po q12h or 200 mg po q8h indefinitely. **OR** **Famciclovir** 500 mg po q12h If acyclovir-resistant: **Foscarnet** 40 mg/kg IV q24h indefinitely.	NOTE: For pts taking acyclovir for chronic suppression who then develop CMV retinitis, stop acyclovir when ganciclovir started—GCV active vs. H. simplex. Valacyclovir (500 mg po q12h) rx of HIV-infected pt: at 6 mos, 65% were recurrence-free vs. 26% receiving placebo *(package insert, Valtrex)*.	**Suppression**, post-treatment, only if recurrences are frequent or severe. *See CID 39 (Suppl. 5):S237, 2004.*

TABLE 12 (18)

TYPE OF INFECTION/ORGANISM/ SITE OF INFECTION	SUGGESTED REGIMENS		COMMENTS
	PRIMARY	ALTERNATIVE	
VIRAL INFECTIONS/Herpes simplex virus (HSV) *(continued)*			
Human herpesvirus 8 **(Kaposi's sarcoma-associated herpesvirus)** *See JCI 113:21, 2004*	*See Table 18, Treatment of HIV-Associated Malignancies.* Effective suppression of HIV-1 replication with ART has best chance of preventing progression of KS or occurrence of new lesions. Castleman's disease responded to ganciclovir 5 mg/kg q12h x 3 weeks *(Blood 103:1632, 2004)* & valganciclovir 900 mg po q12h x 3 weeks *(JID 2006)*.		Virus appears to be spread by saliva *(JID 2007;195:30-36)*. HHV8-associated Castleman disease responds to ART with immune reconstitution, but relapse of disease still occurred. Some case reports of efficacy of sirolimus *(Transplant Proceed 44:2824, 2012)*.
Human papillomavirus (HPV): Condyloma acuminatum (CA) (anogenital warts) *(MMWR 53:46, 2004)* Progression of disease correlates with ↑ HIV RNA in plasma. Rate of recurrence is high, esp. in HIV+ pts, despite rx.	**Patient-applied:** **Podofilox** 0.5% solution or 0.5% gel. Apply to all lesions q12h x 3 consecutive days. Repeat weekly for up to 4 wks. **OR** **Imiquimod** 5% cream; apply to lesions at bedtime & remove in morning on 3 non-consecutive nights, weekly, for up to 16 wks. **OR** **Sinecatechins** 15% ointment TID applied in thin layer to lesions X >16 weeks (until warts clear) NB: No data for use in HIV patients.	**Provider-applied:** Liquid nitrogen cryotherapy—apply until each lesion is thoroughly frozen; repeat every 1–2 wks x 3–4 times. **Trichloroacetic acid (TCA) or bichloracetic acid cauterization 80–95% aqueous solution—apply to each lesion; repeat weekly for 3–6 wks.** Surgical excision or laser surgery Podophyllin resin 10–25% suspension in tincture of benzoin—apply to area & wash off in a few hrs; repeat weekly for up to 3–6 wks.	Do not rx cervical warts until results of Pap smear known. Avoid podophyllin & podofilox in pregnant women. Alternatives: cryotherapy with liquid nitrogen, electrocautery. Cidofovir topical gel + surgical excision 100% effective in achieving complete response in 19 pts but 27% relapsed *(AIDS 16:447, 2002)*. Common Side Effects: • **Podofilox:** Inexpensive and safe (pregnancy safety not established). Mild irritation after treatment. • **Imiquimod:** Mild to moderate redness & irritation. Topical imiquimod effective for treatment of vulvar intraepithelial neoplasms *(NEJM 358:1465, 2008)*. Safety in pregnancy not established. • **Cryotherapy:** blistering and skin necrosis common. • **Podophyllin resin:** Must air dry before treated area contacts clothing. Can irritate adjacent skin. • **TCA:** caustic. Can cause severe pain on adjacent normal skin. Neutralize with soap or sodium bicarbonate. • **Sinecatechins:** Genital, anal, and oral sexual contact should be avoided while the ointment is on the skin. The most common side effects of sinecatechins are erythema, pruritus/burning, pain, ulceration, edema, induration, and vesicular rash.
Molluscum contagiosum virus Typical umbilicated papules with CD4 <100. Effective ART speeds resolution of lesions.	**Treatment:** Usually rx with destructive modalities: cryotherapy with liquid nitrogen, light electrocautery, or curettage.	IV or topical cidofovir (1% cream)	Interferon alfa is not effective. Spontaneous resolution observed in pts with good response to antiretroviral therapy.
	Suppression: Retinoic acid (Retin A) applied once nightly to face may ↓ rate of appearance but does not affect established lesions.		Retinoic acid cannot be used on eyelids or genitalia. Lesions in disseminated cryptococcosis, histoplasmosis may resemble molluscum contagiosum.
Progressive multifocal leukoencephalopathy (PML) (JC virus) Usually in pts with advanced HIV disease *(see Table 11A, page 87)*	**ART** ↑ survival (545 days vs. 60 days, p < 0.001) & either improved (50%) or stabilized (50%) neurological deficits in 12 pts *(AIDS 12:2467, 1999)*. Pts have experienced ↑ neurological manifestations (including death) after initiating ART—possibly due to IRIS. **Watch for IRIS!**		**Cidofovir** effective in some patients. Should be used in conjunction with ART. Cidofovir dose same as for CMV disease (5 mg/kg weekly for 2 weeks, then 5 mg/kg every other week). Must be administered with IV saline hydration and probenecid. Follow renal function.

TABLE 12 (19)

TYPE OF INFECTION/ORGANISM/ SITE OF INFECTION		SUGGESTED REGIMENS		COMMENTS
		PRIMARY	ALTERNATIVE	
VIRAL INFECTIONS (*continued*)				
Varicella zoster virus (VZV) ↑ frequency of zoster reported within 2 mos. of starting ART.				Start treatment within 72 hrs of onset of vesicles. Chronic post-treatment suppression not required. Acyclovir: adjust dose if renal function ↓. Acyclovir-resistant VZV occurs in HIV pts previously rx with acyclovir & is associated with poor prognosis. However, in 11 pts who failed 10 days acyclovir, only 3 had in vitro resistance (mutation of thymidine kinase gene) & no resistance developed on rx. Authors recommend 21 days of rx in such cases (*CID 33:2061, 2001*).
Herpes zoster (shingles) (*CID 44. Suppl: 51, 2007*). Not severe (local dermatomal zoster)		**Famciclovir** 500 mg po tid OR **Valacyclovir** 1 gm po tid[NFDAI] All for 7–10 days.	**Acyclovir** 800 mg po 5 x/day	
Severe (extensive cutaneous, >1 dermatome, trigeminal nerve or visceral involvement)		**Acyclovir** (Zovirax) 10 mg/kg IV (infuse over 1 hr) q8h. Continue until cutaneous & visceral disease clearly resolved.	**Foscarnet** 40 mg/kg IV (infuse over 2 hrs) q8h or 60 mg IV q12h for 14–26 days. *Especially if previous Rx with acyclovir documented acyclovir resistance.*	
Varicella (chickenpox) Mortality high (43%) in AIDS pts (*Int J Inf Dis 6:6, 2002*)		**Acyclovir** 10 mg/kg IV (infuse over 1 hr) q8h x 7 d.	Switch to oral rx (**acyclovir** 800 mg po 5x/day or **famciclovir** 500 mg po q8h or **valacyclovir** 1 gm po q8h) after defervescence if no evidence for visceral involvement (*MMWR 53:99, 2004*).	Adjust acyclovir dosage if renal function ↓.
MISCELLANEOUS CONDITIONS				
Aphthous ulcers, recurrent (RAU) Less of a problem with effective ART		Topical corticosteroids in 60% Orabase may decrease pain and swelling. **Thalidomide** 200 mg po q24h x 14–28 d or 400 mg po q24h x 7 d followed by 200 mg q24h x 7 wks. **CAUTION: Severe teratogenicity—pregnancy category X!** Contraindicated in women who are or have potential to become pregnant. Men must use condoms because drug appears in semen. *Restricted distribution; prescribers must be registered.* Teratogenicity may occur after a single dose. Not an approved indication. Numerous adverse effects including: somnolence, rash (incl. Stevens-Johnson), photosensitivity, neuropathy, ↓ WBC, venous thrombosis.		16/29 pts responded to 200 mg q24h vs. 2/28 placebo. Side effects: somnolence 7/29 & rash 6/29 (*NEJM 336:1487, 1997*). In another study, 8/11 responded to 200 q24h; 4 had somnolence, 2 rash (*JID 180:61, 1999*). 9/10 responded to high-dose (400 mg q24h) but 8/10 developed rash (*CID 28:892, 1999*).
Seborrheic dermatitis	Scalp, mid-moderate	Regular use of dandruff shampoo containing selenium sulfide (Selsun), zinc pyrithione (Head & Shoulders, Danex, Zincon) or sulfur/salicylic acid (Vanseb, Sebulex), or anti-fungal (e.g., 2% ketoconazole) shampoo. Medium potency steroid for short-term may reduce sx, but risk of skin atrophy.		Extremely common in HIV+ patients. Involves hairy areas of scalp, face, chest, back & groin. (*See NEJM 360:387, 2009 for review of seborrheic dermatitis*).
	Facial, trunk, &/or groin	Topical imidazole cream (ketoconazole 2%, clotrimazole 1%) + low potency topical steroid (hydrocortisone 1–2.5%, desonide 0.05%) applied 2x q24h.		Topical rx may cause skin irritation.
Wasting Syndrome Reversed with optimized ART		rhGH 3–6 mg SQ daily. Antiretroviral therapy often sufficient to reverse wasting syndrome in those with advanced HIV disease.	rhGHRF (tesamorelin) 2 mg SQ daily	Modest effects on reduction in VAT (visceral adipose tissue) and increase in lean body mass. AEs consist of metabolic complications (DM; increase in IGF-1) swollen hands, soft tissue swelling, and injection site reactions. Effect is lost once drug discontinued. Expensive.

TABLE 13: DRUGS USED IN TREATMENT &/OR CHRONIC SUPPRESSION OF AIDS-RELATED INFECTIONS: ADVERSE EFFECTS, COMMENTS

DRUG NAME, GENERIC (TRADE)/ USUAL DOSAGE	ADVERSE EFFECTS/COMMENTS
ANTIBACTERIAL DRUGS *(See The Sanford Guide to Antimicrobial Therapy)*	
ANTIFUNGAL DRUGS (of use in HIV patients)	
Non-lipid amphotericin B deoxycholate (Fungizone) 0.3–1 mg/kg/day as single infusion 50 mg Mixing ampho B with lipid emulsion results in precipitation & is discouraged.	**Admin:** Ampho B is a colloidal suspension that must be prepared in electrolyte-free D5W at 0.1 mg/mL to avoid precipitation. No need to protect drug suspensions from light. Ampho B infusions cause chills/fever, myalgia, anorexia, nausea, rarely hemodynamic collapse/hypotension. Postulated due to proinflammatory cytokines but does not appear to be histamine release. Manufacturer recommends a test dose of 1 mg, but often not done (1st few mL of 1st dose is a test dose). Duration of infusion usually 4 or more hrs. No difference found in 1- vs. 4-hr infusions except chills/fever occurred sooner with 1-hr. infusion. Febrile reactions decrease with repeated doses. Rare pulmonary reactions (severe dyspnea & focal infiltrates suggesting pulmonary edema) associated with rapid infusion. Severe rigors respond to meperidine (25–50 mg IV). Premedication with acetaminophen, diphenhydramine, hydrocortisone (25–50 mg) & heparin (1000 units) had no influence on rigors/fever. If cytokine postulate correct, NSAIDs or high-dose steroids may prove efficacious but their use may risk worsening infection under rx or increased risk of nephrotoxicity (i.e., NSAIDs). Clinical side effects ↓ with ↑ age. **Toxicity:** Major concern is nephrotoxicity (15% of 102 pts surveyed). Manifest initially by kaliuresis & hypokalemia, then fall in serum bicarbonate (may proceed to renal tubular acidosis), ↓ in renal erythropoietin & anemia, & rising BUN/serum creatinine. Hypomagnesemia may occur. Can reduce risk of renal injury by **(a) pre- & post-infusion hydration with 500 mL saline (if clinical status will allow salt load),** (b) avoidance of other nephrotoxins, e.g., radiocontrast, aminoglycosides, cis-platinum, (c) use of lipid prep of ampho B. Use of low-dose dopamine did not significantly reduce renal toxicity.
Lipid-based ampho B products:[1,2] Amphotericin B lipid complex (ABLC) (Abelcet) 5 mg/kg/day as single infusion	**Admin:** Consists of ampho B complexed with 2 lipid bilayer ribbons. Compared to standard ampho B, larger volume of distribution, rapid blood clearance & high tissue concentrations (liver, spleen, lung). Dosage: **5 mg/kg q24h;** infuse at 2.5 mg/kg/hr; adult & ped. dose the same. DO NOT use an in-line filter. Do not dilute with saline or mix with other drugs or electrolytes. **Toxicity:** Fever & chills in 14–18%; nausea 9%, vomiting 8%; serum creatinine ↑ in 11%; renal failure 5%; anemia 4%; ↓ K 5%; rash 4%.
Liposomal amphotericin B (L-AMB, AmBisome): 1–5 mg/kg/day as single infusion.	**Admin:** Consists of vesicular bilayer liposome with ampho B intercalated within the membrane. Dosage: **3–5 mg/kg/day** IV as single dose infused over a period of approx. 120 min. 10 mg/kg/d no more efficacious but more toxic than 3 mg/kg/d in a double-blind trials of patients with invasive mold infection *(CID 44:1289, 2007).* If infusion is well tolerated, infusion time can be reduced to 60 min.[2] 1 mg/kg/day was as effective as 4 mg/kg/day (6 mos. survival rates 43% vs. 37%, respectively) in pts with invasive aspergillosis complicating bone marrow transplant &/or neutropenia from malignancy. **Major toxicity:** Generally less than ampho B. Nephrotoxicity 18.7% vs. 33.7% for ampho B, chills 47% vs. 75%, nausea 39.7% vs. 38.7%, vomiting 31.8% vs. 43.9%, rash 24% for both, ↓ Ca 18.4% vs. 20.9%, ↓ K 20.4% vs. 25.6%, ↓ Mg 20.4% vs. 25.6%. Acute infusion-related reactions are common with liposomal ampho B, 20–40%. 86% occurred within 5 min. of infusion, including chest pain, dyspnea & hypoxia or severe abdominal, flank or leg pain; 14% developed flushing & urticaria near the end of 4-hr infusion. All responded to diphenhydramine (1 mg/kg) & interruption of L-AMB infusion. These reactions may be due to complement activation by the liposome.
Caspofungin (Cancidas) 70 mg IV on day 1 followed by 50 mg IV q24h (reduce to 35 mg IV q24h with moderate hepatic insufficiency) Ref: *Ln 362:1142, 2003*	An echinocandin which inhibits synthesis of β-(1, 3)-D-glucan, a critical component of fungal cell walls. Fungicidal against candida (MIC <2 mcg/mL) including those resistant to other antifungals & active against aspergillus (MIC 0.4–2.7 mcg/mL). Serum levels on rec. dosages = peak 12, trough 1.3 (24 hrs) mcg/mL. Approved for rx of candidemia & other candida infections (intra-abdominal abscess, esophageal peritonitis, pleural sponge infection) & refractory aspergillus infections & was successful as salvage Rx in approx. half of pts with invasive aspergillus infections in severely impaired hosts. **Toxicity:** remarkably non-toxic with no nephrotoxicity reported. Only 2% of 263 pts in double-blind trial dc drug due to drug-related adverse event. 14% had ↑ transaminases (similar to triazoles). Most common adverse effect: pruritus at infusion site & headache, fever, chills, vomiting, & diarrhea associated with infusion. Drug metabolized in liver & dosage ↓ to 35 mg in moderate to severe hepatic failure. Class C for pregnancy (embryotoxic in rats & rabbits), so only use if potential benefits outweigh risks. Many drug-drug interactions, esp. cyclosporine (hepatic toxicity) & tacrolimus (drug level monitoring recommended). **No drug in CSF or urine.**

[1] Published data from patients intolerant of or refractory to conventional ampho B deoxycholate (Amp B). **In general ampho B lipid formulations are not superior to ampho B in efficacy in prospective trials although they are less nephrotoxic.**

[2] Comparisons between Abelcet & AmBisome suggest higher infusion-assoc. toxicity (rigors) & febrile episodes with Abelcet (70% vs 36%) but a higher frequency of mild hepatic toxicity with AmBisome (59% vs 38%, p=0.05). Mild elevations in serum creatinine were observed in 1/3 of both.

DRUG NAME, GENERIC (TRADE)/ USUAL DOSAGE	ADVERSE EFFECTS/COMMENTS
ANTIFUNGAL DRUGS (of use in HIV patients) *(continued)*	
Micafungin (Mycamine) 150 mg/day IV for esophageal candidiasis; 100 mg/day IV for candidemia; 50 mg per day for prophylaxis post-bone marrow stem cell transplant	Echinocandin approved by the FDA for rx of esophageal candidiasis & for prophylaxis against candida infections in HSCT recipients. Active against most strains of candida sp. & aspergillus sp. including those resistant to fluconazole such as *C. glabrata* & *C. krusei*. No antagonism seen when combined with other antifungal drugs & occ. synergism with ampho B. No dosage adjustment for severe renal failure or moderate hepatic impairment. Low potential for drug interactions. Micafungin is well tolerated & common adverse events include nausea 7.8%, vomiting 2.4%, & headache 2.4%. Transient ↑ LFTs, BUN, creatinine reported; rare cases of significant hepatitis & renal insufficiency. Few drug-drug interactions. **No drug in CSF or urine.**
Anidulafungin (Eraxis) 200 mg IV on day 1 followed by 100 mg/day IV; for esophageal candidasis 100 mg IV times 1, then 50 mg IV q24h	An echinocandin with antifungal activity (cidal) against candida sp. & aspergillus sp. including ampho B- & triazole-resistant strains. Effective in clinical trials of esophageal candidiasis & in 1 trial was superior to fluconazole in rx of invasive candidiasis/candidemia. Like other echinocandins, remarkably non-toxic; most common side effects: nausea, vomiting, ↓ Mg, ↓ K & headache in 11–13% of pts. No dose adjustments for renal or hepatic insufficiency. Few drug-drug interactions. **No drug in CSF or urine.**
Fluconazole (Diflucan) (available generically) 100 mg tabs 150 mg tabs 200 mg tabs 400 mg IV Oral suspension: 50 mg/5 mL	IV=oral dose because of excellent bioavailability. Pharmacology: absorbed po, water solubility enables IV. Peak serum levels *(see Table 14A)*. T½ 30 hrs (range 20–50 hrs). 12% protein bound. **CSF levels 50–90% of serum in normal,** ↑ in meningitis. No effect on mammalian steroid metabolism. ***Drug-drug interactions common.*** Side effects overall 16% [more common in HIV+ pts (21%)]. Nausea 3.7%, headache 1.9%, skin rash 1.8%, abdominal pain 1.7%, vomiting 1.7%, diarrhea 1.5%, ↑ SGOT 20%. Alopecia (scalp, pubic crest) in 12–20% pts on ≥400 mg po q24h after median of 3 mos (reversible in approx. 6 mos). Rare: severe hepatotoxicity, exfoliative dermatitis. Anaphylaxis, thrombocytopenia, leukopenia.
Flucytosine (Ancobon) 500 mg cap	AEs: Overall 30%. GI 6% (diarrhea, anorexia, nausea, vomiting); hematologic 22% [leukopenia, thrombocytopenia, when serum level >100 mcg/mL (esp. in azotemic pts)]; hepatotoxicity (asymptomatic ↑ SGOT, reversible); skin rash 7%; aplastic anemia (rare—2 or 3 cases). False ↑ in serum creatinine on EKTACHEM analyzer.
Imidazoles, topical For vaginal &/or skin use	Not recommended in 1st trimester of pregnancy. Local reactions: 0.5-1.5%: dyspareunia, mild vaginal or vulvar erythema, burning, pruritus, urticaria, rash. Rarely similar symptoms in sexual partner.
Isavuconazole, Isavuconazonium sulfate	Dosing: 200 mg (372 mg of the Isavuconazonium sulfate), IV or po, q8h x 6 doses (48 hours), THEN 200 mg (372 mg of the Isavuconazonium sulfate), IV or po once daily. Adverse Effects: Most common: nausea, vomiting, diarrhea, headache, elevated liver chemistry tests, hypokalemia, constipation, dyspnea, cough, peripheral edema, and back pain. Hepatic: increased ALT, AST Comments: FDA approved for the treatment of invasive aspergillosis *(Lancet 387:760, 2016)* and mucormycosis infection (*(Lancet Infect Dis 16:828, 2016)*.
Itraconazole (Sporanox) 100 mg cap 10 mg/mL oral solution (fasting state) IV usual dose 200 mg q12h x 4 doses followed by 200 mg q24h for a maximum of 14 days	**Itraconazole tablet & solution forms are not interchangeable, solution preferred.** Many authorities recommend measuring drug serum concentration after 2 wks on prolonged rx to ensured satisfactory absorption. To obtain the highest plasma concentration, the tablet is given with food & acidic drinks (e.g., cola) while the solution is taken in the fasted state; under these conditions, the peak conc. of the capsule is approx. 3 µg/mL & of the solution 5.4 mcg/mL. Peak levels are reached faster (2.2 vs. 5 hrs) with the solution. **Peak plasma concentrations after IV injection (200 mg) compared to oral capsule (200 mg): 2.8 µg/mL (on day 7 of rx) vs. 2 µg/mL (on day 36 of rx).** Protein-binding for both preparations is over 99%, which explains the virtual absence of penetration into the CSF **(do not use to treat meningitis).** Most common adverse effects are dose-related nausea 10%, diarrhea 8%, vomiting 6%, & abdominal discomfort 5.7%. Allergic rash 8.6%, ↑ bilirubin 6%, edema 3.5%, & hepatitis 2.7% reported. ↑ doses may produce hypokalemia 8% & ↑ blood pressure 3.2%. Thrombocytopenia & leukopenia reported. Delirium reported *(Psychosomatics 44:260, 2003)*. Hypokalemia & rhabdomyolysis reported. **Reported to produce impairment in cardiac function.** Potential for significant **drug-drug interactions which can be** life-threatening.

TABLE 13 (3)

DRUG NAME, GENERIC (TRADE)/ USUAL DOSAGE	ADVERSE EFFECTS/COMMENTS
ANTIFUNGAL DRUGS (of use in HIV patients) *(continued)*	
Ketoconazole (Nizoral) 200 mg tab	Gastric acid required for absorption—cimetidine, omeprazole, antacids block absorption. In achlorhydria, dissolve tablet in 4 mL 0.2N HCl, drink with a straw. Coca-Cola ↑ absorption by 65% *(AAC 39:1671, 1995)*. CSF levels "none". **Drug-drug interactions important**. Some interactions can be life-threatening. Dose- dependent nausea & vomiting. Liver toxicity of hepatocellular type reported in about 1:10,000 exposed pts—usually after several days to weeks of exposure. At doses of ≥800 mg/day serum testosterone & plasma cortisol levels fall. With high doses, adrenal (Addisonian) crisis reported.
Posaconazole *(Noxafil)* Suspension: 200 mg po tid with food; Delayed-release 300 mg (3 x 100 mg tabs) po bid x 1 day, then 300 mg po daily; (suspension and delayed-release tabs dosing different) Intravenous: 300 mg IV bid x 1 day, then 300 mg IV daily. FDA approval was for "prophylaxis" of Aspergillus and Candida infections in high risk patients	An oral triazole with activity against a wide range of fungi refractory to other antifungal rx including: aspergillosis, zygomycosis, fusariosis, Scedosporium (Pseudallescheria), phaeohyphomycosis, histoplasmosis, refractory candidiasis, refractory coccidioidomycosis, refractory cryptococcosis, & refractory chromoblastomycosis. Approved for prophylaxis. Posaconazole has similar toxicities as other triazoles: nausea 9%, vomiting 6%, abd. pain 5%, headache 5%, diarrhea, ↑ ALT, AST, & rash (3% each). In pts rx for >6 mos., serious side effects have included adrenal insufficiency, nephrotoxicity, & QTc interval prolongation. Significant drug-drug interactions; inhibits CYP3A4. Measurement of serum concentrations recommended for patients undergoing prolonged courses of therapy: target trough >0.5 to 1.5 mcg/mL.
Voriconazole (Vfend) IV: Loading dose 6 mg/kg q12h x 1 day, then 4 mg/kg q12h IV for invasive aspergillus & serious mold infections; 3 mg/kg q12h IV for serious candida infections **Oral: >40 kg body weight:** 400 mg po q12h x 1 day, then 200 mg po q12h; **<40 kg body weight:** 200 mg po q12h x 1 day, then 100 mg po q12h **Take oral dose 1 hr before or 1 hr after eating.** Oral suspension (40 mg/mL) Oral suspension dosing: Same as for oral tabs. Reduce to ½ maintenance dose for moderate hepatic insufficiency.	A triazole with activity against Aspergillus sp., including Ampho resistant strains of A. terreus. Active vs. Candida sp. (including krusei), Fusarium sp., & various molds. Toxicity similar to other azoles/triazoles including uncommon serious hepatic toxicity (hepatitis, cholestasis & fulminant hepatic failure. Liver function tests should be monitored during rx & drug dc' if abnormalities develop. Rash reported in up to 20%, occ. photosensitivity & rare Stevens-Johnson, hallucinations, & anaphylactoid infusion reactions with fever & hypertension. 1 case of QT prolongation with ventricular tachycardia in a 15 y/o pt with ALL reported. **Approx. 30% experience a transient visual disturbance** following IV or po ("altered/enhanced visual perception", blurred or colored visual change or photophobia) within 30–60 minutes. Visual changes resolve within 30–60 min. after administration & are attenuated with repeated doses **(do not drive at night for outpatient rx).** No persistence of effect reported. Cause unknown. In patients with ClCr <50 mL/min., the drug should be given orally, not IV, since the intravenous vehicle (SBECD-sulfobutylether-B cyclodextrin) may accumulate. Potential for drug-drug interactions high. **NOTE:** Not in urine in active form. Monitor troughs to achieve range of 1 to 1.5 mcg/mL. **Pediatric Dosing** *(Antimicrob Agents 56:3032, 2012)*: **IV DOSING:** **Age <12 years or age 12-14 year old, weighing <50 kg:** 9 mg/kg q12h x 2 doses, then 4-8 mg/kg q12h (higher dose invasive molds and more serious infections); **Age 12-14 year old weighing >50 kg or age >15 years old:** adult dose. **PO DOSING:** **Age <12 years or age 12-14 year old, weighing <50 kg:** 9 mg/kg (max 350 mg) q12h; **Age 12-14 year old weighing >50 kg or age >15 years old:** adult dose.

DRUG NAME, GENERIC (TRADE) USUAL DOSAGE	ADVERSE EFFECTS/COMMENTS

ANTIMYCOBACTERIAL DRUGS (of use in HIV patients)

FIRST LINE DRUGS

DRUG NAME, GENERIC (TRADE) USUAL DOSAGE	ADVERSE EFFECTS/COMMENTS
Isoniazid (INH) (Nydrazid, Laniazid, Teebaconin) 300 mg/day po 300 mg tab 100 mg/mL in 10 mL vials (IM) (Nydrazid, Apothecon)	**Adverse effects:** Overall ~1%. **Peripheral neuropathy** (<1.0%); pyridoxine 25 mg q24h will ↓ incidence; other neurologic sequelae, convulsions, optic neuritis, toxic encephalopathy, psychosis, muscle twitching, dizziness & alterations of sensorium, coma (all rare); allergic skin rashes, lymphadenopathy & vasculitis (SLE-like syndrome), fever, minor disulfiram-like reaction, flushing after Swiss cheese, constipation, **hepatitis** (children 10% mild ↑ SGOT, normalizes with continued rx, age <20 yrs rare, 20–34 yrs 0.3%, 35–40 yrs 1.2%, ≥50 yrs 2.3%) (also ↑ with daily alcohol); acute liver failure (fatal or requiring transplantation) (*Lancet 345:555, 1995*); blood dyscrasias (rare); + antinuclear antibody 20%.
Rifampin (Rifadin, Rimactane, Rifocin) 600 mg/day po 300 mg cap (IV available, Aventis, 600 mg)	**Adverse effects:** Produces an orange-brown discoloration of urine, tears (can stain contact lens), semen, & sweat. Can falsely elevate lab measurements of bilirubin. **Drug-drug interactions:** Many: induces liver cytochrome P450 system (CYP3A) to ↑ drug metabolism, e.g., ↑ Coumadin requirement, ↑ steroid dosage in pts with Addison's disease or asthmatics, ↓ effectiveness of oral contraceptives (uterine bleeding, pregnancies), methadone less effective, reduced levels of azole antifungals, e.g., fluconazole. "Flu syndrome": Manifest as fever, chills, headache, bone pain, dyspnea if rifampin ingestion irregular. Hepatotoxicity: 16 deaths reported in 500,000 recipients. Minor enzyme changes common & resolve while continuing the drug. Alcoholics with preexisting liver disease prone to rifampin-induced toxicity. Interstitial nephritis reported.
Ethambutol (Myambutol) 15–25 mg/kg/day po 400 mg tab	**Adverse effects: Optic neuritis** with decreased visual acuity, central scotomata, & loss of green & red perception at 25 mg/kg/day, not at 15 mg/kg/day; peripheral neuropathy & headache (~1%), rashes (rare), arthralgia (rare), hyperuricemia (rare). Monthly evaluation of visual acuity (>10% loss considered significant), red/green color discrimination; usually reversible if drug discontinued. Anaphylactoid reaction. **Comment:** Disrupts outer cell membrane in M. avium with ↑ activity of other drugs.
Pyrazinamide (PZA) 25 mg/kg/day po 500 mg tab	**Adverse effects: Arthralgia; hyperuricemia** (with or without symptoms); hepatitis (not over 2% if recommended dose not exceeded); gastric irritation; photosensitivity (rare). Serum uric acid if symptomatic gouty attack occurs. **Comment:** Maximum dose 2 gm/day.
Streptomycin 0.75–1 gm/day IM (or IV) 1 gm	**Adverse effects:** Overall 8%. **Ototoxicity,** vestibular dysfunction (vertigo); paresthesias; dizziness & nausea (all less in pts receiving 2–3 doses/wk); tinnitus & high frequency loss 1%; nephrotoxicity (rare); peripheral neuropathy (rare); allergic skin rashes 4–5%; drug fever. Available from Pfizer/Roerig 1-800-254-4445. Reference for IV use: *CID 19:1150, 1994*.
Rifamate® *(see Comment for content)* 2 tablets single dose po q24h (1 hr before meal). 1 tab	**Adverse effects:** Same as individual components. **Comments:** 1 tablet contains 150 mg INH, 300 mg RIF.
Rifater® *(See Comment for content)* If pt not >55 kg: 6 tablets single dose po q24h (1 hr before meal). 1 tab	**Adverse effects:** Same as individual components. **Comments:** 1 tablet contains 50 mg INH, 120 mg RIF, 300 mg PZA. Used in 1st 2 mos of rx (PZA 25 mg/kg). Purpose is convenience in dosing, ↑ compliance (*AnIM 122:951, 1995*) but costs 1.5x more.

TABLE 13 (5)

DRUG NAME, GENERIC (TRADE)/ USUAL DOSAGE	ADVERSE EFFECTS/COMMENTS
ANTIMYCOBACTERIAL DRUGS (of use in HIV patients) *(continued)*	
SECOND LINE DRUGS	
Amikacin (Amikin) 7.5–10 mg/kg/day IV or IM 500 mg vial	**Adverse effects:** Nephrotoxicity; **ototoxicity** [usually high frequency loss—especially with larger total dose (>10 gm), longer duration (>10 days), prior aminoglycosides, pos. family history, assoc. renal impairment & rising trough level (>10 µg/mL). All aminoglycosides may cause or ↑ neuromuscular blockade. Use with caution in pts with myasthenia gravis, Parkinsonism, botulism, with neuromuscular blocking drugs, or with massive transfusion of citrated blood. Avoid concurrent use with ethacrynic acid, furosemide or methoxyflurane. ↑ risk of nephrotoxicity with cis platinum, vancomycin, radiocontrast agents. **Comments:** With edema, ascites, &/or obesity, base calculation of est. creatinine clearance on lean body mass & ideal body weight. For dosing with renal impairment, *see Table 15A.*
Rifabutin (Mycobutin) 300 mg/day po (prophylaxis or treatment) 150 mg	**Adverse effects:** In an anti-MAI trial, rifabutin-related adverse effects occurred in 77% of pts receiving 600 mg (high dose) rifabutin with either clarithro or azithro. Most common was a fall in WBC, then nausea/vomiting/diarrhea in 42%, diffuse polyarthralgia in 19%, & anterior uveitis in 8% *(CID 21:594, 1995).* Uveitis responds to topical steroids & cycloplegics *[CID 22(Suppl. 1):S43, 1996].* Subsequently, max. dose of rifabutin reduced to 300 mg. Other adverse effects similar to rifampin: skin rash 11%, orange-tan to brown skin pigmentation *(CID 21:1515, 1995).* Discolored (reddish) urine 30%. Lab: ↑ SGOT/SGPT 8%.
Rifapentine (Priftin) 600 mg po twice weekly for first 2 mos., then 600 mg po q week 150 mg tabs	**Adverse effects:** Similar to other rifamycins *(see RIF, RFB).* Hyperuricemia seen in 21%. Causes red-orange discoloration of body fluids. Note ↑ prevalence of RIF resistance in pts on weekly rx *(Ln 353:1843, 1999).*
Fluoroquinolones	
Levofloxacin (Levaquin) 250–750 mg po/IV q24h. 750 mg po; 750 mg IV	**Review drug-drug interactions.** **Children:** No FQ approved for use under age 16 based on joint cartilage injury in immature animals. Articular SEs in children est. at 2–3% *(LnID 3:537, 2003).* **CNS toxicity:** Poorly understood. Varies from mild (lightheadedness) to moderate (confusion) to severe (seizures). May be aggravated by NSAIDs. **Photosensitivity**
Moxifloxacin (Avelox) 400 mg po/IV q24h 400 mg po/IV	**QT$_c$ (corrected QT) interval prolongation:** ↑ QT$_c$ (>500 msec or >60 msec from baseline) is considered possible with any FQ. ↑ QT$_c$ can lead to torsades de pointes & ventricular fibrillation. Risk low with current marketed drugs. Risk ↑: women, ↓ K$^+$, ↓ Mg^{++}, bradycardia. (Refs: *NEJM 351:1053 & 1089, 2004*). **Avoid concomitant drugs with potential to prolong QTc:** *For list of such drugs, see SANFORD GUIDE TO ANTIMICROBIAL THERAPY, Table 10C, fluoroquinolones, or www.qtdrugs.org.* **Tendinopathy:** Over age 60, approx. 2–6% of all Achilles tendon ruptures attributable to use of FQ *(ArIM 163:1801, 2003).* ↑ risk with concomitant steroid or renal disease *(CID 36:1404, 2003).*
Clarithromycin (Biaxin) 500 mg po q12h or extended release (Biaxin XL) 2 x 500 mg q24hm 500 mg; 500 mg ER *(FDA approved for MAC; investigational for other atypical mycobacteria, not effective vs. M. tuberculosis)*	**Adverse effects:** Overall ~13%, ~3% discontinued drug secondary to side effects. GI ~13%: diarrhea 3%, nausea 3%, abnormal taste 3%, abdominal pain 2%, dyspepsia 2%. CNS: headache 2%. Lab (each <1%): ↑ SGOT, alk p'tase, ↓ WBC, ↑ prothrombin time 1%, ↑ BUN 4%, ↑ creatinine <1%. Should not be used in pregnant women, has demonstrated adverse effects in animals at blood levels 2–17x higher than achieved in humans. **Check drug-drug interactions.** **Remember** potential prolongation of QTc interval by clarithro, erythro & other macrolides, esp. in combination with other drugs capable of prolonged QTc *(NEJM 312:301, 2005). For list of worrisome drugs: www.qtdrugs.org*
Azithromycin (Zithromax) 250–500 mg po q24h, 1200 mg po once weekly 250 mg; 600 mg *(Investigational in T. gondii, not effective vs. M. tuberculosis)*	**Adverse effects:** Overall 12%, 0.7% discontinued drug secondary to side effects. GI 12.8%: diarrhea 4%, nausea 3%, abdominal pain 2%, vomiting 1%. CNS 1%, ototoxicity (3/21 pts 30–90 days after 500 mg/day, *Lancet 343:241, 1994*). Lab: ↑ SGOT 1.5%, WBC ↓ or ↑ 1%, others <1%. Has not been studied in pregnant women. In rats no embryopathy at dose of 60x human total dose.

DRUG NAME, GENERIC (TRADE), USUAL DOSAGE	ADVERSE EFFECTS/COMMENTS
ANTIPARASITIC DRUGS	
Albendazole (Albenza) Doses vary with indication, 200–400 mg po q12h 200 mg tab	**Adverse effects: Teratogenic, Pregnancy Cat. C.** Give after negative pregnancy test. Abdominal pain, nausea/vomiting, alopecia, ↑ serum transaminase. Rare reports of bone marrow suppression. Take with fatty meal–increases absorption 5-fold.
Atovaquone (Mepron) (Suspension) 750 mg po q12h x 21 days for PJP rx; 1500 mg po q24h for PJP prophylaxis 750 mg/5 mL suspension, cost 210 m_ Ref: *AAC 46:1163, 2002*	**Adverse effects:** Discontinuation rate 9%. Skin rash 23%, only 4% required discontinuation of rx, pruritus 5%. GI: nausea 21%, diarrhea 19%, vomiting 14%, abdominal pain 4%. CNS: headache 16%, insomnia 10%, dizziness 3%. General: fever 14%. Lab: anemia (Hgb <8.0 gm/day, 6%), neutropenia (<750/mm^3, 3%), ↑ AST 4%, ↑ amylase 7%. **Comments:** Has not been evaluated in severe PJP. Better absorbed with meals. Plasma concentration 3x higher when taken with fatty (>23 gm) meal.
Clindamycin (Cleocin) Dose & route varies with indication. 75, 150, 300 mg caps; oral solution 75 mg/5 mL; IV sol'n	**Adverse effects:** Most serious is *C. difficile* toxin-mediated diarrhea; can cause non-toxin mediated diarrhea as well. **Allergic reactions:** Fever, rash, erythema multiforme & even anaphylaxis. Reversible neutropenia, thrombocytopenia & eosinophilia. Liver injury can range from minor to severe.
Dapsone (Dapsone USP, Aczone) 100 mg po q24h or 2x weekly 100 mg tabs	Dose-dependent hemolysis of no consequence at usual doses. Hemolysis enhanced greatly in pts with G6PD deficiency. G-I irritation: anorexia, nausea, vomiting. Dapsone converts 20% of RBC hemoglobin to methemoglobin; only a problem if concomitant pneumonia. High incidence of concomitant rash. Acute poisoning if >1.5 gm po: hemolysis, methemoglobinemia, jaundice, coma *(NEJM 364:957, 2011)*. **Comment:** Usually tolerated even if rash after TMP/SMX.
Ivermectin (Stromectol) Strongyloidiasis: 200 mcg/kg x 1 dose po Onchocerciasis: 150 mcg/kg x 1 po Scabies: 200 mcg/kg x 1 po 3 mg tabs	**Adverse effects:** Post-treatment reaction of pt with onchocerciasis (reaction to dying microfilaria) called Mazzotti-type reaction: pruritus (28%), fever (23%), skin urticaria (23%, tender lymph nodes (10%), arthralgia (9%).
Metronidazole (Flagyl) 500–750 mg po q12h–q8h 500 mg	**Adverse effects: GI:** nausea, vomiting, metallic taste. **Neuro:** headache, paresthesias. Avoid alcohol during & 48 hours post-rx or risk of disulfiram-like reaction: nausea, vomiting, flushing, tachycardia, dypsnea. Peripheral neuropathy possible.
Nitazoxanide (Alinia) Ages 1–4: 100 mg po q12h x 3 days Ages 4–11: 200 mg po q12h x 3 days Adults: 500 mg po q12h 500 mg tabs; peds susp.	**Adverse effects:** Dose dependent, mild and transient G-I disturbance. FDA-approved for otherwise healthy children with infection due to Giardia lamblia or Cryptosporidium parvum. Caution in diabetics: 5 mL suspension contains 1.5 gm sucrose. AEs in <1%. Discolored eyes & urine. Ref: *CID 40:1173, 2005.*
Paromomycin (Humatin, Aminosidine) Dose as 25-35 mg/kg/day po div tid 250 mg caps	**Adverse effects: GI:** doses of >3 gm, nausea, abdominal cramps, diarrhea. CNS: vertigo, headache. Skin: rash. **Comment:** This is an aminoglycoside similar to neomycin ("non-absorbed", ~3% of dose is absorbed). Discontinue promptly if patient complains of tinnitus, ↓ in hearing, or vertigo. Risk of oto-nephrotoxicity if oral drug absorbed due to concomitant inflammatory bowel disease.
Pentamidine isethionate IV (Pentam 300) 4 mg/kg/day IV 300 mg powder	**Adverse effects:** Hypotension with rapid IV administration, rash, nausea, vomiting, nephrotoxicity, cardiac arrhythmia (ventricular tachycardias including torsade de pointes), neutropenia (15%), thrombocytopenia, pancreatitis, hypocalcemia, hypoglycemia followed by hyperglycemia. Sterile abscesses after IM administration. **Comments:** Pentamidine inhibits distal nephron absorption of Na$^+$ with resultant hyperkalemia similar to K-sparing diuretics.

TABLE 13 (7)

DRUG NAME, GENERIC (TRADE)/ USUAL DOSAGE	ADVERSE EFFECTS/COMMENTS
ANTIPARASITIC DRUGS (continued)	
Pentamidine (aerosol) (NebuPent) 300 mg/month (prophylaxis) 300 mg powder	**Adverse effects:** Cough may respond to bronchodilator, upper lobe pneumocystis may occur if given with patient sitting. **Comment:** Risk of extrapulmonary pneumocystis & pneumothorax greater than with systemic prophylaxis. Use aerosol only in patients intolerant of oral drugs.
Primaquine: Primaquine phosphate 26.3 mg = 15 mg of base 15 mg to 30 mg (base) po q24h 26.3 mg	**Adverse effects:** Hemolytic anemia if G6PD deficient; may cause clinically significant methemoglobinemia; nausea/abdominal pain if taken on empty stomach.
Pyrimethamine (Daraprim, Malocide) 50–75 mg po q24h; 25 mg with Leucovorin, tablet 5 mg —see Comments)	**Adverse effects:** Pyrimethamine-induced folate deficiency can cause megaloblastic anemia, ↓ WBC, ↓ platelets, glossitis, stomatitis & exfoliative dermatitis. PO folinic acid, 5 mg/day, will ↓ heme adverse effects & not interfere with efficacy of rx. If high-dose pyrimethamine, ↑ folinic acid to 10–50 mg/day. Pyri + sulfadiazine can cause mental changes due to carnitine deficiency (AJM 95:112, 1993). Other: vomiting, diarrhea, xerostomia
Sulfadiazine 1–1.5 gm po q6h 500 mg tablet	**Adverse effects:** Compared to non-HIV pts, HIV pts have dramatic ↑ in incidence of pruritus, rash, Stevens-Johnson syndrome, myalgia/arthralgia in AIDS pts. Traditionally thought on hypersensitivity basis. Data supports postulate of dose-dependent accumulation of toxic sulfonamide metabolites that fail to clear due to concomitant glutathione deficiency in the AIDS pt (Brit J Pharm 39:621, 1995; JAC 34:1, 1994). In addition, can cause hemolytic anemia in G6PD-def. pts. All sulfonamides can cause crystalluria. Do not use in newborns or late stages of pregnancy as increases risk of kernicterus.
Trimethoprim (Proloprim) 5 mg/kg po q6h 100 mg tabs	**Adverse effects:** Rash, pruritus, marrow suppression rare. Rare cases of aseptic meningitis [fever, headache, CSF ↑ cells (monos), ↑ protein] reported (CID 19:431, 1994). **Comment:** Fewer reactions than TMP/SMX.
Trimethoprim (TMP)-sulfamethoxazole (SMX) (Cotrim, Bactrim, Septra) (Dosage depends on indication) 1 double-strength tab (160 TMP/800 mg SMX); 160/800 mg IV	**Adverse effects:** Compared to non-AIDS pts, AIDS pts have dramatic dose-dependent ↑ in pruritus, skin rash, Stevens-Johnson syndrome. In pts given TMP/SMX + steroids for PJP, % skin reactions ↓ from 47 to 13 (CID 18:319, 1994). Initially thought hypersensitivity was reason; accumulating data support hypothesis of dose-dependent accumulation of toxic sulfonamide metabolites (hydroxylamine). Clearance of metabolites requires glutathione & AIDS pts are deficient (Brit J Pharm 39:621, 1995; JAC 34:1, 1994). May explain ability 2/3 of time to rx through rash (Arch Derm 130:1383, 1994). Beware progressive exanthem— some pts progress to exfoliation &/or Stevens-Johnson syndrome. Tremors associated with high dose (CID 22:598, 1996). **TMP** competes with creatinine for tubular secretion & **can ↑ serum creatinine (reversible); TMP** also blocks distal renal tubular reabsorption of Na⁺ & secretion of K⁺. ↑ **serum K⁺** in 21% of pts (AnIM 124:316, 1996).

DRUG NAME(S) GENERIC (TRADE)	DOSAGE/ROUTE	COMMENTS/ADVERSE EFFECTS
ANTIVIRAL DRUGS (other than antiretrovirals)		
CMV		
Cidofovir (Vistide)	5 mg/kg IV q week x 2 weeks, then once weekly every 2 wks. Properly timed IV prehydration with normal saline & oral probenecid **must be used with each cidofovir infusion** *(see pkg insert for details)*. Renal function (serum creatinine & urine protein) must be monitored prior to each dose *(see pkg insert for details)*.	**Adverse effects: Nephrotoxicity;** dose-dependent proximal tubular injury (Fanconi-like syndrome): proteinuria, glycosuria, bicarbonaturia, phosphaturia, polyuria (nephrogenic diabetic insipidus now reported, *Ln 350:413, 1997*), ↑ creatinine. Concomitant saline prehydration, probenecid, extended dosing intervals allowed use. 25% of pts dc IV cidofovir due to nephrotoxicity. Other toxicities: nausea 48%, fever 31%, alopecia 16%, myalgia 16%, probenecid hypersensitivity 16%, neutropenia 29%. No effect on hematocrit, platelets, LFTs. Other **Black Box** warnings: contraindicated with concomitant nephrotoxic agents, ↓WBC, carcinogenic/teratogenic & ↓sperm in animals, only indicated for rx of CMV retinitis. Contraindicated with serum creatinine >1.5 mg/dL, CrCl ≤55 mL/min or urine protein ≥100 mg/dL. **Comment:** Recommended dosage, frequency or infusion rate of cidofovir must not be exceeded. Dose must be reduced or discontinued if changes in renal function occur during rx. For ↑ of 0.3–0.4 mg/dl in serum creatinine, cidofovir dose must be ↓ from 5 to 3 mg/kg; discontinue cidofovir if ↑ of 0.5 mg/dl above baseline or 3+ proteinuria develops (for 2+ proteinuria, observe pts carefully & consider discontinuation).
Foscarnet (Foscavir)	90 mg/kg q12h IV (induction) 90 mg/kg q24h (maintenance) Dosage adjustment with renal dysfunction *(see Table 15A)*	**Adverse effects: Major clinical toxicity is renal impairment (1/3 of patients)**—↑ creatinine, proteinuria, nephrogenic diabetes insipidus, ↓ K+, ↓ Ca++, ↓ Mg++, ↓ or ↑ phosphate. Other **Black Box** warnings: hydration & frequent monitoring imperative; dose adjustment for renal function *(see label and Table 15A);* **seizures** related to electrolyte/mineral abnormalities. Infusion rate must be controlled: administer by infusion pump over 1.5 to 2 hrs. Prehydrate to establish diuresis before first dose and hydrate concomitantly with subsequent doses. Toxicity ↑ with other nephrotoxic drugs [amphotericin B, aminoglycosides or pentamidine (especially severe ↓ Ca++)]. Other: headache, mild (100%); fatigue (100%); nausea (80%), fever (25%). CNS: seizures. Hematol: ↓ WBC, ↓ Hgb. Hepatic: liver function tests ↑. Neuropathy. Penile ulcers.
Ganciclovir (Cytovene)	IV: 5 mg/kg q12h x 14 days (induction) 5 mg/kg IV q24h daily or 6 mg/kg q24h 5 days per/wk (maintenance). Dosage adjustment with renal dysfunction *(see Table 15A).*	**Adverse effects: Black Box** warnings: cytopenias, carcinogenicity/teratogenicity & aspermia in animals. Absolute neutrophil count dropped below 500/mm³ in 15%, thrombocytopenia 21%, anemia 6%. Fever 48%. GI 50%: nausea, vomiting, diarrhea, abdominal pain 19%, rash 10%. Retinal detachment 11%. (Likely related to underlying disease, not drug). Confusion, headache, psychiatric disturbances & seizures. Neutropenia may respond to granulocyte colony stimulating factor (G-CSF or GM-CSF). Severe myelosuppression may be ↑ with coadministration of zidovudine or azathioprine. 32% dc/interrupted rx, principally for neutropenia. Avoid extravasation.
	Oral: 1 gm q8h with food (fatty meal)	Hematologic less frequent than with IV. Granulocytopenia 18%, anemia 12%, thrombocytopenia 6%. GI, skin same as with IV. Retinal detachment 8%.
Valganciclovir (Valcyte)	900 mg (two 450 mg tabs) po q12h x 21 days for induction, followed by 900 mg po q24h for maintenance. Take with food. Dosage adjustment with renal dysfunction *(see Table 15A)*	A prodrug of ganciclovir with better bioavailability than oral ganciclovir: 60% with food. **Adverse effects:** Similar to ganciclovir.

TABLE 13 (9)

DRUG NAME(S) GENERIC (TRADE)	DOSAGE/ROUTE	COMMENTS/ADVERSE EFFECTS
ANTIVIRAL DRUGS (other than antiretrovirals) *(continued)*		
Herpesvirus (Non-CMV)		
Acyclovir (Zovirax)	Doses: *see Table 12* 200 mg caps, 400 mg and 800 mg tabs IV injection (multiple) Oral suspension 200 mg/5 mL Topical: 5% cream and 5% ointment Dosage adjustment with renal dysfunction *(see Table 15A).*	**Oral:** Generally well-tolerated with occ. diarrhea, vertigo, arthralgia. Less frequent rash, fatigue, insomnia, fever, menstrual abnormalities, acne, sore throat, muscle cramps, lymphadenopathy. **IV:** Phlebitis, caustic with vesicular lesions with IV infiltration, CNS (1%): lethargy, tremors, confusion, hallucinations, delirium, seizures, coma *(CID 21:435, 1995).* Improve 1–2 wks after rx stopped. Renal (5%): ↑ creatinine, hematuria. With high doses may crystallize in renal tubules→ obstructive uropathy (rapid infusion, dehydration, renal insufficiency & ↑ dose ↑ risk). Adequate pre-hydration may prevent such nephrotoxicity. Hepatic: ↑ ALT, AST. Uncommon: neutropenia *(CID 20: 1557, 1995),* rash, diaphoresis, hypotension, headache, nausea.
Famciclovir (Famvir)	Doses: *see Table 12* Tabs: 125 mg, 250 mg, 500 mg.	Pro-drug of penciclovir. **Adverse effects:** similar to acyclovir, included headache, nausea, diarrhea, & dizziness but incidence did not differ from placebo *(JAMA 276:47, 1996).* May be taken without regard to meals. Dose should be reduced if CrCl <60 mL/min *(see package insert & Table 12, page 131 & Table 15A, page 157).*
Penciclovir (Denavir)	Topical 1% cream (1.5 gm tubes)	Apply to area of recurrence of herpes labialis with start of sx, then q2h while awake x 4 days. Well tolerated.
Trifluridine (Viroptic)	Topical 1% solution: 1 drop q2h (max. 9 drops/day) until corneal re-epithelialization, then dose is reduced for 7 additional days (one drop q4h for at least 5 drops/day), not to exceed 21 days total rx.	For HSV keratoconjunctivitis or recurrent epithelial keratitis. **Adverse effects:** Mild burning (5%), palpebral edema (3%), punctate keratopathy, stromal edema.
Valacyclovir (Valtrex)	Doses: *see Table 12.* 500 mg tabs and 1 gm caplets. Dosage adjustment with renal dysfunction *(see Table 15A).*	An ester pro-drug of acyclovir that is well-absorbed, bioavailability 3–5x greater than acyclovir. Can take without regard to meals. **Adverse effects** similar to acyclovir *(see JID 186:S40, 2002).* Thrombotic thrombocytopenic purpura/hemolytic uremic syndrome reported in pts with advanced HIV disease & transplant recipients participating in clinical trials at doses of 8 gm/day.
Hepatitis *(See webedition.sanfordguide.com for currently recommended HCV direct-acting agents)*		
Ribavirin (Rebetol, Copegus)	For use in combination with DAAs for hepatitis C. Available as 200 mg caps and 40 mg/mL oral solution (Rebetol) or 200 mg tabs (Copegus) *(See Comments regarding dosage)*	**Black Box warnings:** ribavirin monotherapy of HCV is ineffective; hemolytic anemia may precipitate cardiac events— use with caution; teratogenic/embryocidal **(Preg Category X).** Drug may persist for 6 mos, avoid pregnancy for at least 6 mos after end of rx of women *or their partners.* Only approved for pts with Ccr >50 mL/min. Also should not be used in pts with severe heart disease or some hemoglobinopathies. ARDS reported *(Chest 124:406, 2003).* **Adverse effects:** hemolytic anemia (may require dose reduction or dc), dental/periodontal disorders, and all adverse effects of concomitant interferon used *(see above).* Dosing depends on: interferon used, weight, HCV genotype, and is modified (or dc) based on side effects (especially degree of hemolysis, with different criteria in those with/without cardiac disease). For example, initial Rebetrol dose with Intron A (interferon alfa-2b) is wt-based: 400 mg am & 600 mg pm for ≤ 75 kg, and 600 mg am & 600 mg pm for wt >75 kg, but with Pegintron approved dose is 400 mg am & 400 mg pm with meals. Doses and duration of Copegus with peg-interferon alfa-2a are less in pts with genotype 2 or 3 (800 mg per day divided into 2 doses, for 24 wks) than with genotypes 1 or 4 (1000 mg per day divided into 2 doses for wt <75 kg and 1200 mg per day divided into 2 doses for ≥ 75 kg for 48 wks). *(See individual labels for details, including initial dosing and criteria for dose modification in those with/without cardiac disease).*

DRUG NAME(S) GENERIC (TRADE)	DOSAGE/ROUTE	COMMENTS/ADVERSE EFFECTS
ANTIVIRAL DRUGS (other than antiretrovirals)/Hepatitis *(continued)*		
Telbivudine (Tyzeka)	One 600 mg tab orally q24h, without regard to food. Dosage adjustment with renal dysfunction, Ccr <50 mL/min *(see label).*	An oral nucleoside analog approved for Rx of Hep B. It has demonstrated higher rates of response and superior viral suppression than lamivudine. **Black Box** warnings regarding lactic acidosis/hepatic steatosis with nucleosides and potential for severe exacerbation of Hep B on dc. Generally well-tolerated with reduced mitochondrial toxicity vs. other nucleosides and no dose limiting toxicity observed *(Ann Pharmacother 40:472, 2006; Medical Letter 49:11, 2007)*. Myalgias and myopathy reported. The genotype resistance rate was 4.7 by one yr increasing to 21.5% by 2 yrs of treatment. It selects for YMDD mutation like lamivudine. Combination with lamivudine was inferior to monotherapy *(Hepatology 45:507, 2007)*.
Tenofovir disoproxil fumarate (TDF) (Viread)	*See Table 6B*	Treatment of Hep B is not an FDA approved indication, but drug is treatment of choice in HIV/HBV co-infected patients requiring therapy for both.
Warts *(See CID 28:S37, 1999)* Regimens are from drug labels specific for external genital and/or perianal condylomata acuminata only *(see specific labels for indications, regimens, age limits).*		
Interferon alfa-2b (IntronA)	Injection of 1 million international units into base of lesion, thrice weekly on alternate days for up to 3 wks. Maximum 5 lesions per course.	Interferons may cause "flu-like" illness and other systemic effects. 88% had at least one adverse effect.
Interferon alfa-N3 (Alferon N)	Injection of 0.05 mL into base of each wart, up to 0.5 mL total per session, twice weekly for up to 8 weeks.	Flu-like syndrome and hypersensitivity reactions. Contraindicated with allergy to mouse IgG, egg proteins, or neomycin.
Imiquimod (Aldara)	5% cream. Thin layer applied at bedtime, washing off after 6-10 hr, thrice weekly to maximum of 16 wks.	Erythema, itching & burning, erosions. Flu-like syndrome, increased susceptibility to sunburn (avoid UV).
Podofilox (Condylox)	0.5% gel or solution twice daily for 3 days, no therapy for 4 days; can use up to 4 such cycles.	Local reactions—pain, burning, inflammation in 50%. Can ulcerate. Limit surface area treated as per label.
Sinecatechins (Veregen)	15% ointment. Apply 0.5 cm strand to each wart three times per day until healing but not more than 16 weeks.	Application site reactions, which may result in ulcerations, phimosis, meatal stenosis, superinfection.

TABLE 14A: SELECTED PHARMACOLOGIC FEATURES OF ANTIMICROBIAL AGENTS USED IN HIV-ASSOCIATED INFECTIONS IN ADULTS

For Cytochrome P450 interactions, see Table 14B. Table terminology key at bottom of each page. Additional footnotes at end of this table, page 151.

DRUG	REFERENCE DOSE/ROUTE	PREG RISK	FOOD EFFECT (PO)[1]	ORAL %AB	PEAK SERUM LEVEL (µg/mL)	PROTEIN BINDING (%)	VOL OF DISTRIB (Vd)	AVER SERUM $T\frac{1}{2}$, hrs[2]	BILE PEN (%)[3]	CSF[4]/ BLOOD (%)	CSF PEN[5]	AUC (µg*hr/mL)	Tmax (hr)
PENICILLINS: Natural													
Benz Pen G	1.2 million units IM	B			0.15 (SD)								
Penicillin G	2 million units IV	B			20 (SD)	65	0.35 L/kg		500	5-10	Yes: Pen-sens S. pneumo		
AMINOPENICILLINS													
AM-SB	3 gm IV	B			109-150/ 48-88 (SD)	28/38		1.2				AM: 120- SB: 71	
CEPHALOSPORINS													
CEPHALOSPORINS—2nd Generation													
Cefotetan	1 gm IV	B			158 (SD)	78-91	10.3 L	4.2	2-21			504	
Cefoxitin	1 gm IV	B			110 (SD)	65-79	16.1 L Vss	0.8	280	3	No		
CEPHALOSPORINS—3rd Generation													
Ceftriaxone	1 gm IV	B			150 (SD), 172-204 (SS)	85-95	5.8-13.5 L	8	200-500	8-16	Yes	1006	
AMINOGLYCOSIDES													
Amikacin, gentamicin, kanamycin, tobramycin		D				0-10	0.26 L/kg	2.5	10-60	0-30	No; intrathecal dose: 5-10 mg		

DRUG	REFERENCE DOSE/ROUTE	PREG RISK	FOOD EFFECT (PO)[1]	ORAL %AB	PEAK SERUM LEVEL (µg/mL)	PROTEIN BINDING (%)	VOL OF DISTRIB (Vd)	AVER SERUM $T_{1/2}$, hrs[2]	BILE PEN (%)[3]	CSF[4]/BLOOD (%)	CSF PEN[5]	AUC (µg*hr/mL)	Tmax (hr)
FLUOROQUINOLONES[7]													
Ciprofloxacin	750 mg po q12h	C	± food	70	3.6 (SS)	20–40	2.4 L/kg	4	2800–4500			31.6 (24 hr)	1-2
	400 mg IV q12h	C	± food		4.6 (SS)	20–40		4	2800–4500	26	1 µg/mL: Inadequate for Strep. sp. (CID 31: 1131, 2000).	25.4 (24 hr)	
	500 mg ER po q24h	C	± food		1.6 (SS)	20–40		6.6				8 (24 hr)	1.5
	1000 mg ER po q24h	C	± food		3.1 (SS)	20–40		6.3				16 (24 hr)	2.0
Gemifloxacin	320 mg po q24h	C	Tab ± food	71	1.6 (SS)	55–73	2-12 L/kg Vss/F	7				9.9 (24 hr)	0.5-2.0
Levofloxacin	500 mg po/IV q24h	C	Tab ± food	99	5.7/6.4 (SS)	24–38	74-112 L Vss	7		30–50		PO:47.5, IV 54.6 (24 hr)	PO: 1.3
	750 mg po/IV q24h	C	Tab ± food / Oral soln: no food	99	8.6/12.1 (SS)	24–38	244 L Vss	7				PO 90.7, IV 108 (24 hr)	PO: 1.6
Moxifloxacin	400 mg po/IV q24h	C	Tab ± food	89	4.2-4.6/4.5 (SS)	30–50	2.2 L/kg	10–14		>50	Yes (CID 49: 1080,2009)	PO 48, IV 38 (24 hr)	PO: 1-3
Ofloxacin	400 mg po/IV q12h	C	Tab ± food	98	4.6/6.2 (SS)	32	1-2.5 L/kg	7				PO 82.4, IV 87 (24 hr)	PO: 1-2
Prulifloxacin[NUS]	600 mg po		± food		1.6 (SD)	45	1231L	10.6-12.1		negligible	no	7.3	1
MACROLIDES, AZALIDES, LINCOSAM DES, KETOLIDES													
Azithromycin	500 mg po	B	Tab/Susp ± food	37	0.4 (SD)	7–51	31.1 L/kg	68	High			4.3	2.5
	500 mg IV	B			3.6 (SD)	7–51	33.3 L/kg	12/68				9.6 (24 hr, pre SS)	
Azithromycin-ER	2 gm po	B	Susp no food	∝ 30	0.8 (SD)	7–50	31.1 L/kg	59	High			20	5.0
Clarithromycin	500 mg po q12h	C	Tab/Susp ± food	50	3-4 (SS)	65–70	4 L/kg	5–7	7000			20 (24 hr)	2.0-2.5
	1000 mg ER po q24h	C	Tab + food	∝ 50	2–3 (SS)	65–70							5-8
Erythromycin Oral (various)	500 mg po	B	Tab/Susp no food / DR Caps ± food	18–45	0.1-2 (SD)	70–74	0.6 L/kg	2–4		2–13	No		Delayed Rel: 3
Lacto/glucep	500 mg IV	B			3-4 (SD)	70–74		2–4					

TABLE 14A (3)

DRUG	REFERENCE DOSE/ROUTE	PREG RISK	FOOD EFFECT (PO)[1]	ORAL %AB	PEAK SERUM LEVEL (µg/mL)	PROTEIN BINDING (%)	VOL OF DISTRIB (Vd)	AVER SERUM $T_{1/2}$, hrs[2]	BILE PEN (%)[3]	CSF[4]/ BLOOD (%)	CSF PEN[5]	AUC (µg*hr/mL)	Tmax (hr)
MACROLIDES, AZALIDES, LINCOSAMIDES, KETOLIDES *(continued)*													
Clindamycin	150 mg po	B	Cap ± food	90	2.5 (SD)	85–94	1.1 L/kg	2.4	250–300		No		0.75
	900 mg IV	B			14.1 (SS)	85–94		2.4	250–300		No		
MISCELLANEOUS ANTIBACTERIALS													
Daptomycin	4–6 mg/kg IV q24h	B			58–99 (SS)	92	0.1 L/kg Vss	8–9		0-8		494-632 (24 hr)	
Doxycycline	100 mg po	B	Tab/cap/susp + food		1.5–2.1 (SD)	93	53-134 L Vss	18	200–3200		No (26%)	31.7	2
Metronidazole	500 mg po/IV q6h	B	ER tab no food, Tab/cap ± food		20–25 (SS)	20	0.6-0.85 L/kg	6–14	100	45–89		560 (24 hr)	Immed Rel: 1.6 ER: 6.8
Rifampin	600 mg po	C	Cap no food	70-90	4–32 (SD)	80	0.65 L/kg Vss	2–5	10,000	7-56	Yes	58	1.5-2
Tetracycline	250 mg po	D	Cap no food		1.5–2.2 (SD)		1.3 L/kg	6–12	200–3200		No (7%)	30	2-4
Trimethoprim (TMP)	100 mg po	C	Tab ± food	80	1 (SD)	44	100-120 V/F	8–15					1-4
TMP-SMX-DS	160/800 mg po q12h	C	Tab/susp ± food	85	1–2/40–60 (SS)	TMP: 44	TMP: 100-120 L	TMP: 11	100–200	50/40			TMP PO: 1-4
	160/800 mg IV q8h	C			9/105 (SS)	SMX: 70	SMX: 12-18 L	SMX: 9	40–70				SMX IV: 1-4
ANTIFUNGALS													
Amphotericin B:													
Standard	0.4–0.7 mg/kg IV	B			0.5–3.5 (SS)		4 L/kg	24		0		17	
Lipid (ABLC)	5 mg/kg IV	B			1–2.5 (SS)		131 L/kg	173				14 (24 hr)	
Cholesteryl complex	4 mg/kg IV	B			2.9 (SS)		4.3 L/kg	39				36 (24 hr)	
Liposomal	5 mg/kg IV	B			83 (SS)		0.1-0.4 L/kg Vss	6.8 ± 2.1				555 (24 hr)	
Fluconazole	400 mg po/IV	D	Tab/susp ± food	90	6.7 (SD)	10	50 L V/F	20–50		50–94	Yes		PO: 1-2
	800 mg po/IV	D	Tab/susp ± food	90	Approx. 14 (SD)			20–50					
Itraconazole	200 mg po soln	C	Soln no food	Low	0.3–0.7 (SD)	99.8	796 L	35		0		29.3 (24 hr)	2.5 Hydroxy: 5.3
Ketoconazole	200 mg po	C	Tab ± food	75	1-4 (SD)	99	1.2 L/kg	6-9	ND	<10	No	12	1-2

<u>**Preg Risk:**</u> **FDA risk categories: A** = no risk in adequate human studies, **B** = animal studies suggest no fetal risk, but no adequate human studies, **C** = adverse fetal effects in animals, but no adequate studies in humans; potential benefit may warrant use despite potential risk, **D** = evidence of human risk, but potential benefit may warrant use despite potential risk **X** = evidence of human risk that clearly exceeds potential benefits; **Food Effect (PO dosing): + food** = take with food, **no food** = take without food, **± food** = take with or without food; **Oral % AB** = % absorbed; <u>**Peak Serum Level: SD**</u> = after single dose, **SS** = steady state after multiple doses; <u>**Volume of Distribution (Vd): V/F**</u> = Vd/oral bioavailability, **Vss** = Vd at steady state, **Vss/F** = Vd at steady state/oral bioavailability; <u>**CSF Penetration:**</u> therapeutic efficacy

DRUG	REFERENCE DOSE/ROUTE	PREG RISK	FOOD EFFECT (PO)[1]	ORAL %AB	PEAK SERUM LEVEL (µg/mL)	PROTEIN BINDING (%)	VOL OF DISTRIB (Vd)	AVER SERUM $T\frac{1}{2}$, hrs[2]	BILE PEN (%)[3]	CSF[4]/BLOOD (%)	CSF PEN[5]	AUC (µg*hr/mL)	Tmax (hr)
ANTIFUNGALS *(continued)*													
Posaconazole	200 mg po	C	Susp + food		0.2-1.0 (SD)	98-99	1774 L	20-66			Yes *(JAC 56: 745, 2005)*	15.1	3-5
Voriconazole	200 mg po q12h	D	Tab/susp no food	96	3 (SS)	58	4.6 L/kg Vss	6		22-100	Yes *(CID 37: 728, 2003)*	39.8 (24 hr)	1-2
Anidulafungin	200 mg IV x 1, then 100 mg IV q24h	C			7.2 (SS)	>99	30-50 L	26.5			No	112 (24 hr)	
Caspofungin	70 mg IV x 1, then 50 mg IV qd	C			9.9 (SD)	97	9.7 L Vss	9-11			No	87.3 (24 hr)	
Flucytosine	2.5 gm po	C	Cap ± food	78-90	30-40 (SD)		0.6 L/kg	3-6		60-100	Yes		2
Micafungin	150 mg IV q24h	C			16.4 (SS)	>99	0.39 L/kg	15-17			No	167 (24 hr)	
ANTIMYCOBACTERIALS													
Bedaquiline	400 mg po qd	B	Tab + food	ND	3.3 (Wk 2)	>99	~ 60x total body water Vss	24-30	ND	ND	ND	22 (24hr)	5
Capreomycin	15 mg/kg IM	C			25-35 (SD)	ND	0.4 L/kg	2-5	ND	<10	No	ND	1-2
Cycloserine	250 mg po	C	Cap, no food	70-90	4-8 (SD)	<20	0.47 L/kg	10	ND	54-79	Yes	110	1-2
Ethambutol	25 mg/kg po	C	Tab + food	80	2-6 (SD)	10-30	6 L/kg Vss/F	4		10-50	No	29.6	2-4
Ethionamide	500 mg po	C	Tab ± food	90	2.2 (SD)	10-30	80 L	1.9	ND	∞100	Yes	10.3	1.5
Isoniazid	300 mg po	C	Tab/syrup no food	100	3-5 (SD)		0.6-1.2 L/kg	0.7-4		Up to 90	Yes	20.1	1-2
Para-aminosalicylic acid (PAS)	4 gm po	C	Gran + food	ND	20 (SD)	50-73	0.9-1.4 L/kg (V/F)	0.75-1.0	ND	10-50	Marg	108	8
Pyrazinamide	20-25 mg/kg po	C	Tab ± food	95	30-50 (SD)	5-10		10-16		100	Yes	500	2
Rifabutin	300 mg po	B	Cap + food	20	0.2-0.6 (SD)	85	9.3 L/kg (Vss)	32-67	300-500	30-70	ND	8.6	2.5-4.0
Rifampin	600 mg po	C	Cap no food	70-90	4-32 (SD)	80	0.65 L/kg Vss	2-5	10,000	7-56	Yes	58	1.5-2
Rifapentine	600 mg po q72h	C	Tab + food	ND	15 (SS)	98	70 L	13-14	ND	ND	ND	320 over 72hrs	4.8
Streptomycin	1 gm IV	D			25-50 (SD)	0-10	0.26 L/kg	2.5	10-60	0-30	No; Intrathecal: 5-10 mg		

Preg Risk: FDA risk categories: A = no risk in adequate human studies, **B** = animal studies suggest no fetal risk, but no adequate human studies, **C** = adverse fetal effects in animals, but no adequate studies in humans; potential benefit may warrant use despite potential risk, **D** = evidence of human risk, but potential benefit may warrant use despite potential risk **X** = evidence of human risk that clearly exceeds potential benefits; **Food Effect (PO dosing): + food** = take with food, **no food** = take without food, **± food** = take with or without food; **Oral % AB** = % absorbed; **Peak Serum Level: SD** = after single dose, **SS** = steady state after multiple doses; **Volume of Distribution (Vd): V/F** = Vd/oral bioavailability, **Vss** = Vd at steady state, **Vss/F** = Vd at steady state/oral bioavailability; **CSF Penetration:** therapeutic efficacy comment based on dose, usual susceptibility or target organism & penetration into CSF; **AUC** = area under drug concentration curve; **24hr** = AUC 0-24; **Tmax** = time to max plasma concentration.

TABLE 14A (5)

DRUG	REFERENCE DOSE/ROUTE	PREG RISK	FOOD EFFECT (PO)[1]	ORAL %AB	PEAK SERUM LEVEL (µg/mL)	PROTEIN BINDING (%)	VOL OF DISTRIB (Vd)	AVER SERUM $T_{1/2}$, hrs[2]	BILE PEN (%)[3]	CSF[4]/ BLOOD (%)	CSF PEN[5]	AUC (µg*hr/mL)	Tmax (hr)
ANTIPARASITICS													
Albendazole	400 mg po	C	Tab + food		0.5–1.6	70							Sulfoxide: 2-5
Artemether/ Lumefantrine	4 tabs po: 80/480 mg	C	Tab + food		Art: 9 (SS), D-Art: 1, Lum: 5.6-9 (not SS)			Art: 1.6, D-Art: 1.6, Lum: 101					Art: 1.5-2.0 Lum: 6-8
Atovaquone	750 mg po bid	C	Susp + food	47	24 (SS)	99.9	0.6 L/kg Vss	67		<1	No	801 (750 mg x1)	
Dapsone	100 mg po q24h	C	Tab ± food	70-100	1.1 (SS)	70	1.5 L/kg	10–50					2-6
Ivermectin	12 mg po	C	Tab no food		0.05–0.08 (SD)		9.9 L/kg						4
Mefloquine	1.25 gm po	C	Tab + food		0.5–1.2 (SD)	98	20 L/kg	13–24 days					17
Miltefosine	50 mg po tid	X	Cap + food		31 (SD)	95		7-31 (long) *AAC 52:2855, 2008*					
Nitazoxanide	500 mg po tab	B	Tab/susp + food		9–10 (SD)	99						41.9 Tizoxanide	Tizoxanide: 1-4
Proguanil[8]	100 mg	C	Tab + food		No data	75	1600-2000 L V/F						
Pyrimethamine	25 mg po	C	Tab ± food	"High"	0.1–0.3 (SD)	87	3 L/kg	96					2-6
Praziquantel	20 mg per kg po	B	Tab + food	80	0.2–2.0 (SD)		8000 L V/F	0.8-1.5				1.51	1-3
Tinidazole	2 gm po	B	Tab + food	48	48 (SD)	12	50 L	13				902	1.6
ANTIVIRAL DRUGS—NOT HIV													
Acyclovir	400 mg po bid	B	Tab/cap/susp ± food	10–20	1.21 (SS)	9–33	0.7 L/kg	2.5–3.5				7.4 (24 hr)	
Adefovir	10 mg po	C	Tab ± food	59	0.02 (SD)	≤4	0.37 L/kg Vss	7.5				0.22	1.75
Cidofovir w/Probenecid	5 mg/kg IV	C			19.6 (SD)	<6	0.41 L/kg (VSS)	2.2	ND	0	No	40.8	1.1
Entecavir	0.5 mg po q24h	C	Tab/soln no food	100	4.2 ng/mL (SS)	13	>0.6 L/kg V/F	128–149				0.14	0.5-1.5
Famciclovir	500 mg po	B	Tab ± food	77	3–4 (SD)	<20	1.1 L/kg*	2-3				8.9 Penciclovir	Penciclovir: 0.9
Foscarnet	60 mg/kg IV	C			155 (SD)	4	0.46 L/kg	<1				2195 µM*hr	No

Preg Risk: FDA risk categories: A = no risk in adequate human studies, **B** = animal studies suggest no fetal risk, but no adequate human studies, **C** = adverse fetal effects in animals, but no adequate studies in humans; potential benefit may warrant use despite potential risk, **D** = evidence of human risk, but potential benefit may warrant use despite potential risk **X** = evidence of human risk that clearly exceeds potential benefits; **Food Effect (PO dosing): + food** = take with food, **no food** = take without food, **± food** = take with or without food; **Oral % AB** = % absorbed; **Peak Serum Level: SD** = after single dose, **SS** = steady state after multiple doses; **Volume of Distribution (Vd): V/F** = Vd/oral bioavailability, **Vss** = Vd at steady state, **Vss/F** = Vd at steady state/oral bioavailability; **CSF Penetration:** therapeutic efficacy

DRUG	REFERENCE DOSE/ROUTE	PREG RISK	FOOD EFFECT (PO)[1]	ORAL %AB	PEAK SERUM LEVEL (µg/mL)	PROTEIN BINDING (%)	VOL OF DISTRIB (Vd)	AVER SERUM $T\frac{1}{2}$, hrs[2]	BILE PEN (%)[3]	CSF[4]/BLOOD (%)	CSF PEN[5]	AUC (µg*hr/mL)	Tmax (hr)
ANTIVIRAL DRUGS—NOT HIV *(continued)*													
Ganciclovir	5 mg/kg IV	C			8.3 (SD)	1–2	0.7 L/kg Vss	3.5				24.5	
Oseltamivir	75 mg po bid	C	Cap/susp ± food	75	0.065/0.35[9] (SS)	3	23-26 L/kg Vss*	1–3				5.4 (24 hr) Carboxylate	
Peramivir	600 mg IV	?			35-45 (SD)	<30	ND	7.7-20.8	ND	ND	ND	90-95	ND
Ribavirin	600 mg po	X	Tab/cap/soln + food	64	0.8 (SD)		2825 L V/F	44				25.4	2
Rimantadine	100 mg po	C	Tab ± food		0.05-0.1 (SD)		17-19 L/kg	25				3.5	6
Telbivudine	600 mg po q24h	B	Tab/soln ± food		3.7 (SS)	3.3	>0.6 L/kg V/F	40-49				26.1 (24 hr)	2
Valacyclovir	1000 mg po	B	Tab ± food	55	5.6 (SD)	13–18	C.7 L/kg	3				19.5 Acyclovir	
Valganciclovir	900 mg po q24h	C	Tab/soln + food	59	5.6 (SS)	1–2	C.7 L/kg	4				29.1 Ganciclovir	Ganciclovir: 1-3
ANTIRETROVIRAL DRUGS													
Abacavir (ABC)	600 mg po q24h	C	Tab/soln ± food	83	4.3 (SS)	50	0.86 L/kg	1.5	12–26	Low	No	12 (24 hr)	
Atazanavir (ATV)	400 mg po q24h	B	Cap + food	Good	2.3 (SS)	86	88.3 L V/F	7		Intermed	?	22.3 (24 hr)	2.5
Darunavir (DRV)	(600 mg+ 100 mg RTV) bid	B	Tab + food	82	3.5 (SS)	95	2 L/kg	15		Intermed	?	116.8 (24 hr)	2.5-4.0
Delavirdine (DLV)	400 mg po tid	C	Tab ± food	85	19 ± 11(SS)	98		5.8	3			180 µM*hr	1
Didanosine (ddI)	400 mg EC[10] po	B	Cap no food	30–40	?	<5	308-363 L	1.4	25–40	Intermed	?	2.6	2
Dolutegravir	50 mg po	B	± food		3.67 (SS)	>99	17.4 (V/F)	14				53.6	2-3
Efavirenz (EFV)	600 mg po q24h	D	Cap/tab no food	42	4.1 (SS)	99	252 L V/F	52–76	3			184 µM*hr (24 hr)	3-5
Elvitegravir (with cobicistat, TDF and FTC, as Stribild)	150 mg (EVG) 150 mg (Cobi) 200 mg (FTC) 300 mg (TDF)	B	Tab + Food	No data	EVG: 1.7 Cobi: 1.1	98-99 (EVG, cobi)		EVG: 12.9 Cobi: 3.5				EVG: 23 Cobi: 8.3	EVG: 4 Cobi: 3
Emtricitabine (FTC)	200 mg po q24h	B	Cap/soln ± food	93	1.8 (SS)	<4		10	39	Intermed	?	10 (24 hr)	1-2
Enfuvirtide (ENF)	90 mg sc bid	B		84	5 (SS)	92	5.5 L	4				97.4 (24 hr)	

Preg Risk: FDA risk categories: A = no risk in adequate human studies, **B** = animal studies suggest no fetal risk, but nc adequate human studies, **C** = adverse fetal effects in animals, but no adequate studies in humans; potential benefit may warrant use despite potential risk, **D** = evidence of human risk, but potential benefit may warrant use despite potential risk **X** = evidence of human risk that clearly exceeds potential benefits; **Food Effect** (PO dosing): **+ food** = take with food, **no food** = take without food, **± food** = take with or without food; **Oral % AB** = % absorbed; **Peak Serum Level: SD** = after single dose, **SS** = steady state after multiple doses; **Volume of Distribution (Vd): V/F** = Vd/oral bioavailability, **Vss** = Vd at steady state, **Vss/F** = Vd at steady state/oral bioavailability; **CSF Penetration:** therapeutic efficacy comment based on dose, usual susceptibility or target organism & penetration into CSF; **AUC** = area under drug concentration curve; **24hr** = AUC 0-24; **Tmax** = time to max plasma concentration.

TABLE 14A (7)

DRUG	REFERENCE DOSE/ROUTE	PREG RISK	FOOD EFFECT (PO)[1]	ORAL %AB	PEAK SERUM LEVEL (µg/mL)	PROTEIN BINDING (%)	VOL OF DISTRIB (Vd)	AVER SERUM $T_{1/2}$, hrs[2]	BILE PEN (%)[3]	CSF[4]/ BLOOD (%)	CSF PEN[5]	AUC (µg*hr/mL)	Tmax (hr)
ANTI RETROVIRAL DRUGS (continued)													
Etravirine (ETR)	200 mg po bid	B	Tab + food		0.3 (SS)	99.9		41	2			9 (24 hr)	2.5-4.0
Fosamprenavir (FPV)	(700 mg po+ 100 mg RTV) bid	C	Boosted ped susp + food Adult susp no food Tab ± food	No data	6 (SS)	90		7.7	No data	Intermed	?	79.2 (24 hr)	2.5
Indinavir (IDV)	800 mg po tid	C	Boosted cap + food, Cap alone no food	65	9 (SS)	60		1.2–2		High	Yes	92.1 µM*hr (24 hr)	0.8
Lamivudine (3TC)	300 mg po	C	Tab/soln ± food	86	2.6 (SS)	<36	1.3 L/kg	5–7	18–22	Intermed	?	11	
Lopinavir/RTV (LPV/r)	400 mg po bid	C	Soln + food	No data	9.6 (SS)	98–99		5–6 (LPV)		Intermed	?	186 LPV	LPV: 4
Maraviroc (MVC)	300 mg po bid	B	Tab ± food	33	0.3–0.9 (SS)	76	194 L	14-18		Intermed	?	3 (24 hr)	0.5-4.0
Nelfinavir (NFV)	1250 mg po bid	B	Tab/powd + food	20–80	3–4 (SS)	98	2-7 L/kg V/F	3.5–5		Low	No	53 (24 hr)	
Nevirapine (NVP)	200 mg po	C	Tab/susp ± food	>90	2 (SD)	60	1.2 L/kg Vss	25–30	4	High	Yes	110 (24 hr)	
Raltegravir (RAL)	400 mg po bid	C	Tab ± food	No data	5.4 (SS)	83	287 L Vss/F	9		Intermed	?	28.6 µM*hr (24 hr)	3
Rilpivirine	25 mg po	B	Tab + food	No data	0.1-0.2 (SD)	99.7	152L	45-50	ND	-	-	2.4 (24 hr)	-
Ritonavir (RTV)	600 mg po bid	B	Cap/soln + food	65	11.2 (SS)	98–99	0.41 L/kg V/F	3–5		Low	No		Soln: 2-4
Saquinavir (SQV)	(1000 +100 RTV) mg po bid	B	Tab/cap + food	4	0.37 min (SS conc)	97	700 L Vss	1–2		Low	No	29.2 (24 hr)	
Stavudine (d4T)	40 mg bid	C	Cap/soln ± food	86	0.54 (SS)	<5	46L	1	3-5	Low	No	2.6 (24 hr)	1
Tenofovir disoproxil fumarate (TDF)	300 mg po	B	Tab ± food	25 fasted 39 w/food	0.3 (SD)	<1–7	1.3 L/kg Vss	17	>60	Low	No	2.3	1

Preg Risk: FDA risk categories: **A** = no risk in adequate human studies, **B** = animal studies suggest no fetal risk, but no adequate human studies, **C** = adverse fetal effects in animals, but no adequate studies in humans; potential benefit may warrant use despite potential risk, **D** = evidence of human risk, but potential benefit may warrant use despite potential risk **X** = evidence of human risk that clearly exceeds potential benefits; **Food Effect** (PO dosing): **+ food** = take with food, **no food** = take without food, **± food** = take with or without food; **Oral % AB** = % absorbed; **Peak Serum Level: SD** = after single dose, **SS** = steady state after multiple doses; **Volume of Distribution (Vd): V/F** = Vd/oral bioavailability, **Vss** = Vd at steady state, **Vss/F** = Vd at steady state/oral bioavailability; **CSF Penetration:** therapeutic efficacy

DRUG	REFERENCE DOSE/ROUTE	PREG RISK	FOOD EFFECT (PO)[1]	ORAL %AB	PEAK SERUM LEVEL (µg/mL)	PROTEIN BINDING (%)	VOL OF DISTRIB (Vd)	AVER SERUM $T\frac{1}{2}$, hrs[2]	BILE PEN (%)[3]	CSF[4]/ BLOOD (%)	CSF PEN[5]	AUC (µg*hr/mL)	Tmax (hr)
ANTI RETROVIRAL DRUGS *(continued)*													
Tipranavir (TPV)	(500 + 200 RTV) mg po bid	C	Cap/soln + food		47–57 (SS)	99.9	7.7-10 L	5.5–6		Low	No	1600 µM*hr (24 hr)	3
Zidovudine (ZDV)	300 mg po	C	Tab/cap/syrup ± food	60	1–2	<38	1.6 L/kg	0.5–3	11	High	Yes	2.1	0.5-1.5

FOOTNOTES

1. Refers to adult oral preparations unless otherwise noted.
2. Assumes CrCl >80 mL per min.
3. Peak concentration in bile/peak concentration in serum x 100. If blank, no data.
4. CSF levels with inflammation.
5. Judgment based on drug dose & organism susceptibility. CSF concentration ideally ≥10 above MIC.
6. Concern over seizure potential
7. Take all po FQs 2–4 hours before sucralfate or any multivalent cations: Ca++, Fe++, Zn++.
8. Given with atovaquone as Malarone for malaria prophylaxis.
9. Oseltamivir/oseltamivir carboxylate.
10. EC = enteric coated.

Preg Risk: FDA risk categories: A = no risk in adequate human studies, **B** = animal studies suggest no fetal risk, but no adequate human studies, **C** = adverse fetal effects in animals, but no adequate studies in humans; potential benefit may warrant use despite potential risk, **D** = evidence of human risk, but potential benefit may warrant use despite potential risk **X** = evidence of human risk that clearly exceeds potential benefits; **Food Effect (PO dosing): + food** = take with food, **no food** = take without food, **± food** = take with or without food; **Oral % AB** = % absorbed; **Peak Serum Level: SD** = after single dose, **SS** = steady state after multiple doses; **Volume of Distribution (Vd): V/F** = Vd/oral bioavailability, **Vss** = Vd at steady state, **Vss/F** = Vd at steady state/oral bioavailability; **CSF Penetration:** therapeutic efficacy comment based on dose, usual susceptibility or target organism & penetration into CSF; **AUC** = area under drug concentration curve; **24hr** = AUC 0-24; **Tmax** = time to max plasma concentration.

TABLE 14B: CYTOCHROME P450 INTERACTIONS OF ANTIMICROBIALS

Cytochrome P450 isoenzyme terminology:
e.g., 3A4: **3** = family, **A** = subfamily, **4** = gene; **PGP** = P-glycoprotein; **UGT** = uridine diphosphate glucuronosyltransferase; **OATP** = organic anion transporter polypeptide;
OCT = organic cation transporter; **BCRP** = breast cancer resistance protein

DRUG	Substrate	Inhibits	Induces	DRUG	Substrate	Inhibits	Induces
Antibacterials				**Antiretrovirals**			
Azithromycin (all)	PGP	PGP (weak)		Atazanavir	3A4	1A2, 2C9, 3A4	
Clarithromycin (all)	3A4	3A4, PGP		Cobicistat	3A4, 2D6	3A4, 2D6, PGP, BCRP, OATP1B1, OATP1B3	
Metronidazole		2C9					
Rifampin	PGP		1A2, 2C9, 2C19, 2D6 (Weak), 3A4, PGP	Darunavir	3A4	3A4	
				Delavirdine	2D6, 3A4	2C9, 2C19, 3A4	
TMP-SMX	SMX: 2C9 (major), 3A4	SMX: 2C9 TMP: 2C8		Efavirenz	2B6, 3A4	2B6, 2C9, 2C19	2C19, 3A4
				Elvitegravir	CYP3A, UGT		2C9
Trimethoprim		2C8		Etravirine	2C9, 2C19, 3A4	2C9, 2C19 (weak)	3A4
Antifungals				Fosamprenavir	3A4	2C19, 3A4	Fosamprenavir
Fluconazole (400 mg)	3A4 (minor), PGP	2C9, 2C19, 3A4, UGT		Indinavir	3A4, PGP	3A4, PGP	
Itraconazole	3A4, PGP	3A4, PGP		Lopinavir	3A4	3A4	
Ketoconazole	3A4	3A4, PGP		Maraviroc	3A4, PGP	2D6	
Posaconazole	PGP, UGT	3A4, PGP		Nelfinavir	2C9, 2C19, 3A4, PGP	3A4, PGP	3A4
Terbinafine	2D6			Nevirapine	2B6, 3A4		3A4
Voriconazole	2C9, 2C19, 3A4	2C9, 2C19 (major), 3A4		Raltegravir	UGT		
Antimycobacterials (Also Rifampin, above)				Ritonavir	2D6, 3A4, PGP	2B6, 2C9, 2C19, 2D6, 3A4, PGP	3A4, 1A2 (?), 2C9 (?), PGP (?)
Bedaquiline	3A4						
Ethionamide	3A4 (?)			Saquinavir	3A4, PGP	3A4, PGP	
Isoniazid	2E1	2C19, 3A4		Tipranavir	3A4, PGP	1A2, 2C9, 2C19, 2D6	3A4, PGP (weak)
Rifabutin	3A4						
Rifapentine		2C9, 3A4	3A4, UGT				

Refs: Hansten PD, Horn JR. The top 100 drug interactions: a guide to patient management 2012; E. Freeland (WA): H&H Publications; 2010; and package inserts.

TABLE 15A: DOSAGE OF ANTIMICROBIAL DRUGS IN ADULT PATIENTS WITH RENAL IMPAIRMENT

- For listing of drugs with NO need for adjustment for renal failure, *see Table 15B.*
- Adjustments for renal failure are based on an estimate of creatinine clearance (CrCl) which reflects the glomerular filtration rate.
- **Different methods for calculating estimated CrCl are suggested for non-obese and obese patients.**
  - Calculations for ideal body weight (IBW) in kg:
    - *Men:* 50 kg plus 2.3 kg/inch over 60 inches height.
    - *Women:* 45 kg plus 2.3 kg/inch over 60 inches height.
  - Obese is defined as 20% over ideal body weight or body mass index (BMI) >30

- Calculations of estimated CrCl *(References, see (NEJM 354:2473, 2006 (non-obese), AJM 84:1053, 1988 (obese))*
  - **Non-obese patient—**
    - Calculate ideal body weight (IBW) in kg (as above)
    - Use the following formula to determine estimated CrCl

$$\frac{(140 \text{ minus age})(\text{IBW in kg})}{72 \times \text{serum creatine}} = \begin{array}{l}\text{CrCl in mL/min for men.} \\ \text{Multiply answer by 0.85} \\ \text{for women (estimated)}\end{array}$$

  - **Obese patient—**
    - Weight ≥20% over IBW or BMI >30
    - Use the following formulas to determine estimated CrCl

$$\frac{(137 \text{ minus age}) \times [(0.285 \times \text{wt in kg}) + (12.1 \times \text{ht in meters}^2)]}{51 \times \text{serum creatine}} = \text{CrCl (obese male)}$$

$$\frac{(146 \text{ minus age}) \times [(0.287 \times \text{wt in kg}) + (9.74 \times \text{ht in meters}^2)]}{60 \times \text{serum creatine}} = \text{CrCl (obese female)}$$

- If estimated CrCl ≥90 mL/min, *see Tables 10A and 10D for dosing.*
- What weight should be used to calculate dosage on a mg/kg basis?
  - If less than 20% over IBW, use the patient's actual weight for all drugs.
  - **For obese patients** (≥20% over IBW or BMI >30).
    - **Aminoglycosides:** (IBW plus 0.4(actual weight minus IBW) = adjusted weight.
    - **Vancomycin:** actual body weight whether non-obese or obese.
    - **All other drugs:** insufficient data *(Pharmacotherapy 27:1081, 2007).*
- For slow or sustained extended daily dialysis **(SLEDD)** over 6-12 hours, adjust does as for CRRT. For details, *see CID 49:433, 2009; CCM 39:560, 2011.*
- General reference: Drug Prescribing in Renal Failure, 5th ed., Aronoff, et al. (eds.) *(Amer College Physicians, 2007 and drug package inserts).*

Abbreviations: **HEMO** = hemodialysis; **CAPD** = chronic ambulatory peritoneal dialysis; **ESRD** = endstage renal disease; **NUS** = not available in the U.S.

TABLE 15A (2)

ANTIMICROBIAL	HALF-LIFE (NORMAL/ ESRD) hr	DOSE FOR NORMAL RENAL FUNCTION	METHOD *(see footer)*	ADJUSTMENT FOR RENAL FAILURE Estimated creatinine clearance (CrCl), mL/min			HEMODIALYSIS, CAPD	COMMENTS & DOSAGE FOR CRRT
				>50–90	10–50	<10		
ANTIBACTERIAL ANTIBIOTICS								
Aminoglycoside Antibiotics: Traditional multiple daily doses—adjustment for renal disease								
Amikacin	1.4–2.3/17–150	7.5 mg per kg q12h or 15 mg per kg once daily (see below)	I	7.5 mg/kg q24h or 15 mg/kg once daily	30-50: 7.5 mg/kg q24h **Same dose for CRRT** 10-30: 7.5 mg/kg q48h	7.5 mg/kg q72h	HEMO: 7.5 mg/kg AD CAPD: 15–20 mg lost per L dialysate per day *(see Comment)*	**High flux hemodialysis** membranes lead to unpredictable amino-glycoside clearance, measure post-dialysis drug levels for efficacy and toxicity. With **CAPD,** pharma-cokinetics highly variable—**check serum levels.** Usual method for CAPD: 2 liters of dialysis fluid placed qid or 8 liters per day (give 8Lx20 mg lost per L = 160 mg of amikacin supplement IV per day) Adjust dosing weight for obesity: [ideal body weight + 0.4 (actual body weight – ideal body weight)] *(CID 25:112, 1997).* **Gent SLEDD dose** in critically ill: 6 mg/kg IV q48h starting 30 min before start of SLEDD (daily SLEDD; q48h Gent) *(AAC54:3635, 2010).*
Streptomycin	2–3/30–80	15 mg per kg (max. of 1 gm) q24h. Once daily dosing below	I	15 mg/kg q24h	15 mg/kg q24-72h **Same dose for CRRT**	15 mg/kg q72-96h	HEMO: 7.5 mg/kg AD CAPD: 20–40 mg lost per L dialysate per day	

ONCE-DAILY AMINOGLYCOSIDE THERAPY: ADJUSTMENT IN RENAL INSUFFICIENCY

Creatinine Clearance (mL per min.) Drug	>80	60–80	40–60	30–40	20–30	10–20	<10–0
	Dose q24h (mg per kg)				*Dose q48h (mg per kg)*	*Dose q72h and AD*	
Amikacin	15	12	7.5	4	7.5	4	3

ANTIMICROBIAL	HALF-LIFE (NORMAL/ ESRD) hr	DOSE FOR NORMAL RENAL FUNCTION	METHOD	>50–90	10–50	<10	HEMODIALYSIS, CAPD	COMMENTS & DOSAGE FOR CRRT
Fluoroquinolone Antibiotics								
Levofloxacin	6–8/76	750 mg q24h IV, PO	D&I	750 mg q24h	**20-49:** 750 q48h	**<20:** 750 mg once, then 500 mg q48h	HEMO/CAPD: Dose for CrCl <20	CRRT 750 mg once, then 500 mg q48h, although not FDA-approved.
Macrolide Antibiotics								
Clarithromycin	5–7/22	500-1000 mg q12h	D	500 mg q12h	500 mg q12-24h	500 mg q24h	HEMO: Dose AD CAPD: None	CRRT as for CrCl 10-50

TABLE 15A (3)

ANTIMICROBIAL	HALF-LIFE (NORMAL/ ESRD) hr	DOSE FOR NORMAL RENAL FUNCTION	METHOD (see footer)	ADJUSTMENT FOR RENAL FAILURE Estimated creatinine clearance (CrCl), mL/min			HEMODIALYSIS, CAPD	COMMENTS & DOSAGE FOR CRRT
				>50–90	10–50	<10		
Miscellaneous Antibacterial Antibiotics								
Metronidazole	6–14/7–21	7.5 mg per kg q6h	D	100%	100% **Same dose for CRRT**	50%	HEMO: Dose as for CrCl <10 AD CAPD: Dose for CrCl <10	
Sulfamethoxazole (SMX)	10/20–50	1 gm q8h	I	q12h	q18h Same dose for CAVH	q24h	HEMO: Extra 1 gm AD CAPD: 1 gm q24h	
Trimethoprim (TMP)	11/20–49	100–200 mg q12h	I	q12h	**>30:** q12h **10-30:** q18h **Same dose for CRRT**	q24h	HEMO: Dose AD CAPD: q24h	CRRT dose: q18h
Trimethoprim-sulfamethoxazole-DS (Doses based on TMP component)								
Treatment (based on TMP component)	As for TMP	5–20 mg/kg/day divided q6-12h	D	No dose adjustment	**30-50:** No dose adjustment **10-29:** Reduce dose by 50%	Not recommended; but if used: 5–10 mg/kg q24h	Not recommended; but if used: 5–10 mg/kg q24h AD CRRT: 5-7.5 mg/kg q8h	
TMP-SMX Prophylaxis	As for TMP	1 tab po q24h or 3 times per week	No change	100%	100%	100%		
ANTIFUNGAL ANTIBIOTICS								
Amphotericin B & Lipid-based ampho B	24h-15 days//unchanged	Non-lipid: 0.4– 1 mg/kg/day ABLC: 5 mg/kg/day LAB: 3–5 mg/kg/day	I	q24h	q24h **Same dose for CRRT**	q24h	HEMO/CAPD/CRRT: No dose adjustment	For ampho B, toxicity lessened by saline loading; risk amplified by concomitant cyclosporine A, aminoglycosides, or pentamidine
Fluconazole	37/100	100–400 mg q24h	D	100%	50%	50%	HEMO: 100% of recommended dose AD CAPD: Dose for CrCl <10	CRRT: 200-400 mg q24h
Flucytosine	3–6/75–200	37.5 mg per kg q6h	I	q12h	q12–24h **Same dose for CRRT**	q24h	HEMO: Dose AD CAPD: 0.5–1 gm q24h	Goal is peak serum level >25 mcg per mL and <100 mcg per mL
Itraconazole, po soln	21/25	100–200 mg q12h	D	100%	100% **Same dose for CRRT**	50%	HEMO/CAPD: oral solution: 100 mg q12-24h	
Itraconazole, IV	21/25	200 mg IV q12h	–	200 mg IV bid	Do not use IV itra if CrCl <30 due to accumulation of carrier: cyclodextrin			
Terbinafine	36–200/?	250 mg po per day	–	q24h	Use has not been studied. Recommend avoidance of drug.			
Voriconazole, IV	Non-linear kinetics	6 mg per kg IV q12h times 2, then 4 mg per kg q12h	–	No change	If CrCl <50 mL per min., accum. of IV vehicle (cyclodextrin). Switch to po or DC **For CRRT:** 4 mg/kg po q12h			

Abbreviation Key: Adjustment Method **D** = dose adjustment, **I** = interval adjustment; **CAPD** = continuous ambulatory peritoneal dialysis; **CRRT** = continuous renal replacement therapy; **HEMO** = hemodialysis; **AD** = after dialysis; **"Supplement"** or **"Extra"** is to replace drug lost during dialysis – additional drug beyond continuation of regimen for CrCl <10 mL/min.

TABLE 15A (4)

ANTIMICROBIAL	HALF-LIFE (NORMAL/ ESRD) hr	DOSE FOR NORMAL RENAL FUNCTION	METHOD (see footer)	ADJUSTMENT FOR RENAL FAILURE Estimated creatinine clearance (CrCl), mL/min			HEMODIALYSIS, CAPD	COMMENTS & DOSAGE FOR CRRT
				>50–90	10–50	<10		
ANTIPARASITIC ANTIBIOTICS								
Pentamidine	3-12/73-18	4 mg per kg per day	I	q24h	q24h **Same dose for CRRT**	q24–36h	HEMO: 4 mg/kg q48h AD CAPD: Dose for CrCl<10	
ANTITUBERCULOUS ANTIBIOTICS *(See http://11ntcc.ucsd.edu/TB)*								
Amikacin/ Streptomycin								
Capreomycin		15 mg/kg q24h	I	15 mg/kg q24h	15 mg/kg q24h CRRT: 25 mg/kg q24h (max 2.5 gm q24h)	15 mg/kg AD 3x/wk	HEMO: 15 mg/kg AD 3x/wk	
Ethambutol	4/7-15	15–25 mg per kg q24h	I	15-25 mg/kg q24h	**CrCl 30-50:**15 mg/kg q24–36h **Same dose for CRRT** **For CrCl 10-20:** 15-25 mg/kg q24-48h	15-25 mg/kg q48h	HEMO: 20 mg/kg 3x/wk AD CAPD: 25 mg/kg q48h	If possible, do serum levels on dialysis pts.
Isoniazid	0.7–4/8-17	5 mg per kg per day (max. 300 mg)	D	100%	100% **Same dose for CRRT**	100%	HEMO: Dose AD CAPD/: Dose for CrCl <10	
Pyrazinamide	9/26	25 mg per kg q24h (max. dose 2.5 gm q24h)	D	25 mg/kg q24h	**CrCl 21-90:** 25 mg/kg q24h **Same dose for CRRT** **For CrCl 10-20:** 25 mg/kg q48h	12-25 mg per kg 3x/wk	HEMO: 25 mg/kg 3x/wk AD CAPD: No reduction	
Rifampin	1.5–5/1.8-11	600 mg per day	D	600 mg q24h	300–600 mg q24h **Same dose for CRRT**	300–600 mg q24h	HEMO: No adjustment CAPD/: Dose for CrCl <10	Biologically active metabolite
ANTIVIRAL AGENTS FOR ANTIRETROVIRALS *(See CID 40:1559, 2005)*								
Acyclovir, IV	2-4/20	5–12.4 mg per kg q8h	D&I	100% q8h	100% q12–24h	50% q24h	HEMO: Dose AD CAPD: Dose for CrCl <10	Rapid IV infusion can cause ↑ Cr. CRRT dose: 5-10 mg/kg q24h
Adefovir	7.5/15	10 mg po q24h	I	10 mg q24h	10 mg q48–72h[1]	10 mg q72h[1]	HEMO: 10 mg q week AD	CAPD: No data; CRRT: Dose?
Amantadine	12/500	100 mg po bid	I	q12h	q24-48h	q 7 days	HEMO/CAPD: Dose for CrCl<10	CRRT: Dose for CrCl 10-50
Atripla	See each drug	200 mg emtricitabine + 300 mg tenofovir + 600 mg efavirenz	I	Do not use if CrCl <50				

ANTIMICROBIAL	HALF-LIFE (NORMAL/ ESRD) hr	DOSE FOR NORMAL RENAL FUNCTION	METHOD (see footer)	ADJUSTMENT FOR RENAL FAILURE Estimated creatinine clearance (CrCl), mL/min			HEMODIALYSIS, CAPD	COMMENTS & DOSAGE FOR CRRT
				>50–90	10–50	<10		
ANTIVIRAL AGENTS FOR ANTIRETROVIRALS (continued)								
Cidofovir: Complicated dosing—see package insert								
Induction	2.5/unknown	5 mg per kg once per wk for 2 wks	–	5 mg per kg once per wk	Contraindicated in pts with CrCl ≤55 mL/min.			Major toxicity is renal. No efficacy, safety, or pharmacokinetic data in pts with moderate/severe renal disease.
Maintenance	2.5/unknown	5 mg per kg q2wks	–	5 mg per kg q2wks	Contraindicated in pts with CrCl ≤55 mL/min.			
Didanosine tablets[2]	0.6–1.6/4.5	125–200 mg q12h buffered tabs	D	200 mg q12h	200 mg q24h	<60 kg: 150 mg q24h >60 kg: 100 mg q24h	HEMO: Dose AD CAPD/CRRT: Dose for CrCl <10	Based on incomplete data. Data are estimates.
		400 mg q24h enteric-coated tabs	D	400 mg q24h	125–200 mg q24h	**Do not use EC tabs**	HEMO/CAPD: Dose for CrCl <10	**If <60 kg & CrCl <10 mL per min, do not use EC tabs**
Emtricitabine (CAPS)	10/>10	200 mg q24h	I	200 mg q24h	**30–49:** 200 mg q48h **10–29:** 200 mg q72h	200 mg q96h	HEMO: Dose for CrCl <10	See package insert for oral solution.
Emtricitabine + Tenofovir	See each drug	200-300 mg q24h	I	No change	**30–50:** 1 tab q48h	**CrCl <30:** Do not use		
Entecavir	128–149/?	0.5 mg q24h	D	0.5 mg q24h	0.15–0.25 mg q24h	0.05 mg q24h	HEMO/CAPD: 0.05 mg q24h	Give after dialysis on dialysis days
Famciclovir	2.3–3/10–22	500 mg q8h	D&I	500 mg q8h	500 mg q12–24h	250 mg q24h	HEMO: Dose AD CAPD: No data	CRRT: Not applicable

Foscarnet (CMV dosage). Dosage adjustment based on est. CrCl divided by wt (kg). Normal half-life ($T\frac{1}{2}$) 3 hrs with terminal $T\frac{1}{2}$ of 18-88 hrs. $T\frac{1}{2}$ very long with ESRD.

		CrCl (mL/min per kg body weight—only for Foscarnet							
		>1.4	>1-1.4	>0.8-1	>0.6-0.8	>0.5-0.6	>0.4-0.5	<0.4	See package insert for further details
Induction: 60 mg/kg IV q8h x 2-3 wks		60 q8h	45 q8h	50 q12h	40 q12h	60 q24h	50 q24h	Do not use	
Maintenance: 90-120 mg/kg/day IV		120 q24h	90 q24h	65 q24h	105 q48h	80 q48h	65 q48h	Do not use	

ANTIMICROBIAL	HALF-LIFE	DOSE FOR NORMAL RENAL FUNCTION	METHOD	>50–90	10–50	<10	HEMODIALYSIS, CAPD	COMMENTS & DOSAGE FOR CRRT
Ganciclovir	3.6/30	IV: Induction 5 mg per kg q12h IV	D&I	**70-90:** 5 mg per kg q12h **50-60:** 2.5 mg/kg q12h	**25-49:** 2.5 mg per kg q24h **10-24:** 1.25 mg/kg q24h	1.25 mg per kg 3 times per wk	HEMO: Dose AD CAPD: Dose for CrCl <10	
		Maintenance 5 mg per kg q24h IV	D&I	2.5–5.0 mg per kg q24h	0.6-1.25 mg per kg q24h	0.625 mg per kg 3 times per wk	HEMO: 0.6 mg per kg AD CAPD: Dose for CrCl <10	
		po: 1 gm tid po	D&I	0.5–1 gm tid	0.5–1 gm q24h	0.5 gm 3 times per week	HEMO: 0.5 gm AD	

[2] Ref: for NRTIs and NNRTIs: *Kidney International 60:821, 2001*

<u>Abbreviation Key</u>: Adjustment Method: **D** = dose adjustment, **I** = interval adjustment; **CAPD** = continuous ambulatory peritoneal dialysis; **CRRT** = continuous renal replacement therapy; **HEMO** = hemodialysis; **AD** = after dialysis; **"Supplement"** or **"Extra"** is to replace drug lost during dialysis – additional drug beyond continuation of regimen for CrCl <10 mL/min.

TABLE 15A (6)

ANTIMICROBIAL	HALF-LIFE (NORMAL/ ESRD) hr	DOSE FOR NORMAL RENAL FUNCTION	METHOD (see footer)	ADJUSTMENT FOR RENAL FAILURE Estimated creatinine clearance (CrCl), mL/min			HEMODIALYSIS, CAPD	COMMENTS & DOSAGE FOR CRRT
				>50–90	10–50	<10		
ANTIVIRAL AGENTS FOR ANTIRETROVIRALS (continued)								
Maraviroc	14–18/No data	300 mg bid		300 mg bid				Risk of side effects increased if concomitant CYP3A inhibitor
Lamivudine	5–7/15–35	300 mg po q24h	D&I	300 mg po q24h	50–150 mg q24h	25–50 mg q24h	HEMO: Dose AD; CAPD: Dose for CrCl<10. CRRT: 100 mg 1st day, then 50 mg/day.	
Oseltamivir, therapy	6-10/>20	75 mg po bid – treatment	I	75 mg q12h	**30-60:** 30 mg bid **<30:** 30 mg once daily	No data	HEMO: 30 mg after each HEMO[3]; CAPD: 30 mg after each exchange	Dose for prophylaxis if CrCl <30: 30 mg once daily CRRT: ND
Peramivir		600 mg once daily	P&I	600 mg q24h	**31-49:** 150 mg q24h **10-30:** 100 mg q24h	100 mg (single dose) then 15 mg q24h	HEMO: 100 mg (single dose) then 100 mg 2 hrs AD (dialysis days only)	CRRT: http://www.cdc.gov/h1n1flu/ eva/peramivir.htm
Ribavirin	Use with caution in patients with creatinine clearance <50 mL per min.							
Rimantadine	13–65/Prolonged	100 mg bid po	I	100 mg bid	100 mg q24h–bid	100 mg q24h	HEMO/CAPD: No data	Use with caution, little data
Stavudine, po	1-1.4/5.5-8	30–40 mg q12h	D&I	100%	50% q12–24h	≥60 kg: 20 mg per day <60 kg: 15 mg per day	HEMO: Dose as for CrCl <10 AD CAPD: No data CRRT: Full dose	
Stribild		1 tab daily		If CrCl <70: contraindicated	If CrCl <50: discontinue			
Telbivudine	40-49/No data	600 mg po daily	I	600 mg q24h	**30-49:** 600 mg q48H **<30:** 600 mg q72h	600 mg q96h	HEMO: As for CrCl <10 AD	
Tenofovir, po	17/?	300 mg q24h		300 mg q24h	**30-49:** 300 mg q48h **10-29:** 300 mg q72-96h	No data	HEMO: 300 mg q7d or after 12 hrs of HEMO.[4]	
Valacyclovir	2.5–3.3/14	1 gm q8h	D&I	1 gm q8h	1 gm q12–24h **Same dose for CRRT**	0.5 gm q24h	HEMO: Dose AD CAPD: Dose for CrCl <10	CAVH dose: As for CrCl 10–50
Valganciclovir	4/67	900 mg po bid	D&I	900 mg po bid	450 mg q24h to 450 mg every other day	DO NOT USE	*See package insert*	
Zidovudine	1.1–1.4/1.4–3	300 mg q12h	D&I	300 mg q12h	300 mg q12h **Same dose for CRRT**	100 mg q8h	HEMO: Dose for CrCl <10 AD CAPD: Dose for CrCl <10	

[3] HEMO wt-based dose adjustments for children age >1 yr (dose after each HEMO): ≤15 kg: 7.5 mg; 16-23 kg: 10 mg; 24-40 kg: 15 mg; >40 kg: 30 mg (CID 50:127, 2010).

[4] Acute renal failure and Fanconi syndrome reported.

Abbreviation Key: Adjustment Method: **D** = dose adjustment, **I** = interval adjustment; **CAPD** = continuous ambulatory peritoneal dialysis; **CRRT** = continuous renal replacement therapy; **HEMO** = hemodialysis; **AD** = after dialysis; **"Supplement"** or **"Extra"** is to replace drug lost during dialysis — additional drug beyond continuation of regimen for CrCl <10 mL/min.

TABLE 15B: NO DOSAGE ADJUSTMENT WITH RENAL INSUFFICIENCY

Antibacterials	Antifungals	Anti-TBc	Antivirals	
Azithromycin	Anidulafungin	Ethionamide	Abacavir	Lopinavir
Moxifloxacin	Caspofungin	Isoniazid	Atazanavir	Nelfinavir
Pyrimethamine	Itraconazole oral solution	Rifampin	Darunavir	Nevirapine
	Ketoconazole	Rifabutin	Delavirdine	Raltegravir
	Micafungin	Rifapentine	Efavirenz	Ribavirin
	Voriconazole, **po only**		Enfuvirtide[1]	Saquinavir
			Fosamprenavir	Tipranavir
			Indinavir	

[1] Enfuvirtide: Not studied in patients with CrCl <35 mL/min. DO NOT USE

TABLE 15C: DOSAGE OF ANTIRETROVIRAL DRUGS IN PATIENTS WITH IMPAIRED HEPATIC FUNCTION

See CID 40:174, 2005. Dose reduction may be indicated in the presence of liver disease.

DRUG GENERIC (TRADE)	STANDARD DOSE	DOSING IF HEPATIC IMPAIRMENT CHILD-PUGH SCORE*	ADJUSTED DOSE	COMMENTS
Protease inhibitors				
Atazanavir (Reyataz)	300–400 mg po q24h	7-9 >9	300 mg q24h Do not use	No ritonavir boosting if hepatic impairment
Darunavir	600 mg po bid with ritonavir	Use with caution. No specific dose suggested		
Fosamprenavir (Lexiva)	1400 mg po q12h	5-9 10-15	700 mg q12h 350 mg bid	
Indinavir (Crixivan)	800 mg po q8h	Mild to moderate hepatic insufficiency	600 mg q8h	
Lopinavir/ritonavir (Kaletra)	400 mg/ 100 mg po q12h	No dosage recommendations; use with caution if hepatic impairment		
Nelfinavir (Viracept)	1250 mg po q12h	No dosage recommendations; use with caution if hepatic impairment		
Ritonavir (Norvir)	600 mg po q12h	No dosage recommendations; use with caution if hepatic impairment		
Saquinavir (Invirase)	1000 mg po + 100 mg ritonavir bid	No dosage recommendations; use with caution if hepatic impairment		
Stribild	once daily	3 (Child-Pugh column)	Do not use	
Tipranavir	500 mg + 200 mg ritonavir po bid	5-9 >9	No dosage adjustment Do not use	
Fusion & Entry Inhibitors				
Enfuvirtide (Fuzeon)	90 mg subQ q12h	No dosage adjustment recommendations		
Maraviroc (Selzentry)	300 mg po bid; *See page 35.*	No dosage recommendations; use caution if hepatic impairment		
Other Antiretrovirals				
Abacavir	600 mg po q24h	5-6 >6	200 mg bid Avoid	Use oral solution
Delavirdine	400 mg po tid	Metabolized in liver	No dosage adjustment data	
Efavirenz/Rilpivirine	600 mg po q24h	Metabolized in liver	No dosage adjustment data	
Etravirine	200 mg po bid	Up to 9 >9	No dose adjustment No data; **Caution**	
Nevirapine	200 mg po bid	Up to 6 >6	**Caution** **Contraindicated**	

*CALCULATION OF CHILD-PUGH SCORE—Classification below

CLINICAL FEATURE	SCORE GIVEN		
	1	2	3
Encephalopathy *(see below)***	None	Grade 1–2	Grade 3–4
Albumin	>3.5 gm/dl	2.8–3.5 gm/dl	<2.8 gm/dl
Total bilirubin	<2 mg/dl	2–3 mg/dl	>3 mg/dl
If taking indinavir or if Gilbert's syndrome	<4 mg/dl	4–7 mg/dl	>7 mg/dl
Prothrombin time or	<4	4–6	>6
INR	<1.7	1.7–2.3	>2.3

CLASSIFICATION

Score	Class
5–6	A
7–9	B
>9	C

****GRADE OF ENCEPHALOPATHY**

Grade	Clinical Criteria
1	Mild confusion, anxiety, restlessness, fine tremor, slow coordination
2	Drowsiness, asterixis
3	Somnolent but arousable, marked confusion, speech incomprehensible, incontinent, hyperventilation
4	Coma, decerebrate posturing, flaccidity

TABLE 16: DRUG-DRUG INTERACTIONS BETWEEN NON-NUCLEOSIDE REVERSE TRANSCRIPTASE INHIBITORS (NNRTIs), PROTEASE INHIBITORS, CCR-5 ANTAGONIST

(Adapted from *Guidelines for the Use of Antiretroviral Agents in HIV-Infected Adults & Adolescents; see www.aidsinfo.nih.gov*)
For multiple drug-drug interactions, *see The Sanford Guide to Antimicrobial Therapy 2019, Table 22A; https://www.hiv-druginteractions.org (University of Liverpool)*

NAME (Abbreviation, Trade Name)	Atazanavir (ATV, Reyataz)	Darunavir (DRV, Prezista)	Fosamprenavir (FOS-APV, Lexiva)	Indinavir (IDV, Crixivan)	Lopinavir/Ritonavir (LP/R, Kaletra)	Nelfinavir (NFV, Viracept)	Saquinavir (SQV, Invirase)	Tipranavir (TPV)
Delavirdine (DLV, Rescriptor)	No data	No data	**Co-administration not recommended**	IDV levels ↑ 40%. Dose: IDV 600 mg q8h, DLV standard	Expect LP levels to ↑. No dose data	NFV levels ↑ 2X; DLV levels ↓ 50%. Dose: No data	SQV levels ↑ 5X. Dose: SQV 800 mg q8h, DLV standard	No data
Efavirenz (EFV, Sustiva)	ATV AUC ↓ 74%. Dose: EFV standard; ATA/RTV 300/100 mg q24h with food	Standard doses of both drugs	FOS-APV levels ↓. Dose: EFV standard; FOS-APV 1400 mg + RTV 300 mg q24h or 700 mg FOS-APV + 100 mg RTV q12h	Levels: IDV ↓ 31%. Dose: IDV 1000 mg q8h. EFV standard	Level of LP ↓ 40%. Dose: LP/R 533/133 mg q12h, EFV standard	Standard doses	Level: SQV ↓ 62%. Dose: SQV 400 mg + RTV 400 mg q12h	No dose change necessary
Etravirine (ETR, Intelence)	↑ ATV & ↑ ETR levels.	Standard doses of both drugs	↑ levels of FOS-APV.	↓ level of IDV.	↑ levels of ETR, ↓ **levels of LP/R.**	↑ levels of NFV.	↓ ETR levels 33%; SQV/R no change. Standard dose of both drugs.	↓ levels of ETR, ↑ levels of TPV & RTV. **Avoid combination.**
Nevirapine (NVP, Viramune)	Avoid combination. ATZ increases NVP concentrations >25%; NVP decreases ATZ AUC by 42%	Standard doses of both drugs	Use with caution. NVP AUC increased 14% (700/100 Fos/rit; NVP AUC inc 29% (Fos 1400 mg bid).	IDV levels ↓ 28%. Dose: IDV 1000 mg q8h or combine with RTV; NVP standard	LP levels ↓ 53%. Dose: LP/R 533/133 mg q12h; NVP standard	Standard doses	Dose: SQV + RTV 400/400 mg, both q12h	**Standard doses**

TABLE 17: ANTIMICROBICS IN PREGNANCY

Partial list with emphasis on anti-retrovirals and drugs used for opportunistic infections.
For more complete list, *see Table 8, The Sanford Guide to Antimicrobial Therapy.*

Drug	FDA Pregnancy Categories*	Placental Transfer (%)	Breastfeeding	Adverse Effects: Fetus, Mother
Antibacterial Agents				
Fluoroquinolones	C	80–90	No	Potential arthropathy
Macrolides:				
Azithromycin	B	ND	ND	None
Clarithromycin	C	ND	OK	Fetal toxicity in primates
Metronidazole	B	+	No	None: do not use in 1st trimester
Antifungal Agents:				
Amphotericin B	B	+	OK	None
Echinocandins:				
Anidulafungin	C			
Caspofungin:	C			
Micafungin	C			
Fluconazole, itraconazole	C	ND	ND	NHS
Flucytosine	C			
Posaconazole	C	ND	ND	
Voriconazole	D			**Risk of birth defects**
Antiparasitic Agents:				
Pentamidine	C	+	No	NHS
Pyrimethamine	C	+	No	None: do not use in 1st trimester
Sulfonamides	C	70–90	No	Potential kernicterus & hem-G6PD
Trimethoprim	C	30–100	OK	None
Antimycobacterial Agents:				
Ethambutol	ND	30	OK	None
Isoniazid	C	100	OK	None
Pyrazinamide	C	ND	OK	None
Rifabutin	B	ND	ND	–
Rifampin	C	33	OK	Postnatal bleeding in infant
Streptomycin	D	10–40	OK	Ototoxicity (16% deafness)
Thalidomide	**X**	Presumably	ND	**Major risk birth defects**
Antiviral Agents (Non- HIV Drugs):				
Acyclovir, valacyclovir	B	70	OK ?	None. No data with vala—administer with caution to breast feeding mother
Adefovir	C	ND	No	Not recommended in pregnancy
Cidofovir	C	ND	No	Not recommended in pregnancy
Entecavir	C	ND	ND	
Famcyclovir	B	ND	ND	
Ganciclovir, valganciclovir	C	No	No	Carcinogenic in animals, NHS
Interferons	C	ND	ND	
Ribavirin	**X**	ND	No	**Major risk of birth defects**
Antiretroviral Drugs:				
Nucleoside and nucleotide analogue reverse transcriptase inhibitors (NRTIs):				
Abacavir	C	>80	No	Teratogen in rats at 35x human exposure
Didanosine	B	50	No	No evidence of teratogenicity
Emtricitabine	B	ND	No	No evidence of teratogenicity
Lamivudine	C	100	No	No evidence of teratogenicity
Stavudine	C	76	No	Tumors in rodents
Tenofovir	B	ND	No	
Zalcitabine	C	30-50	No	Tumors in rodents
Zidovudine	C	85	No	Tumors in rodents
Non-nucleoside reverse transcriptase inhibitors (NNRTIs):				
Delavirdine	C	ND	No	Teratogenic in rats; rodent tumors
Efavirenz	C	ND	No	
Etravirine	B	ND	No	
Nevirapine	C	100	No	Tumors in rodents
Rilpivirine	B	ND	No	No evidence of teratogenicity

TABLE 17 (2)

Drug	FDA Pregnancy Categories*	Placental Transfer (%)	Breastfeeding	Adverse Effects: Fetus, Mother
Protease Inhibitors (PIs):				
Fosamprenavir	C	ND	No	Tumors in rodents
Atazanavir	B	ND	No	Tumors in female mice
Darunavir	B	ND	No	Negative
Etravirine	B	ND	No	
Indinavir/	C	ND	No	Tumors in rodents
Lopinavir/ritonavir	C	ND	No	Tumors in rodents
Nelfinavir	B	ND	No	Tumors in rodents
Ritonavir	B	15-100	No	Tumors in rodents
Saquinavir	B	Minimal	No	No evidence of teratogenicity
Tipranavir	C	No		No evidence of teratogenicity
Fusion Inhibitors:				
Enfuvirtide	B	ND	No	No evidence of teratogenicity
Chemokine Receptor Antagonist:				
Maraviroc	B	ND	No	
Integrase Inhibitor:				
Dolutegravir	B	ND	No	
Elvitegravir	B	ND	No	
Raltegravir	C	ND	No	
Combinations:				
Stribild	B			

* **FDA Pregnancy Risk Categories:**

A = Adequate studies in pregnant women, no risk

B = Animal reproduction studies, no fetal risk; no controlled studies in pregnant women

C = Animal reproduction studies have shown fetal adverse effect; no controlled studies in humans; potential benefit may warrant use despite potential risk

D = Evidence of human fetal risk; potential benefit may warrant use despite potential risk

X = Animal and human studies demonstrate fetal abnormalities; risks in pregnant women clearly exceed potential benefits

TABLE 18: SPECTRUM & TREATMENT OF HIV/AIDS-ASSOCIATED MALIGNANCIES

I. **Spectrum of associated malignancies: AIDS-defining neoplasms: Incidence decreasing with ART**
   A. **Kaposi's sarcoma** & other KSHV/HHV8 related neoplasms:
      1. Primary body cavity lymphoma (primary effusion lymphoma)
      2. Multicentric Castleman disease

   B. **HIV-associated lymphoma**
      1. Primary CNS lymphoma (EBV)
      2. Non-Hodgkin's lymphoma (EBV)
      3. Body cavity lymphoma; primary effusion lymphoma (HHV8/EBV)
      4. Plasmablastic lymphoma of the oral cavity

   C. **Cervical, oropharyngeal & anogenital cancer due to human papillomavirus (HPV)**
   D. **Other neoplasms with increased incidence in AIDS patients** –not AIDS-defining neoplasms
      1. Basal cell carcinoma of the skin (EBV implicated in many patients)
      2. Hodgkin's disease
      3. Seminoma
      4. Pediatric leiomyosarcoma
      5. Breast & lung cancer at earlier age
      6. Neuroendocrine (Merkel cell) carcinoma (Polyoma virus implicated)

II. **Kaposi's sarcoma (KS)—Epidemiology, pathophysiology & treatment**
   A. **Etiology & pathogenesis**
      1. Human herpesvirus type 8 (HHV8); also called Kaposi's sarcoma-associated herpesvirus (KSHV)
      2. HHV8/KSHV
         a. Viral DNA found in all KS tumors
         b. Infection precedes KS
         c. Seropositivity rate predicts KS rate
         d. Virus latent in most cells; lytic in <5% of cells
         e. Targets spindle cells

   B. **Diagnosis**
      1. Clinical appearance & then biopsy
      2. HHV8/KSHV serology; can now quantitate HHV8 in plasma by PCR

   C. **HHV8 (KSHV) is etiology of 3 tumors:**
      1. Kaposi's sarcoma
      2. Primary effusion lymphoma
      3. Multicentric Castleman's disease
      4. Can manifest as KSHV-inflammatory syndrome (CID 62:730, 2016): distinct increase in IL-6 & IL-10; high mortality

   D. **Treatment**
      1. **Immune reconstitution** (improvement) with effective antiretroviral therapy of HIV infection leads to:
         a. Reports of clearance of HHV8 from circulating cells; 60–80% response rate
         b. Protease inhibitors have anti-tumor activity in mice & patients: *Nature Med 8:225, 2002*
         c. Reports of success with sirolimus in renal transplant pts with KS *(Transplant Proceed 44:2824, 2012)*.
         d. Ref: *Cochrane Database Rev 9:CD003256, 2014.*
      2. **Suggest oncology consultation for best local and systemic therapy.**

III. **Primary body cavity lymphoma; primary effusion lymphoma**
   A. Etiology: HHV8/KSHV; some cells also positive for EBV
   B. Diagnosis: Biopsy of tumor masses in pleural space, pericardial space, intra-abdominal cavity
   C. Treatment: rmCHOP (rituximab-methotrexate CHOP). Suggest oncology consult
   D. Concomitant ART prolongs survival *(CID 47:410, 418, 1209, 2008)*

IV. **Multicentric Castleman disease**
   A. Rare lymphoproliferative disorder
   B. Etiology: HHV8/KSHV
   C. Clinical: Fever, lymphadenopathy, splenomegaly
   D. Treatment: Very effective--Vinblastine or etoposide or rituximab

TABLE 18 (2)

V. **HIV-associated lymphoma**
    A. **General**
        1. Compared to immunocompetent pts, present in advanced stage
        2. ART can unmask lymphoma *(IRIS phenomenon) (CID 59:279, 2014)*
        3. HIV-associated non-Hodgkin's lymphomas virtually all of B-cell origin
        4. Viral association
            a. Systemic lymphomas—no viral association
            b. CNS lymphoma—EBV DNA present in 100% but predictive value low *(CID 38:1629, 2004)*
            c. Body-cavity lymphomas—HHV8 genome present in virtually all
        5. Prognosis improving coincident with effective antiretroviral therapy

    B. **Primary CNS lymphoma**: can involve brain, leptomeninges, eyes or spinal cord
        1. Usually in patients with very low CD4 counts
        2. Detection of EBV DNA by PCR in CSF in >90% pts but predictive value low *(CID 38:1629, 2004)*
        3. Treatment
            a. Consensus for use of high dose methotrexate *(Neurology 83:235, 2014)*
            b. No consensus on management beyond methotrexate: combination of chemotherapy, marrow transplant & irradiation. Consultation advised.

    C. **Non-Hodgkin's lymphoma**
        1. Consultation suggested. Treatment is complex.
        2. Influence of HIV on treatment outcome *(Ann Oncology 26:958, 2015)*.

VI. **Cervical carcinoma**
    A. Epidemiology: More frequent, more severe in HIV patients
    B. Etiology: Human papilloma virus

    C. **Recommendations** *(Int J Gyn Obstet 132:252, 2016)*
        1. Pap smears x 2 in year one & then annually if normal initially; every 3 yrs if CD4 >500/mm^3
        2. More frequent Pap smears if:
            a. Previous abnormal Pap smear
            b. History of papilloma (wart) virus infection
            c. Post-treatment for cervical intraepithelial neoplasia
            d. Symptomatic AIDS or CD4 count <200/mm^3
        3. If Pap smear abnormal, refer for colposcopy &/or biopsy
        4. If CD4 count >200 and under age 26, suggest human papilloma virus vaccine.

VII. **Anal neoplasia**. Prevalence of risk factors, *see NEJM 365:1576, 2011*
    A. Epidemiology
        1. HIV-infected immunodeficient patients at increased risk of human papillomavirus (HPV)-related anal neoplasia: 47% in one series of pts with anal warts *(CID 51:107, 2010)*
        2. ART may also slow progression *(CID 52:1174, 2011)*
    B. Recommendations for HIV-infected pts with history of anal intercourse
        1. Anal Pap smear
        2. Routine anoscopy with biopsy as indicated
        3. Wide surgical resection for established neoplasia
        4. Anal high grade squamous intraepithelial lesions commonly found in HIV positive women regardless of sexual practices *(CID 64:289, 2017)*.

VIII. **Hepatocellular carcinoma**
    A. HIV/HBV or HIV/HCV co-infection leads to more rapid progression of liver disease
    B. Concomitant increased risk of hepatocellular carcinoma

IX. **Incidence of Non-AIDS Defining Neoplasms.** In areas of high prevalence of use of effective ART: Increased incidence of Non-AIDS defining neoplasms and decreased incidence of AIDS-defining neoplasms *(AnIM 163:507, 2015)*

TABLE 19: IMMUNIZATION OF ADULTS AND ADOLESCENTS WITH HIV INFECTION

Reference:
https://aidsinfo.nih.gov/guidelines/html/4/adult-and-adolescent-opportunistic-infection/365/figure--immunization

Recommended immunization schedule for adults and adolescents with HIV infection, United States, 2017

Vaccine	Age					CD4 Cell Count (cells/µl)	
	13-18 years	19-26 years	27-59 years	60-64 years	≥65 years	<200	≥200
Influenza[1]	1 dose annually					1 dose annually	
Tdap/Td[2]	1 dose Tdap, then Td booster every 10 yrs					1 dose Tdap, then Td booster every 10 yrs	
MMR[3]	2 doses if CD4 cell count ≥200					Contraindicated	2 doses if born in 1957 or later
VAR[4]	2 doses if CD4 cell count ≥200					Contraindicated	2 doses
HZV[5]						Contraindicated	
HPV[6]	3 doses					3 doses through age 26 yrs	
PCV13[7]	1 dose					1 dose	
PPSV23[7]	2 doses				1 dose	Up to 3 doses depending on age	
HepA[8] *	2 or 3 doses depending on vaccine					2 or 3 doses depending on vaccine	
HepB[9]	3 doses					3 doses	
MenACWY[10]	2 doses, then booster every 5 yrs					2 doses, then booster every 5 yrs	
MenB[10]*	2 or 3 doses depending on vaccine					2 or 3 doses depending on vaccine	
HIB[11]*	1 or 3 doses depending on indication					1 or 3 doses depending on indication	

* Persons with HIV and other indication

Abbreviations used for vaccines					
HepA	hepatitis A vaccine	IIV	inactivated influenza vaccine	RIV	recombinant influenza vaccine
HepA-HepB	hepatitis A and hepatitis B vaccine	MenACWY	serogroups A, C, W, and Y meningococcal vaccine	Td	tetanus and diphtheria toxoids
HepB	hepatitis B vaccine	MenB	serogroup B meningococcal vaccine	Tdap	tetanus toxoid, reduced diphtheria toxoid, and acellular pertussis vaccine
HiB	*Haemophilus influenzae* type b vaccine	MMR	measles, mumps, and rubella vaccine (live)	VAR	varicella vaccine (live)
HPV vaccine	human papillomavirus vaccine	PCV13	13-valent pneumococcal conjugate vaccine		
HZV	herpes zoster vaccine (live)	PPSV23	23-valent pneumococcal polysaccharide vaccine		

Footnotes. Recommended immunization schedule for adults and adolescents with HIV infection, United States, 2017

1. **Influenza vaccination**
   Administer age-appropriate inactivated influenza vaccine (IIV) or recombinant influenza vaccine (RIV) to adults and adolescents annually. Administer IIV or RIV to pregnant women. For adults and adolescents with a history of hives-only egg allergy, administer IIV or RIV. Those with a history of egg allergy other than hives (e.g., angioedema or respiratory distress) may receive IIV or RIV in a medical setting under supervision of a health care provider who can recognize and manage severe allergic conditions. A list of currently available influenza vaccines is available at www.cdc.gov/flu/protect/vaccine/vaccines.htm.

2. **Tetanus, diphtheria, and pertussis vaccination**
   Administer 1 dose of tetanus toxoid, reduced diphtheria toxoid, and acellular pertussis vaccine (Tdap) to adults and adolescents who were not previously vaccinated with Tdap, followed by a tetanus and diphtheria toxoids (Td) booster every 10 years. Administer 1 dose of Tdap to women during each pregnancy, preferably in the early part of gestational weeks 27–36. Information on the use of Tdap or Td as tetanus prophylaxis in wound management is available at www.cdc.gov/mmwr/preview/mmwrhtml/rr5517a1.htm.

3. **Measles, mumps, and rubella vaccination**
   Administer a 2-dose series of measles, mumps, and rubella vaccine (MMR) at least 1 month apart to adults and adolescents with a CD4 cell count ≥200 cells/µL who do not have evidence of immunity to measles, mumps, and rubella (born before 1957, documentation of receipt of MMR, or laboratory evidence of immunity or disease). Pregnant women with a CD4 cell count ≥200 cells/µL who do not have immunity to rubella should receive a 2-dose series of MMR at least 1 month apart after pregnancy. Adults and adolescents with a CD4 cell count <200 cells/µL should not receive MMR.

4. **Varicella vaccination**
   Administer a 2-dose series of varicella vaccine (VAR) 3 months apart to adults and adolescents with a CD4 cell count ≥200 cells/µL who do not have evidence of immunity to varicella (documented receipt of 2 doses of VAR, born in the United States before 1980, diagnosis of varicella or zoster by a healthcare provider, or laboratory evidence of immunity). Those with a CD4 cell count <200 cells/µL should not receive VAR.

TABLE 19 (2)

5. **Herpes zoster vaccination**
   There is no recommendation for herpes zoster vaccine (HZV) for adults and adolescents with a CD4 cell count ≥200 cells/μL. Those with a CD4 cell count <200 cells/μL should not receive HZV.

6. **Human papillomavirus vaccination**
   Administer a 3-dose series of human papillomavirus (HPV) vaccine at 0, 1–2, and 6 months to adults and adolescents through age 26 years. Pregnant women are not recommended to receive HPV vaccine.

7. **Pneumococcal vaccination**
   Administer 1 dose of 13-valent pneumococcal conjugate vaccine (PCV13) followed by 1 dose of 23-valent pneumococcal polysaccharide vaccine (PPSV23) at least 2 months later. Administer a second dose of PPSV23 at least 5 years after the first dose of PPSV23. If the most recent dose of PPSV23 was administered before age 65 years, at age 65 years or older, administer another dose of PPSV23 at least 5 years after the last dose of PPSV23.

8. **Hepatitis A vaccination**
   Administer a 2-dose series of single antigen hepatitis A vaccine (HepA) at 0 and 6–12 months or 0 and 6–18 months, depending on the vaccine, or a 3-dose series of combined hepatitis A and hepatitis B vaccine (HepA-HepB) at 0, 1, and 6 months to adults and adolescents who may not have a specific risk but wants protection against hepatitis A infection. Administer a HepA-containing vaccine series to adults and adolescents at risk which includes chronic liver disease, receive clotting factor concentrates, men who have sex with men, inject illicit drugs, and travel in countries with endemic hepatitis A.

9. **Hepatitis B vaccination**
   Administer a 3-dose series of single-antigen hepatitis B vaccine (HepB) or combined hepatitis A and hepatitis B vaccine (HepA-HepB) at 0, 1, and 6 months.

10. **Meningococcal vaccination**
    Administer a 2-dose primary series of serogroup A, C, W, and Y meningococcal vaccine (MenACWY) at least 2 months apart, and revaccinate every 5 years. Serogroup B meningococcal vaccine (MenB) is not routinely recommended. Young adults and adolescents age 16 through 23 years (preferred age range is 16 through 18 years) may receive MenB (a 2-dose series of MenB-4C at least 1 month apart or a 3-dose series of MenB-FHbp at 0, 1–2, and 6 months) based on individual clinical decision.

11. **Haemophilus influenzae type b vaccination**
    Adults and adolescents with HIV infection are not routinely recommended to receive Haemophilus influenzae type b vaccine (Hib). Administer Hib to those with asplenia, hematopoietic stem cell transplant, and other indications.

**TABLE 20A: MEASURES TO BE TAKEN BY PHYSICIANS IN PREPARING HIV+ PATIENTS
& INDIVIDUALS LIKELY TO HAVE "RISKY" BEHAVIOR FOR OVERSEAS TRAVEL**

The likelihood of developing an illness during international travel is 22-64% depending on destination
(NEJM 2016; 375:247).

Since illnesses are likely to be more serious &/or become chronic in the HIV+ patient, there is advice to be given
& measures to be taken to minimize risks. These include:

If the traveler is likely to engage in risky behavior during travel, ascertain the HIV antibody status before travel,
especially if travel is planned to a developing country. Condom use is an absolute requirement. Recommendations
revised so that TDF/FTC PrEP should be considered for high risk individuals. See: *https://www.cdc.gov/hiv/pdf/
risk/prep/cdc-hiv-prep-guidelines-2017.pdf*

Ensure sufficient supplies of medications and information about need for refrigeration or special storage.

Review planned itinerary & activities in light of the patient's immune status & review the added risks for travel,
especially to developing or tropical countries. In some instances, it may be prudent to recommend a change
in itinerary or activities because of serious risks that cannot be eliminated or reduced.

Recommend the following measures to reduce exposure to pathogens:

- Assiduously avoid food & beverages that may be contaminated, especially raw or undercooked shellfish,
  fish, meat, or eggs; raw, unpeeled fruits & vegetables; tap water & ice; as well as unpasteurized milk
  & milk products (cheese).
- Insist on eating only well-cooked foods & on drinking only very hot or bottled beverages.
- Reduce contact with vectors, for example, by using insect repellent & avoiding outdoor exposure at dusk
  or other times & places of increased insect activity.
- Frequent handwashing, ideally with alcohol based hand cleanser gels.

Urge the patient to obtain prompt evaluation of symptoms of illness & early treatment of infection. Where possible,
identify a physician knowledgeable about HIV infection at the destination prior to departure[1]. Arrange for
continuation of medical management during travel (for example, prophylaxis for Pneumocystis jirovecii pneumonia).

Use vaccine & prophylactic therapy as indicated by the planned itinerary & activities. Avoid live vaccines in pts
with profound immunodeficiency not on ARV therapy. Assure most recent influenza vaccines have been
administered, including H1N1 vaccine (regardless of time of year). Prescribe antimicrobial agents (with or without
antimotility drugs) & counsel the patient on their use for early treatment of diarrheal disease[2].

For overview of considerations in immunocompromised individuals see: *https://www.cdc.gov/travel/yellowbook/
2018/advising-travelers-with-specific-needs/immunocompromised-travelers#5040*

For a list of English-speaking doctors abroad & health information: International Association for Medical
Assistance to Travelers (IAMAT), 417 Center St., Lewiston, NY 14092. *See https://www.iamat.org/*

For suggestions regarding a medical kit & advice (for all travelers): *https://wwwnc.cdc.gov/travel/page/pack-
smart#travelhealthkit*

TABLE 20B: IMMUNIZATION OF HIV+ ADULTS TRAVELING TO DEVELOPING COUNTRIES[*]

| VACCINE/TOXOID | STAGE OF HIV INFECTION | | COMMENTS |
	ASYMPTOMATIC HIV+[*]	SYMPTOMATIC (AIDS)[*]	
"Routine" for All Developing Countries			
eIPV	Yes	Yes	*See Table 19.* OPV contraindicated
Hepatitis A	Yes	Yes	*See Table 19*
Typhoid Vi polysaccharide vaccine (Connaught)	Yes	Yes	Boosters recommended q2 yrs. Live attenuated (eg, Ty21a) oral typhoid vaccine contraindicated
Immune globulin (IG)	Yes	Yes	For 2–3 mos travel, 0.02 mL/kg IM single dose
"Special" Depending on Itinerary: Country & Activity			
Cholera (inactivated vaccine)	*See Comments*	*See Comments*	Vaccine does not prevent transmission, efficacy ~50%, risk to U.S. travelers very low. WHO does not recommend, but some countries require (check with Health Dept.). If required, have vaccination completed, signed, dated & validated to avoid risk of revaccination & quarantine.
Rabies (pre-exposure) (inactivated vaccine)	Yes, if indicated (Animal handlers, travelers spending 1 mo or more in country where rabies is a constant threat)	Yes, if indicated	Course: Three 1 mL of HDCV or RVA IM on days 0, 7, 28. Test serum for antibodies 2 wks after 3rd dose.
Meningococcal (polysaccharide vaccine) (Menomune) or polysaccharide-protein conjugate (Menactra)	New 2016 recs *MMWR 65:1189, 2016:* All HIV+ individuals >2 mo should be vaccinated		
Yellow Fever (live attenuated)	Yes (±); offer choice if potential exposure unavoidable	No (contraindicated)	
Japanese Encephalitis	Yes, if indicated: travel to Asia, in monsoon (summer) months, staying in rural areas		Requires 3 injections: day 0, 7, & 30. An abbreviated schedule at days 0, 7, 14 can be used but less effective.
Plague (inactivated)	Yes, if indicated: to areas of endemic plague, esp. if staying in rural areas, not in tourist hotels		
BCG (Bacillus Calmette-Guerin) vaccine	No	No	Live attenuated vaccine.

[*] All travelers should have current routine immunizations, *see https://aidsinfo.nih.gov/guidelines/html/4/adult-and adolescent-opportunistic-infection/365/figure--immunization*

For further information, *see www.travmed.com; www.fitfortravel.scot.nhs.uk.*

TABLE 21: STIMULATING RBCs, WBCs & PLATELETS IN HIV PATIENTS*

DRUG NAME, GENERIC (TRADE) COST	COMMENTS ON USE, ADVERSE EFFECTS
Erythropoietin (Epogen, Procrit) **Darbepoetin** (Aranesp, Nesp) = long-acting erythropoietin **Peginesatide** (Omontys) Meta-analysis of use in dialysis pts: increased risk of stroke, increased BP, vascular access thrombosis *(An Int Med 153:23, 2010).*	**FDA approved for Rx of anemia in HIV. FDA advisory warning:** ↑ risk of death, thromboembolic, and cardiovascular events. Monitor hemoglobin dose to maintain the hemoglobin level of ≤11 gm/dL. Antibody to erythropoietin can lead to red cell aplasia *(AJG 100:1415, 2005).* **Erythropoietin Dose:** 40,000–60,000 units subQ once weekly equal efficacy as 3x/wk. rx. *(AIDS Res Human Retroviruses 20:1037, 2004).* **Dose of darbepoetin:** 0.45 mcg/kg IV or subQ **q wk.** **Peginesatide Dose:** 0.04 mg/kg IV or sc once per month.
Granulocyte-CSF or G-CSF, Filgrastim (Neupogen), Pegfilgrastim (Neulasta), **Granulocyte-monocyte CSF or GM-CSF,** Sargramostim (Leukine)	**G-CSF:** Standard dose 5 mcg/kg/day subQ; lower doses may work in HIV pts, i.e., 1 mcg/kg/day subQ until ANC >1000 cells/dl, then 1–2x/wk. No effect on HIV replication. Pegylated G-CSF—pegfilgrastim: 6 mg subQ once per chemotherapy cycle. **GM-CSF:** Dose 5 mcg/kg/day subQ → ↑ PMNs. Trend toward ↑ CD4 and slightly lower VL. Adverse effects: fever, myalgia, fatigue, malaise, headache, bone pain.
Intravenous immune serum globulin (IVIG) (Gamimune N, Gammar, & others) General dosage: (1) Adults: 200–400 mg/kg q21 days; (2) Children: 400 mg/kg/month	Few indications in the era of ART. For immune thrombocytopenia use IVIG if pt bleeding or for immediate invasive procedure; rapid but transient effects. Dose 1-2 gm/kg for 2-5 days. Rho (D) immune globulin more cost effective and may be more effective. *(See Immunol Allergy Clin N Am 28:851, 2008).*
Rho (D) Immune Globulin (Anti-Rh immunoglobulin), intravenous (human) (WinRho) 1500 intl units (equals 300 mcg)	Treatment for **HIV-induced ITP** in non-splenectomized Rh+ pts. Coats Rh+ RBC with antibody; competes with antibody-coated platelets for binding sites on splenic macrophages. Some RBC hemolysis. Effective AIDS pts. Dose: 25–50 mcg/kg/day x 7 days, then q3 wks. One small study of 9 pts. found that rho immune globulin produced higher platelet counts and a longer duration of effect than IVIG *(Am J Hematol 82:335, 2007).*

NOTE: Majority of hematologic problems resolve, or substantively improve, with control of HIV replication. In general, treat HIV first before using drugs outlined above.

TABLE 22: AIDS INFORMATION & REFERRAL SERVICES

- AIDS/HIV Clinical Trials conducted by National Institutes of Health & FDA-approved efficacy trials: 1-800-874-2572

- For a wide variety of AIDS/HIV information, resources, publications, call the National AIDS Clearinghouse: 1-800-458-5231

- To find out about AIDS resources in your area, call the National AIDS Hotline: 1-800-342-2437

- The AIDS/HIV Treatment Directory is published by the American Federation for AIDS Research (AmFAR) & is updated semi-annually; 733 Third Ave., 12th Floor, New York, NY 10017-3204. Telephone: 1-800-392-6327

- The HIV/AIDS Treatment Information Service (Public Health Coordinating Group): 1-800-HIV-0440

- Travel information for patients: *www.travmed.com* & *www.fitfortravel.scot.nhs.uk*

- The National Clinicians' Post-Exposure Prophylaxis Hotline, for the latest information on post-exposure protocols and preventative therapy: *http://www.nccc.ucsf.edu/about_nccc/pepline/*

- The Francis J. Curry National Tuberculosis Center, for information on educational programs and phone consultation (415-502-4700 or 877-390-NOTB(6682)) on prevention and management of tuberculosis: *http://www.nationaltbcenter.edu/*

Helpful Websites for Information / Questions About HIV/AIDS:

CDC National Information Prevention Network: *www.cdcnpin.org*
AmFAR (American Foundation for AIDS Research): *www.amfar.org*
International Antiviral Society USA: *http://www.iasusa.org*
NATAP (National AIDS Treatment Advocacy Project) *www.natap.org*
San Francisco General Hospital: *http://hivinsite.ucsf.edu*
Stanford HIV Drug Resistance Database: *http://hivdb.stanford.edu*
University of Liverpool HIV Drug Interactions Assessment: *www.hiv-druginteractions.org*
WHO Treatment Guidelines: *www.who.org*
HHS HIV Treatment Guidelines for ART in Adults, Adolescents, and Children. Plus OI Guidelines: *www.aidsinfo.nih.gov*

TABLE 23: LIST OF GENERIC & COMMON TRADE NAMES

GENERIC NAME: TRADE NAMES

Abacavir: Ziagen
Abacavir + Lamivudine: Epzicom
Abacavir + Lamivudine + Zidovudine:
   Trizivir
Abacavir + Dolutegravir + Lamivudine:
   Triumeq
Acyclovir: Zovirax
Adefovir: Hepsera
Albendazole: Albenza
Amikacin: Amikin
Amphotericin B: Fungizone
Ampho B-liposomal: AmBisome
Ampho B-lipid complex: Abelcet
Ampicillin + sulbactam: Unasyn
Artemether + Lumefantrine: Coartem
Atazanavir: Reyataz
Atazanavir + Cobi: Evotaz
Atovaquone: Mepron
Atovaquone + Proguanil: Malarone
Azithromycin: Zithromax
Azithromycin ER: Zmax
Aztreonam: Azactam, Cayston
Bedaquiline: Sirturo
Bictegravir + FTC + TAF: Biktarvy
Caspofungin: Cancidas
Cefotetan: Cefotan
Cefoxitin: Mefoxin
Ceftriaxone: Rocephin
Chloroquine: Aralen
Cidofovir: Vistide
Ciprofloxacin: Cipro, Cipro XR
Clarithromycin: Biaxin, Biaxin XL
Clindamycin: Cleocin
Clofazimine: Lamprene
Cycloserine: Seromycin
Darunavir: Prezista
Darunavir + Cobi: Prezcobix
Darunavir + Cobi + FTC + TAF:
   Symtuza
Delavirdine: Rescriptor
Didanosine: Videx
Diethylcarbamazine: Hetrazan
Diloxanide furoate: Furamide
Dolutegravir: Tivicay
Dolutegravir + RPV: Juluca
Doravirine: Pifeltro
Doravirine + 3TC + TDF: Delstrigo
Doxycycline: Vibramycin
Efavirenz: Sustiva
Efavirenz + Emtricitabine + Tenofovir:
   Atripla
Efavirenz + 3TC + TDF: Symfi/Symfi Lo
Elvitegravir: Vitekta
Elvitegravir + Cobicistat +
   Emtricitabine + Tenofovir: Stribild
Elvitegravir + Cobi + Emtricitabine +
   TAF: Genvoya
Emtricitabine: Emtriva
Emtricitabine + TAF: Descovy
Emtricitabine + TDF: Truvada
Emtricitabine + TDF + rilpivirine:
   Complera
Emtricitabine + Rilpivirine + TAF:
   Odefsey
Enfuvirtide (T-20): Fuzeon

Entecavir: Baraclude
Etravirine: Intelence
Erythromycin (s): Ilotycin
   Ethyl succinate: Pediamycin
   Glucoheptonate: Erythrocin
   Estolate: Ilosone
Erythro+sulfisoxazole: Pediazole
Ethambutol: Myambutol
Ethionamide: Trecator
Famciclovir: Famvir
Fluconazole: Diflucan
Flucytosine: Ancobon
Fosamprenavir: Lexiva
Foscarnet: Foscavir
Ganciclovir: Cytovene
Gatifloxacin: Tequin
Gemifloxacin: Factive
Gentamicin: Garamycin
Halofantrine: Halfan
Idoxuridine: Dendrid, Stoxil
INH + RIF: Rifamate
INH + RIF + PZA: Rifater
Interferon alfa: Intron A
Interferon, pegylated: PEG-Intron,
   Pegasys
Interferon + Ribavirin: Rebetron
Imiquimod: Aldara
Indinavir: Crixivan
Isavuconazole: Cresemba
Itraconazole: Sporanox
Iodoquinol: Yodoxin
Ivermectin: Stromectol, Sklice
Kanamycin: Kantrex
Ketoconazole: Nizoral
Lamivudine: Epivir, Epivir-HBV
Lamivudine + Abacavir: Epzicom
Lamivudine + TDF: Cimduo
Levofloxacin: Levaquin
Lopinavir + Ritonavir: Kaletra
Mafenide: Sulfamylon
Maraviroc: Selzentry
Mebendazole: Vermox
Mefloquine: Lariam
Meropenem: Merrem
Mesalamine: Asacol, Pentasa
Metronidazole: Flagyl
Micafungin: Mycamine
Minocycline: Minocin
Moxifloxacin: Avelox
Nelfinavir: Viracept
Nevirapine: Viramune
Nitazoxanide: Alinia
Nitrofurantoin: Macrobid, Macrodantin
Nystatin: Mycostatin
Ofloxacin: Floxin
Oseltamivir: Tamiflu
Paromomycin: Humatin
Pentamidine: NebuPent, Pentam 300
Podophyllotoxin: Condylox
Posaconazole: Noxafil
Praziquantel: Biltricide
Primaquine: Primachine
Proguanil: Paludrine
Pyrantel pamoate: Antiminth
Pyrimethamine: Daraprim

Pyrimethamine+sulfadoxine: Fansidar
Raltegravir: Isentress
Ribavirin: Virazole, Rebetol
Rifabutin: Mycobutin
Rifampin: Rifadin, Rimactane
Rifapentine: Priftin
Rilpivirine: Edurant
Ritonavir: Norvir
Saquinavir: Invirase
Spectinomycin: Trobicin
Stavudine: Zerit
Stibogluconate: Pentostam
Sulfamethoxazole: Gantanol
Sulfasalazine: Azulfidine
Sulfisoxazole: Gantrisin
Telavancin: Vibativ
Telbivudine: Tyzeka
Tenofovir disoproxil fumarate: Viread
Tenofovir alafenamide fumarate:
   Tenofovir-AF
Terbinafine: Lamisil
Thalidomide: Thalomid Thiabendazole
   Mintezol
Tipranavir: Aptivus
Trifluridine: Viroptic
Trimethoprim: Primsol
Trimethoprim + Sulfamethoxazole:
   Bactrim, Septra
Valacyclovir: Valtrex
Valganciclovir: Valcyte
Voriconazole: Vfend
Zalcitabine: HIVID
Zanamivir: Relenza
Zidovudine (ZDV): Retrovir
Zidovudine + 3TC: Combivir
Zidovudine + 3TC + Abacavir: Trizivir

TABLE 23 (2)

TRADE NAME: GENERIC NAME

Abelcet: Ampho B-lipid complex
Albenza: Albendazole
AmBisome: Ampho B-liposomal
Amikin: Amikacin
Ancobon: Flucytosine
Antiminth: Pyrantel pamoate
Aptivus: Tipranavir
Aralen: Chloroquine
Atripla: Efavirenz + Emtricitabine + Tenofovir
Augmentin, Augmentin ES-600 Avelox: Moxifloxacin
Azactam: Aztreonam
Azulfidine: Sulfasalazine
Bactrim: Trimethoprim + Sulfamethoxazole
Baraclude: Entecavir
Biaxin, Biaxin XL: Clarithromycin
Biktarvy: Bictegravir + FTC + TAF
Biltricide: Praziquantel
Cancidas: Caspofungin
Cayston: Aztreonam (inhaled)
Cefotan: Cefotetan
Cimduo: 3TC + TDF
Cipro, Cipro XR: Ciprofloxacin & extended release
Coartem: Artemether/Lumefantrine
Combivir: ZDV + 3TC
Complera: Emtricitabine + TDF + Rilpivirine
Cresemba: Isavuconazole
Crixivan: Indinavir
Cytovene: Ganciclovir
Daraprim: Pyrimethamine
Delstrigo: DOR + 3TC + TDF
Descovy: Emtricitabine + TAF
Diflucan: Fluconazole
Edurant: Rilpivirine
Emtriva: Emtricitabine
Epivir, Epivir-HBV: Lamivudine
Epzicom: Lamivudine + Abacavir
Evotaz: Atazanavir + Cobi
Factive: Gemifloxacin
Famvir: Famciclovir
Fansidar: Pyrimethamine + Sulfadoxine
Flagyl: Metronidazole
Floxin: Ofloxacin
Foscavir: Foscarnet
Fulvicin: Griseofulvin
Fungizone: Amphotericin B
Fuzeon: Enfuvirtide (T-20)
Gantanol: Sulfamethoxazole
Gantrisin: Sulfisoxazole
Garamycin: Gentamicin
Genvoya: Elvitegravir + Cobi + Emtricitabine + TAF
Halfan: Halofantrine
Hepsera: Adefovir
Herplex: Idoxuridine
Hiprex: Methenamine hippurate
HIVID: Zalcitabine
Humatin: Paromomycin
Iosone: Erythromycin estolate
Ilotycin: Erythromycin
Intelence: Etravirine
Intron A: Interferon alfa
Invanz: Ertapenem

Invirase: Saquinavir
Isentress: Raltegravir
Juluca: DTG + RPV
Kantrex: Kanamycin
Kaletra: Lopinavir + Ritonavir
Lamprene: Clofazimine
Lariam: Mefloquine
Levaquin: Levofloxacin
Lexiva: Fosamprenavir
Malarone: Atovaquone + Proguanil
Maxaquin: Lomefloxacin
Mefoxin: Cefoxitin
Mepron: Atovaquone
Minocin: Minocycline
Mintezol: Thiabendazole
Myambutol: Ethambutol
Mycamine: Micafungin
Mycobutin: Rifabutin
Nebcin: Tobramycin
NebuPent: Pentamidine
Nizoral: Ketoconazole
Norvir: Ritonavir
Noxafil: Posaconazole
Odefsey: Emtricitabine + Rilpivirine + TAF
Omnicef: Cefdinir
Pediamycin: Erythro. ethyl succinate
Pediazole: Erythro. ethyl succinate + Sulfisoxazole
Pegasys, PEG-Intron: Interferon, pegylated
Pentam 300: Pentamidine
Pifeltro: Doravirine
Pipracil: Piperacillin
Polycillin: Ampicillin
Polymox: Amoxicillin
Prezcobix: Darunavir + Cobi
Prezista: Darunavir
Priftin: Rifapentine
Primaxin: Imipenem + Cilastatin
Primsol: Trimethoprim
Rebetol: Ribavirin
Rebetron: Interferon + Ribavirin
Relenza: Zanamivir
Rescriptor: Delavirdine
Retin A: Tretinoin Retrovir: Zidovudine (ZDV)
Reyataz: Atazanavir
Rifadin: Rifampin
Rifamate: INH + RIF
Rifater: INH + RIF + PZA
Rimactane: Rifampin
Rocephin: Ceftriaxone
Selzentry: Maraviroc
Septra: Trimethoprim + Sulfa
Seromycin: Cycloserine
Silvadene: Silver sulfadiazine
Sirturo: Bedaquiline
Sklice: Ivermectin lotion
Sporanox: Itraconazole
Stoxil: Idoxuridine
Stribild: Elvitegravir + Cobicistat + Emtricitabine + Tenofovir
Stromectol: Ivermectin
Sulfamylon: Mafenide
Sulperazon[NUS]: Cefoperazone-sulbactam
Sustiva: Efavirenz

Symfi/Symfi Lo: EFV + 3TC + TDF
Symmetrel: Amantadine
Symtuza: DRV + Cobi + FTC + TAF
Synagis: Palivizumab
Synercid: Quinupristin + Dalfopristin
Tamiflu: Oseltamivir
Tazicef: Ceftazidime
Teflaro: Ceftaroline
Tegopen: Cloxacillin
Tequin: Gatifloxacin
Thalomid: Thalidomide
Tienam: Imipenem
Tinactin: Tolnaftate
Tindamax: Tinidazole
Tivicay: Dolutegravir
Trecator SC: Ethionamide
Triumeq: Abacavir + Dolutegravir + Lamivudine
Trizivir: Abacavir + ZDV + 3TC
Trobicin: Spectinomycin
Truvada: Emtricitabine + TDF
Tyzeka: Telbivudine
Unasyn: Ampicillin/sulbactam
Unipen: Nafcillin
Valcyte: Valganciclovir
Valtrex: Valacyclovir
Vancocin: Vancomycin
Vermox: Mebendazole
Vfend: Voriconazole
Vibativ: Telavancin
Vibramycin: Doxycycline
Videx: Didanosine
Viracept: Nelfinavir
Viramune: Nevirapine
Virazole: Ribavirin
Viread: Tenofovir-DF
Vistide: Cidofovir
Vitekta: Elvitegravir
Yodoxin: Iodoquinol
Zerit: Stavudine
Ziagen: Abacavir
Zinacef: Cefuroxime
Zithromax: Azithromycin
Zmax: Azithromycin ER
Zovirax: Acyclovir
Zosyn: Piperacillin + Tazobactam
Zyvox: Linezolid

172

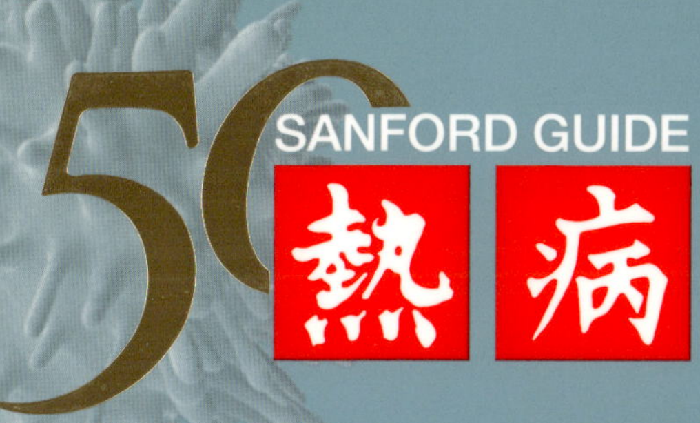

THE SANFORD GUIDE

HIV/AIDS & Hepatitis Therapy

2019

Michael S. Saag, M.D.
David N. Gilbert, M.D.
Henry F. Chambers, M.D.
George M. Eliopoulos, M.D.
Andrew T. Pavia, M.D.

Douglas Black, Pharm.D.
David O. Freedman, M.D.
Kami Kim, M.D.
Brian S. Schwartz, M.D.

HIV/AIDS RAPID REFERENCE

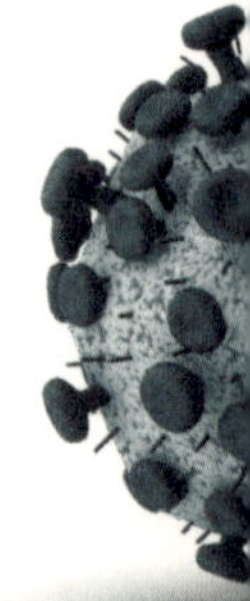

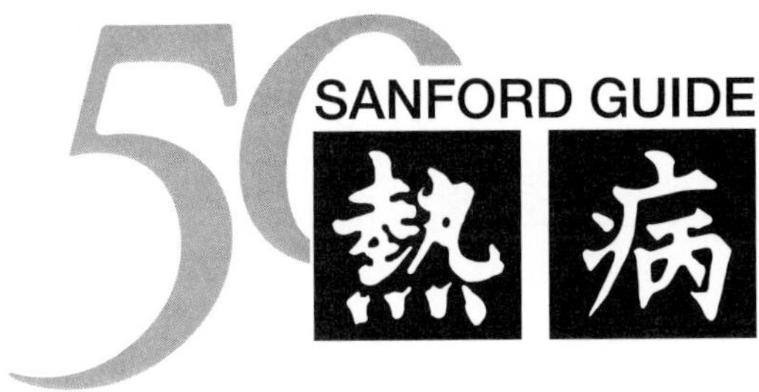

THE SANFORD GUIDE

Hepatitis Therapy
2019

3rd Edition

Michael S. Saag, M.D.
David N. Gilbert, M.D.
Henry F. Chambers, M.D.
George M. Eliopoulos, M.D.
Andrew T. Pavia, M.D.

Douglas Black, Pharm.D.
David O. Freedman, M.D.
Kami Kim, M.D.
Brian S. Schwartz, M.D.

— TABLE OF CONTENTS —

— LIST OF FIGURES —

— ABBREVIATIONS —

3TC = Lamivudine
ABC = abacavir
AD = after dialysis
AIDS = acquired immune deficiency syndrome
ALT = Alanine aminotransferase
APRI = AST-platelet ratio
AST = Aspartate transaminase
AUC = Area under the curve
bDNA = Branched-chain DNA amplification
BOC = Boceprevir
CAPD = continuous ambulatory peritoneal dialysis
cccDNA = covalently closed circular DNA
CrCl = creatinine clearance
CRRT = continuous renal replacement therapy
DAAs = Direct acting (antiviral) agents
DBV = Dasabuvir
dc = discontinue
DCV = daclatasvir
ddI = didanosine
EBR = elbasvir
EIA = Enzyme linked immunosorbent assay
ELF = Enhanced liver fibrosis (Score)
ESRD = endstage renal disease
ETR = End of Treatment Response
Flu = fluconazole
FTC = emtricitabine
G = generic
GGT = Gamma-glutamyltransferase
GLE = Glecaprevir
gm = gram
GZR = grazoprevir
HAV = Hepatitis A Virus
HBcAb (Anti-HBc) = Hepatitis B core antibody
HBeAb (Anti-HBe) = Hepatitis B e antibody
HBeAg = Hepatitis B e antigen
HBsAb (anti-HBS) = Hepatitis B surface antibody
HBsAg = Hepatitis B surface antigen
HBV = Hepatitis B Virus
HCC = Hepatocellular carcinoma
HCV = Hepatitis C Virus
HDV = Hepatitis D (Delta) Virus
HE = Homing endonucleases
HEV = Hepatitis E Virus
HIV = Human immunodeficiency virus
HSV = Herpes simplex virus
IFN = Interferon
IL-28B = Interleukin 28-B locus
IM = intramuscular
INR = International normalized ratio (clotting scale)
IDU = Intravenous drug user
IVIG = intravenous immune globulin
kg = kilogram
kPa = kilo-Pascals

LDV = Ledipasvir
mcg = microgram
MELD Score = Model for End Stage Liver Disease Score
mg = milligram
mL = milliliter
MSM = Men who have sex with men
NNRTI = non-nucleoside reverse transcriptase inhibitor
NS3 = Serine protease gene
NS4a = Serine Protease Co-factor
NS5a = Inhibition of viral particle assembly gene product
NS5b = RNA-Dependent/RNA Polymerase gene product
NUC = Nucleoside (or Nucleotide) agent
OBV = Ombitasvir
PCR = polymerase chain reaction
PCT = Porphyria cutanea tarda
PEG-IFN = Pegylated interferon
PI = protease inhibitor
PIB = Pibrentasvir
po = orally (by mouth)
PTV/r = Paritaprevir + ritonavir
RBV = Ribavirin
RR = Relative risk
RT-PCR = Reverse transcriptase -Polymerase chain reaction
RTV = ritonavir
Rx/rx = Treatment
SBP = Spontaneous Bacterial Peritonitis
sc = subcutaneous
SD = serum drug level after single dose
sgRNA = single guide RNA
siRNA = Short-interfering RNA
SMV = Simeprevir
SOF = Sofosbuvir
Spy Cas9 = Strept pyogenes CRISPR-associated protein 9
SS = steady state serum level
STD = sexually transmitted disease
SVR = Sustained virologic response
TAF = Tenofovir Alafenamide
TALENs = Transcription-activator-like effector nucleases
TDF = tenofovir
TLR 7 = Toll-like receptor 7
TNF = Tumor necrosis factor
TVR = Telaprevir
ULN = Upper Limit of Normal
VEL = velpatasvir
VL = viral load
ZFN = Zinc Finger Nucleases
µg = microgram

— JOURNALS AND OTHER REFERENCES —

AJM = American Journal of Medicine
Amer College Physicians = American College of Physicians
Am J Pub Health = American Journal of Public Health
Ann Trop Med Parasitol = Annals of Tropical Medicine & Parasitology
CCM = Critical Care Medicine
CID = Clinical Infectious Diseases
Cleveland Clinic J Med = Cleveland Clinic Journal of Medicine
Curr HIV/AIDS Rep = Current HIV/AIDS Reports
Gastro = Gastroenterology
Hpt = Hepatology
JAMA = Journal of the American Medical Association
JID = Journal of Infectious Diseases
J Virology = Journal of Virology
Ln = Lancet
Methods in Molec Biology = Methods in Molecular Biology
MMWR = Morbidity & Mortality Weekly Report
Nature Rev Microbiol = Nature Reviews: Microbiology
NEJM = New England Journal of Medicine

TABLE 1: HEPATITIS A VIRUS (HAV)

HAV Treatment: No therapy recommended.

HAV Prophylaxis Post-exposure:

If within 2 wks of exposure, prophylactic IVIG 0.02 mL/kg IM x 1 is protective. Hep A vaccine equally effective as IVIG in randomized trial and is emerging as preferred therapy *(NEJM 357:1685, 2007)*.

HAV Superinfection: 40% of pts with chronic Hepatitis C virus (HCV) infection who developed superinfection with HAV developed fulminant hepatic failure *(NEJM 338:286, 1998)*. Similar data in pts with chronic Hepatitis virus (HBV) infection that suffer acute HAV *(Ann Trop Med Parasitol 93:745, 1999)*. **Hence, need to vaccinate a HBV and HCV pts with HAV vaccine.**

HAV Immunization (See also, *Table 10*):

Recommended for:

1) high risk groups, e.g., MSM, homeless populations, and injection drug users;
2) persons working with HAV-infected primates in research labs;
3) persons with chronic liver disease and clotting factor recipients;
4) travel to endemic areas; and
5) persons with close contact with adoptees from endemic areas.

Single antigen vaccine (Havrix) administered in 2 doses at 0 and 6-12 months.

Combined HAV/HBV vaccine (Twinrix) administered in 3 doses at 0, 1 and 6 months.

TABLE 2: HEPATITIS B VIRUS (HBV)

TABLE 2A: EPIDEMIOLOGY OF HBV INFECTION

Caseload. 350,000,000 cases worldwide, at least 1.25 million in US; defined as persons Hepatitis B surface antigen (HBsAg) positive for more than 6 months *(Am J Pub Health 89:14-18, 1994; MMWR 54 (RR-16): 1- 31, 2005)*. 15-40% of Carriers will develop complications, including cirrhosis, hepatic decompensation, and/or hepatocellular carcinoma.

Risk of Transmission. Hepatitis B virus (HBV) replicates to high titers in the blood, especially during initial (acute) infection. Any parenteral or mucosal exposure can transmit the virus. HBV is transmitted via perinatal, percutaneous, sexual exposure, and close person-to-person contact (e.g., open cuts or sores). It is ~ 100-fold more efficiently transmitted than HIV. HBV is present in most tissues and body fluids (serum, saliva, semen, vaginal secretions) and can survive for long periods of time on environmental surfaces. HBV is not spread, however, through food or water, sharing eating utensils, breastfeeding, hugging, kissing, hand holding, coughing or sneezing.

Virology & Life Cycle. DNA virus: HBV is a partially double stranded hepadnavirus. Once within the cell nucleus, the HBV DNA causes the liver cell to produce surface (HBs) proteins, the core (HBc) protein, DNA polymerase, the HBe protein, HBx protein and other as yet undetected proteins and enzymes. HBV has a unique mechanism of replication via reverse transcription of pregenomic RNA by its DNA polymerase. The lack of proofreading function leads mutant virions that can fuel antiviral resistance. Produces full virion (42 nm complete virus; Dane Particle) and smaller (22 nm) HBsAg particles in large quantities. Primarily infects hepatocytes, although believed to infect lymphocytes as well. HBV amplifies via reverse transcription of an RNA intermediate. Enters nucleus; forms covalently closed circular (CCC) DNA. May, but does not always, integrate into host DNA.

Eight Genotypes

- o   **A** (N. America / Europe / Parts of Africa): More responsive to IFN Rx
- o   **B** (Asia): More responsive to IFN Rx
- o   **C** (Asia): More severe liver disease; slower HBsAg clearance; more HCC; Less responsive to IFN Rx
- o   **D** (India / Middle East / Mediterranean / Africa): Less responsive to IFN Rx
- o   **E** (Africa)
- o   **F** (S. America)
- o   **G** (Undetermined)
- o   **H** (Undetermined)

TABLE 2B: NATURAL HISTORY OF HBV

Acute HBV Infection. Usually asymptomatic (incubation period of 1 – 4 months). If symptomatic, usually abates in days to weeks; rarely associated with hepatic failure (unless co-infected with Hepatitis Delta Virus, HDV). Factors associated with natural clearance include: Cellular Immune Responses (NK cell; NK T-cell; and virus specific CD4 T cells and CD8 cytotoxic T lymphocytes). Those who resolve the acute infection maintain broad and strong CTL responses.

Note: HBV DNA can persist at low levels for > 20 years and those who seem to clear infection likely are not truly cured of HBV infection. Subsequent chemotherapy or immune suppressive therapy: risk factors for re-emergence of HBV replication *(Hpt 61:703, 2015).*

FIGURE 1   Lifecycle of Hepatitis B Virus

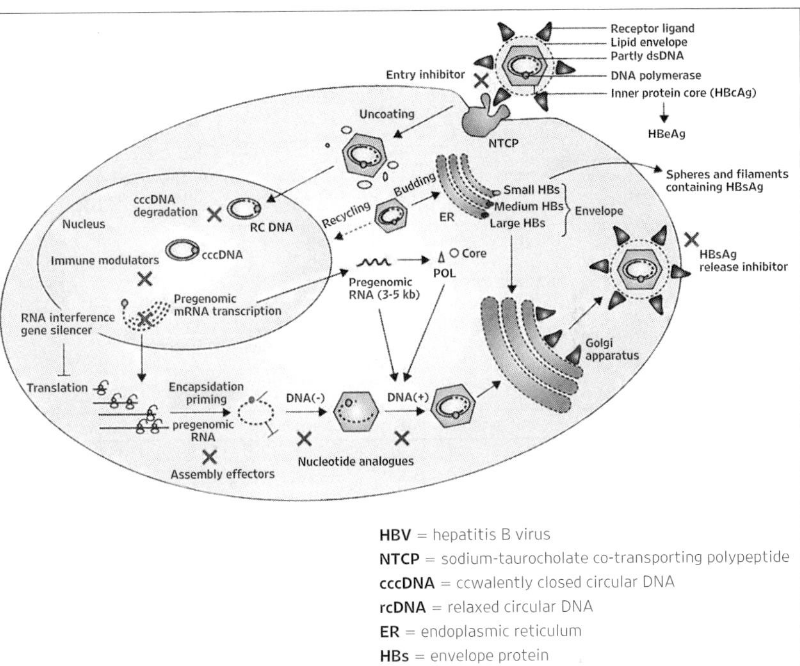

HBV = hepatitis B virus
NTCP = sodium-taurocholate co-transporting polypeptide
cccDNA = ccwalently closed circular DNA
rcDNA = relaxed circular DNA
ER = endoplasmic reticulum
HBs = envelope protein

Figure: The HBV lifecycle and potential therapeutic targets

After HBV virions attach to the NTCP receptor, they are uncoated and transported to the nucleus, in which cccDNA serves as a template for viral transcription of pregenomic RNA, which then directs the synthesis of viral DNA and mRNA encoding all viral proteins and securing HBV persistence. Genomic replication of HBV happens via virally encoded polymerase and a reverse transcriptase. Encoded polymerase uses pregenomic RNA as a template to synthesise the minus-strand viral DNA via its RN A-dependent DNA polymerisation activity, which is then used by the encoded polymerase as the template for the plus strand DNA synthesis. The process eventually leads to nucleocapsid maturation as rcDNA is formed which can be either enveloped or secreted out of the cell as a virion particle or be delivered into the nucleus to amplify the cccDNA pool. Potential targets of the HBV lifecycle (indicated by red crosses) include entry inhibitors, cccDNA degradation, immune modulation, RNA interference, assembly effectors, HBV DNA polymerase inhibitors, and HBsAg release inhibitors.

Ref: Lancet ID 16: e12, 2016

TABLE 2B (2)

Three Phases of Infection. The presence of HBsAg establishes the diagnosis of chronic hepatitis B. Not all patients successfully make it through all 3 phases: Immune tolerant phase (+HBeAg, +HBsAg, High level HBV DNA); Inflammatory phase (reduction in HBV DNA; Elevated transaminases); Non-Replicative phase (loss of HBeAg; reduction of HBV DNA; Normalization of ALT/AST).

FIGURE 2   Phases of HBV infection

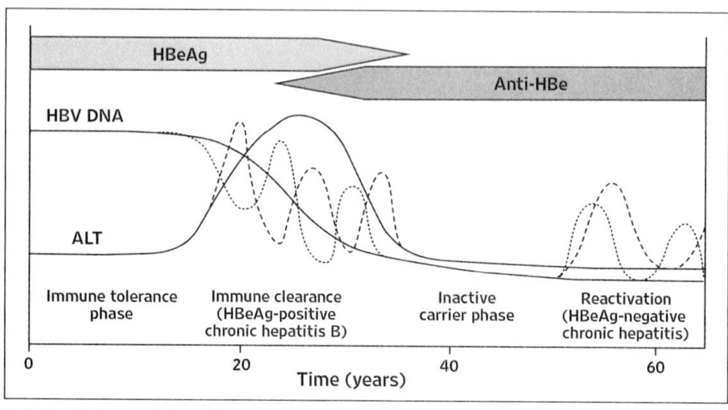

Ref: Clin Gastro Hep 12:16, 2014

Diagnostic Test Panels

Interpretation of Diagnostic Test Panels						
	Acute HBV	Inactive chronic HBV	Active Chronic HBV	Vaccinated / Immune	Cleared / Latent Infection	Occult HBV
HBsAg	+++	+	++	-	-	-
Anti-HBs	-	-	-	++	++	-
Anti-HBc (IgM)	++	-	-	-	-	-
Anti-HBc (IgG)	+++	+	+	-	+	+
HBeAg	+++	-	+/-	-	-	-
Anti-HBe	-	-	+/-	-	+/-	+/-
HBV DNA	+++	+	++/+++	-	-	+/-
ALT / AST	Elevated	Normal	Elevated	Normal	Normal	Normal

Chronic HBV. Chronic HBV is a dynamic disease and individuals with CHB can transition through different clinical phases with variable levels of serum ALT activity, HBV DNA, and HBV antigens. The levels of serum ALT and HBV DNA as well as liver fibrosis are important predictors of long-term outcome that inform decisions for treatment initiation as well as treatment response. Therefore, serial testing of ALT and HBV-DNA levels are needed to guide treatment decisions *(see HBV Guidelines: Hepatology 67: 1560, 2018)*.

Progression of Disease. The following factors are associated with faster progression (and higher rates of HCC): level of HBV DNA (strongest predictor of development of cirrhosis), family history of HCC or cirrhosis, older age, male, alcohol use, HIV co-infection, HCV co-infection.

TABLE 2C: CLINICAL PRESENTATION OF HBV

Symptoms. Patients with HBV are usually asymptomatic. When symptomatic, common complaints include: fatigue, nausea, anorexia, myalgias, arthralgias, asthenia, weight loss (except where ascites). Poor correlation between symptoms and disease stage or transaminase elevation.
Note: For patients with cirrhosis, abrupt change in clinical symptoms or lab findings suggests spontaneous bacterial peritonitis (SBP): tap ascites!

Signs. Depends on stage of disease. Skin disorders: spider angiomas. Stigmata of cirrhosis: ascites, jaundice, hepatomegaly, splenomegaly, peripheral edema, hemorrhoids, caput medusa.

Laboratory Abnormalities. Transaminase elevation: 1/3 normal transaminase levels, only 25% have > 2x ULN, poor correlation between transaminase elevation and liver history. Otherwise, no specific lab abnormalities except when cirrhotic or hepatic decompensation: low albumin, elevated bilirubin, AST/ALT ratio>1, low platelet count, cryoglobulinemia.

Extrahepatic Manifestations.

- Lymphoma
- mixed cryoglobulinemia
- glomerulonephritis (membranoproliferative)
- auto-antibody disorders (e.g., thyroiditis)
- PCT and Lichen planus
- diabetes mellitus
- polyarteritis nodosum

Staging. Current treatment recommendations depend, in part, on the amount of liver fibrosis and hepatic inflammation.
    a. **Liver biopsy is the gold standard.** *See Table 3D, page 13,* for Metavir Classification System (staging and histologic activity score).
    b. **Inflammation and fibrosis.** Battery of enzymes and serum proteins are used as a surrogate marker of hepatic inflammation and fibrosis. One example is the Fibrosure Index. Correlation with liver biopsy fibrosis is shown in Figure 2. Accuracy of Fibrosure result is best at the lower (<0.2) or higher (>0.8) values.
    c. **Child-Pugh Score and Model for End Stage Liver Disease (MELD).** *See Table 3D, page 14.*

FIGURE 3   Fibrosure Index Correlation to Fibrosis Stage

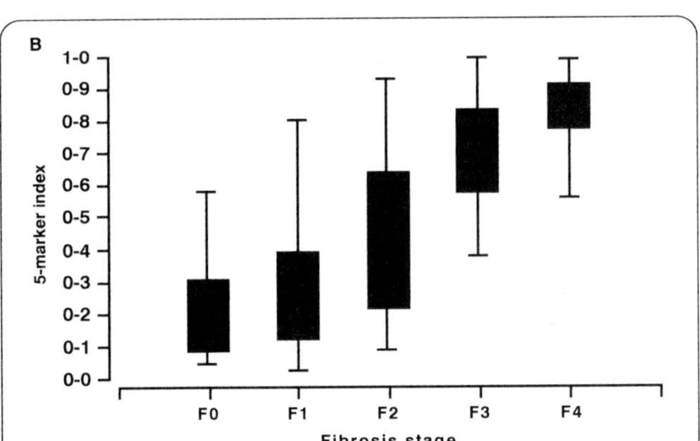

Ref: Imbert-Bismut, Lancet 2001

TABLE 2D: TREATMENT OF HBV (WITH & WITHOUT HIV CO-INFECTION)

Indications for Treatment. Decision to treat HBV infection is based on evidence of HBV viral replication (as evidenced by viral load and positive HBe antigen) and magnitude of liver fibrosis. Emerging trend toward using long-term nucleoside Rx for viremic patients with HBV. Reductions in progression and some reduction in risk of Hepatocellular Carcinoma *(Gastroenterology 147: 143-161, 2014)*.

When to Treat. The following are key indicators: HBeAg status, HBV viral load (HBV DNA), elevated liver enzymes (ALT level), cirrhosis. For HBeAg+ patients, treatment is typically deferred for 3-6 months to observe spontaneous seroconversion from HBeAg+ to negative.

When to Treat HBV					
HBeAg status	HBV DNA: "viral load"	ALT	Fibrosis*	Treatment** IFN = interferon; NUC = nucleoside/tide analogue	Comments
+	> 20,000	< 2x ULN	F0 – F2	Observe	Low efficacy with current Rx; biopsy helpful in determining whether to Rx. Lean toward Rx if older age or + Family Hx HCC
+	> 20,000	< 2x ULN	F3 - F4	Treat: IFN or NUC	No IFN if decompensated cirrhosis
+	> 20,000	> 2x ULN	Any	Treat: IFN or NUC	INF has higher chance of seroconversion to HBeAg Negative and HBsAg Negative status.
-	< 2000	< 1x ULN	Any	Observe	Might Treat if F4; **No IFN if decompensated cirrhosis.**
-	2000-20,000	< 2x ULN	F0 – F2	Observe	
-	2000-20,000	< 2x ULN	F3 – F4	Treat: NUC or (IFN)	NUCs favored if HBeAg negative; Treatment duration ill-defined. Certainly >1 yr, likely chronic Rx (indefinitely)
-	> 2,000	> 2x ULN	Any	Treat: NUC or IFN	NUCs favored if HBeAg negative; Treatment duration chronic / indefinite

References: *AASLD HBV Treatment Guidelines (Hepatology 67:1560, 2018; www.aasld.org); and EASL Guidelines (Hpt 57:167, 2012)*
* Liver Biopsy or fibrosure assay is helpful in determining when and how to treat
** Treatment options listed below

Treatment Regimens
- **If infected with HBV alone:** single drug therapy is usually sufficient.
- **If HBV-HIV coinfection:** combination therapy recommended; one of the agents should be a tenofovir derivative (TAF or TDF). If the patient cannot take tenofovir, then entecavir should be used.
- **If HBV-HCV co-infected:** watch closely for HBV flare when treating HCV. HCV treatment can lead to fulminant liver failure in rare cases.

	Drug/Dose	Comments
Preferred Regimens Many fewer AEs with oral regimens	**Entecavir** 0.5 mg po once daily OR **TDF** 300 mg po once daily OR **Pegylated-Interferon-alpha 2a** (PEG-IFN)180 µg sc once weekly	Entecavir: Do not use Entecavir if Lamivudine resistance present. Use 1 mg daily if cirrhosis present. Entecavir/Tenofovir: Treat for at least 24-48 weeks after seroconversion from HBeAg to anti-HBe. Indefinite chronic therapy for HBeAg negative patients. Renal impairment dose adjustments necessary. PEG-IFN: Treat for 48 weeks
Alternative Regimens	**Lamivudine** 100 mg po once daily OR **Telbivudine** 600 mg po once daily OR **Emtricitabine** 200 mg po once daily (investigational) OR **Adefovir** 10 mg po once daily	These alternative agents are rarely used except in combination. **When used, restrict to short term therapy owing to high rates of development of resistance.** Not recommended as first-line therapy. Use of Adefovir has mostly been replaced by Tenofovir. **Do not use adefovir in HIV infected patients.**
Preferred Regimen for HIV-HBV Co-Infected Patient	**Truvada or Descovy** (TDF 300 mg OR TAF 25 mg + **Emtricitabine** 200 mg) po once daily + another anti-HIV drug	ALL patients if possible as part of a fully suppressive anti-HIV/anti-HBV regimen. Tenofovir alafenamide (TAF) equally effective as tenofovir DF (TDF). Continue therapy indefinitely.

TDF = tenofovir disoproxil fumarate; **TAF** = tenofovir alafenamide fumarate

TABLE 2D (2)

Treatment Regimens *(continued)*

- The goal of therapy for HBeAg+ patients is seroconversion from positive to negative (but this rarely occurs). For HBeAg negative patients, the goal is suppression of HBV DNA viral load to < 50 IU/mL.

Summary of Sustained Viral Response After One Year of Therapy Note: low frequency of loss of HBeAg loss.						
	PEG-INF 2a	Lamivudine	Adefovir	Entecavir	Telbivudine	Tenofovir
HBeAg Seroconversion	27%	16-21%	12%	21%	22%	21%
HBV DNA <50 IU/mL	25-63%	60-73%	51-64%	67-90%	60-88%	80-95%
ALT normalization	39%	41-75%	48-61%	68%	60%	77%
HBeAg loss	3%	<1%	0	2%	<1%	3%
Viral Resistance	0	15-30%	Minimal	0	6%	0

Ref: Hpt 45:507, 2007.

Comments

- **All patients with HBV infection should be vaccinated against Hepatitis A.**
- **All patients with HBV should be evaluated for presence of Hepatitis D (HDV or Delta) virus infection.**
- Interferon best used in HBeAg+ patients; much higher conversion rates from HBeAg+ to HBeAg- and from HBsAg+ to HBsAg- with IFN compared to nucleoside regimens, if patient can tolerate IFN side effects.
- **IFN therapy** favored in **Genotype A (and B)** patients; and those who have lower HBV DNA, higher ALT, younger age, and women, all have higher seroconversion response rates.
- For those who seroconvert from HBeAg to anti-HBe, if consolidation therapy for one additional year, 20% will serorevert back to HBeAg+ status within 1 – 3 years. Ongoing monitoring is required for all patients.
- **NOTE: Return to active HBV replicative state, including HBsAg seroreversion, spikes in HBV DNA, and liver inflammation/damage, can occur when HBV infected patients receive chemotherapy or immunomodulating agents!** This is especially a concern when using Rituxan or for those patients receiving Stem Cell Transplantation. Use of a nucleoside agent recommended prior to the initiation of chemotherapy and /or immunotherapy in HBsAg positive patients and in selected HBsAg-, anti-HBS+, anti-HBc+ patients *(Hpt 61:763, 2015; JAMA 312:2505 & 2521, 2014).*
- All patients with cirrhosis, HBeAg+ status, older patients, and those with a positive family history of hepatocellular carcinoma (HCC) should have periodic (every 6 – 12 month) screening for HCC with an ultrasound (alpha-fetoprotein assay not recommended).
- **Resistance:** Lamivudine, Telbivudine, and Adefovir, when used as monotherapy are associated with high level resistance. Frequency of emergence of mutations increases with duration of therapy (> 6 months). Reviewed in *Lancet Inf Dis. 12: 341, 2012.*
- **Combination Therapy:** Under investigation. Early studies demonstrate higher rates of virologic success (HBV DNA < 50 IU/ml), HBeAg seroconversion, and possibly less emergence of resistance. Not yet recommended as primary mode of therapy except where resistance already exists, in patients with HIV-HBV co-infection, and for those with advanced disease and decompensated cirrhosis.
- Tenofovir alafenamide fumarate (TAF) formulation 25 mg ~equally active as standard tenofovir (TDF) against HBV. Used regularly in HIV-HBV co-infected patients, but not yet recommended as mono-therapy for mono-infected persons with HBV.

TABLE 2E: HEPATITIS B DRUGS IN DEVELOPMENT

New Drugs for Hepatitis B

- Most of the focus of newer drugs for HBV infection is to achieve cure. The barrier to cure is the elimination of the covalently closed-circular (ccc) DNA component of HBV. The targets for new therapeutic agents are shown in this figure from Lok *(J Hepatology 67: 487, 2017)*.

FIGURE 4   HBV Drug Development Targets

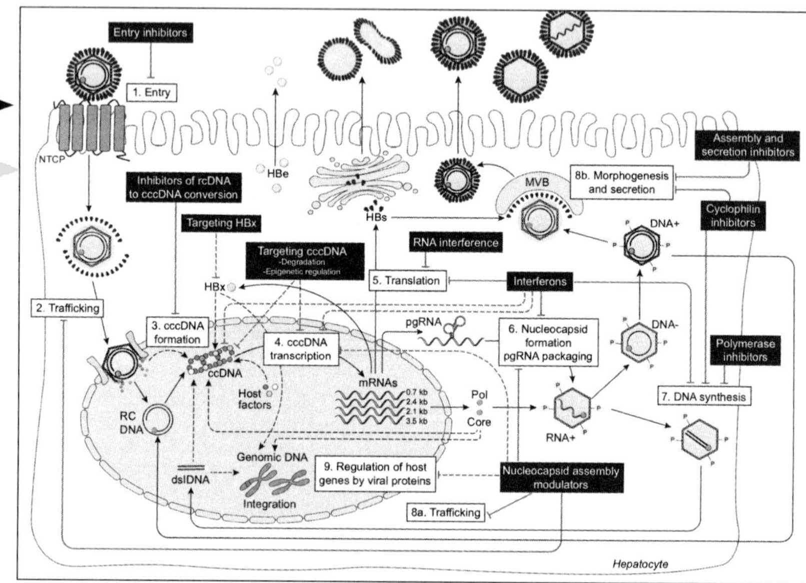

Ref: J Hepatology 67: 487, 2017

TABLE 2F: HEPATITIS D (DELTA) VIRUS

Hepatitis D (Delta) Virus

- Hepatitis D virus (HDV) is also known as "Delta" hepatitis
  - HDV is an incomplete RNA virus; missing envelop proteins
- Small circular RNA virus; replication defective. **Requires hepatitis B virus co-infection in order to survive and propagate in humans**
- Transmitted by blood and blood products or sexual transmission; Risk factors similar to those for HBV infection
- Infection with HDV can occur at the same time infection with HBV (leads to persistent infection < 10%) or can occur as a 'super-infection' of HBV at a later time (persistent infection ~80%)
- Super-infection of HBV can lead to dramatic deterioration of clinical status, including rapid liver failure and death in patients with pre-existing HBV.

Diagnosis: Antibody tests (Presence of IgM antibodies indicates acute infection) or HDV RNA PCR.

Treatment:

- **Acute infection / illness:** Supportive Care. Liver transplant may be required in cases of fulminant hepatitis.
- **Chronic infection: Alfa interferon 2b** (5 million units/m^2 3x/wk x 4 mos, then 3 million units/m^2 x additional 8 mos) can be used. Most effective when used early in course of therapy.
- It is unclear if successful treatment of HBV consistently eliminates HDV.

Prevention: HBV vaccination also protects against infection with HDV, owing to the requirement of HBV co-infection for Hepatitis D virus to survive and propagate

TABLE 3: HEPATITIS C VIRUS (HCV)

TABLE 3A: EPIDEMIOLOGY OF HEPATITIS C (HCV)

Caseload

180 million cases of Hepatitis C virus (HCV) worldwide. Highest rates in Africa and Asia. Egypt > 15% prevalence. 4.1 million cases in the U.S. (1.6%). Most patients infected prior to 1990 *(Hpt 49:1335, 2009)*. Approximately 20,000 new infections/year in the U.S. Most HCV infected persons do not know their status.

Risk of Transmission. Intravenous drug users (IDU) > blood products recipients > homosexual > heterosexual.

Sexual transmission	Number of sexual partners (2.2-2.9 relative risk (RR)). For persons with preexisting Herpes simplex (HSV) (3.85RR). Preexisting trichomonas (3.3 RR)
HIV	1.9-4.4 RR
Healthcare workers	Primary needle stick injury. Risk of HBV ≥ HCV > HIV, if not vaccinated for HBV.
Vertical transmission	

FIGURE 5   **Risk of Transmission of HCV**

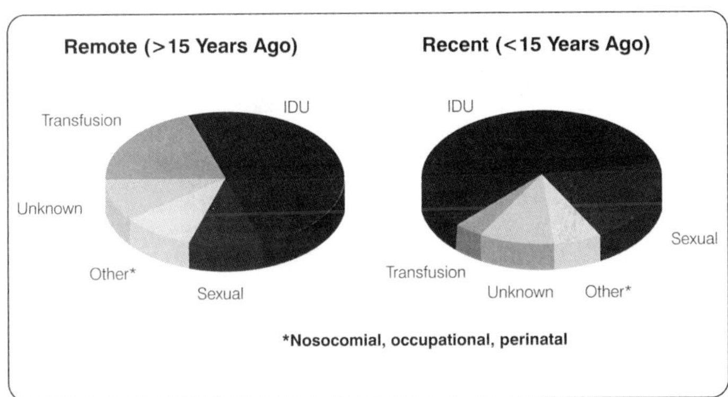

Ref: Alter MJ. N Engl J Med. 1999;341 ;556-562. CDC. MMWR. 1998;47:1

TABLE 3B: DIAGNOSIS OF HCV

Testing

Categories of HCV diagnostic tests and test type:
- HCV Antibody Test: EIA assay.
- HCV Quantitative Viral Load (HCV RNA): PCR.
- HCV Genotype 1-6: Sequencing.

HCV Quantitation Tests:

Assay (Mfg)	Method	Genotypes Detected	Linear Range (IU/mL)	Limit of Detection (Genotype 1 in Plasma)(IU/mL)	Lower Limit of Quantitation (IU/mL)
COBAS® TaqMan® HCV Test v2 (For use with High Pure System) (Roche Diagnostics)	Semi-automated RT-PCR	1-6	43-69,000,000	15	25
COBAS® AmpliPrep COBAS® TaqMan® HCV Test	Automated RT-PCR	1-6	25-300,000,000	7.1	43
Versant HCV RNA 3.0 Assay (Siemens Health Care Diagnostics)	Semi-automated bDNA signal amplification		615-7,700,000		615
Abbott RealTime HCV (Abbott Diagnostics)	Semi-automated RT-PCR		12-100,000,000		12

TABLE 3B (2)

FIGURE 6   HCV Testing Algorithm

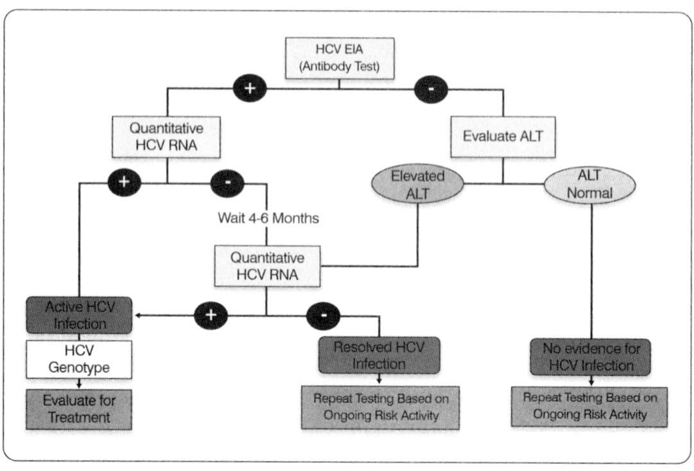

Ref: Cleveland Clinic J Med 70:S7, 2003

TABLE 3C: NATURAL HISTORY OF HCV INFECTION

Acute HCV

- Usually asymptomatic. If symptomatic, usually abates in days to weeks; rarely associated with hepatic failure. Typically leads to chronic infection–in 60-80% of cases (elevated transaminases).
- Factors associated with natural clearance include:
  - HLA-DRB1*1101 and DQB1*0301 haplotypes
  - Favorable IL-28B genetic status
  - Gene locus on chromosome 19 predicts response to IFN therapy
  - Low HCV viral load.
- Treatment of acute HCV usually results in "cure" (sustained virologic response–SVR). Therefore, Rx should be initiated within first 6 mos of infection when possible.

FIGURE 7   Chronic HCV Progression

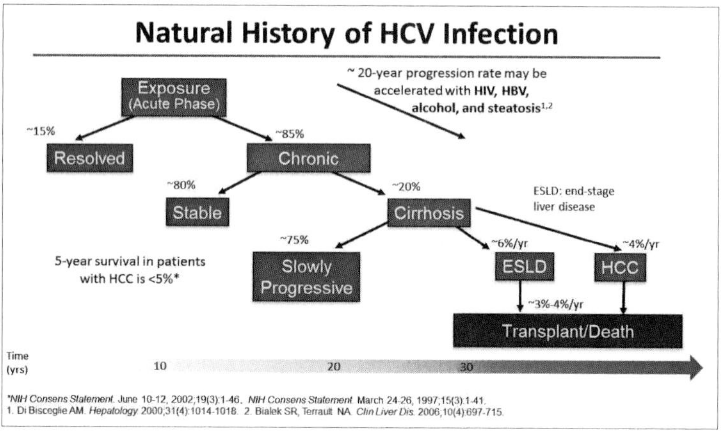

TABLE 3C (2)

Chronic HCV

Associated With Faster Progression	Survival
• Older age at time of infection • Male gender • Alcohol use • HIV Co-infection • HBV Co-infection • Acquisition or re-infection post-transplant	• With compensated cirrhosis: 5 years survival = 91% (10 year = 79%) • With decompensated cirrhosis: 5 years survival = 50%.

TABLE 3D: CLINICAL PRESENTATION OF HCV

Symptoms. Usually asymptomatic. When symptomatic, common complaints include: fatigue, nausea, anorexia, myalgias, arthralgias, asthenia, Weight loss (except where ascites). Note: there is poor correlation between symptoms and disease stage or transaminase elevations

Signs. Depends on stage of disease. Skin disorders: spider angiomas, porphyria cutanea tarda (PCT). Stigmata of cirrhosis: ascites, jaundice, hepatomegaly, splenomegaly, peripheral edema, hemorrhoids

Laboratory Abnormalities. Transaminase elevation: 1/3 normal transaminase levels, only 25% have > 2X ULN, poor correlation between transaminase elevation and liver histology. Otherwise, no specific lab abnormalities except when cirrhotic or hepatic decompensation: low albumin, elevated bilirubin, AST/ALT ratio > 1, low platelet count, cryoglobulinemia

Extrahepatic Manifestations.

- Lymphoma
- mixed cryoglobulinemia
- glomerulonephritis membranoproliferative)
- auto-antibody disorders (e.g. thyroiditis)
- PCT and Lichen planus
- diabetes mellitus

Staging
- **Liver Biopsy.** Liver Biopsy is the gold standard for HCV staging.

Metavir Classification System		
	F0	No scarring
	F1	Minimal scarring
Staging	F2	Scarring outside immediate area that contains blood vessels
	F3	Bridging fibrosis; spreading and connecting to other areas containing scarring
	F4	Cirrhosis; advance scarring of liver

Non-Invasive Tests
- **Most Commonly Used Liver Staging Tests:**
    - **FIB-4** = Age (yrs) x AST (U/L) / (Plt count (109/L) x √ (ALT (U/L))
        - FIB-4 value< 1.45 (fibrosis unlikely); > 3.25 (fibrosis likely)
    - **APRI** = AST (IU/L) / AST (Upper limit of Normal) (IU/L) /Platelet Count (109/L)
        - APRI value< 0.7 (fibrosis unlikely); > 1.0 (fibrosis likely)
    - **Fibroscan**: Optimal cut-offs: F0< 4.5 kPa; F2 ~ 7.1 kPa; F4: > 12.5 kPa
- The following is a **list of available non-invasive HCV tests,** i.e., in lieu of liver biopsy. AUC = area under ROC curve: indicates relative correlation with biopsy findings (F0-F4).

TABLE 3D (2)

Non-Invasive Tests *(continued)*

Score	Serum Markers	≥ F2 (%)	AUC ≥ F2	F4 (%)	AUC F4
Fibrosure (US) & Fibrotest (outside US)	GGT Haptoglobin Bilirubin Apolipoprotein A1 alpha-2-macroglobulin	33-74	0.74-0.89	3-25	0.82-0.92
Foms	Age GGT Cholesterol Platelets	32-59	0.75-0.91	3-20	-
APRI	AST Platelets	27-74	0.69-0.88	3-25	0.61-0.94
FIB-4	Age ALT AST Platelets	21-36	0.74-0.85	7	0.91
Hepascore	Age Sex alpha-2-macroglobulin Hyaluronate Bilirubin GGT	39-79	0.74-0.86	6-34	0.80-0.94
Fibrometer	Platelets Prothrombin time Macroglobulin AST Hyaluronate Age Urea	41-56	0.78-0.89	4-15	0.94
ELF	N-terminal propeptide of collagen type III Hyaluronic acid TIMP-1 Age	27-64	0.77-0.87	12-16	0.87-0.90
Fibroscan	Transient elastography	37-74	0.72-0.91	8-25	0.87-0.98

Modified from Martinez, Hpt 53:325, 2011.

Model for End-Stage Liver Disease (MELD) / Child-Pugh Score (A, B, or C)
- MELD score used to determine End-Stage Liver Disease

    MELD = 3.78 × $\log_e$ (bilirubin in mg/dl) + 11.2 × $\log^e$ (INR) + 9.57 × $\log_e$ (creatinine in mg/dL) + 6.43.
- If MELD score > 10, refer to hepatologist for transplantation evaluation

Child-Pugh Score (Add score from each Clinical Feature below)

Clinical Feature	Score: 1	Score: 2	Score: 3
Encephalopathy *(see below)*	None	Grade 1-2	Grade 3-4
Albumin	>3.5 gm/dL	2.8–3.5 gm/dL	<2.8 gm/dL
Total bilirubin	<2 mg/dL	2–3 mg/dL	>3 mg/dL
(If taking indinavir or if Gilbert's syndrome)	<4 mg/dL	4–7 mg/dL	>7 mg/dL
INR	<1.7	1.7-2.3	>2.3

Grade of Encephalopathy

Grade	Description
1	Mild confusion, anxiety, restlessness, fine tremor, slow coordination
2	Drowsiness, asterixis
3	Somnolent but arousable, marked confusion, speech incomprehensible, incontinent, hyperventilation
4	Coma, decerebrate posturing, flaccidity

Child-Pugh score Classification

Child-Pugh Total Score	Class
5-6	A
7-9	B
>9	C

TABLE 3E: HCV TREATMENT REGIMENS & RESPONSE

Indications for Treatment

- Treatment is indicated for all patients with chronic HCV. Rx should be initiated urgently for those with more advanced fibrosis (F3 / F4) and those with underlying co-morbid conditions due to HCV.
- Type and duration of Rx is based on genotype and stage of fibrosis. All DAA regimens with or without ribavirin are the preferred choice.
  - o Pegylated interferon (Peg-IFN) is no longer a recommended regimen.

Definitions of Response to Therapy

- **End of Treatment Response (ETR):** Undetectable at end of treatment.
- **Relapse:** Undetectable at end of therapy (ETR) but rebound (detectable) virus within 12 weeks after therapy stopped.
- **Sustained Virologic Response (SVR):** CURE! Still undetectable at end of therapy and beyond 12 weeks after therapy is stopped.

HCV Treatment Regimens

- Biopsy is a 'gold standard' for staging HCV infection and is helpful in some settings to determine the ideal timing of HCV treatment. When bx not obtained, "non-invasive" tests are often employed to assess the relative probability of advanced fibrosis or cirrhosis. Fibroscan (elastography) is now approved in the US and most of the world as a means of assessing liver fibrosis. Elastography values of >10 kPa (Kilopascals) correlates with significant fibrosis (F3 or F4 disease).
- **Resistance tests:** Genotypic resistance assays are available that can determine polymorphisms associated with reduction in susceptibility to some DAAs (Direct Acting Agents, e.g., protease inhibitors). However, resistance tests are recommended only for those who have failed treatment with a prior NS5A or protease inhibitor regimen.
- Patients with decompensated cirrhosis should only be treated by hepatologists owing to the risk of rapid clinical deterioration while receiving treatment for HCV.
- **Black Box Warning for ALL Direct Acting Agents (DAA):** Cases of HBV reactivation, occasionally fulminant, during or after DAA therapy have been reported in HBV/HCV coinfected patients who were not already on HBV suppressive therapy. See U.S. FDA Drug Safety Announcement, Oct 4, 2016. For HCV/HBV coinfected patients who are HBsAg+ and are not already on HBV suppressive therapy, monitoring HBV DNA levels during and immediately after DAA therapy for HCV is recommended and antiviral treatment for HBV should be given if treatment criteria for HBV are met. See HBV treatment.

DAAs for Initial Treatment

- See also *www.hcvguidelines.org* and *webedition.sanfordguide.com* for updates.
- Suffixes Matter:
  - o "______ previr" = Protease (NS3-4a) Inhibitor
  - o "______ asvir" = NS5a inhibitor
  - o "______ buvir" = Nucleoside / Non-nucleoside (NS5b) inhibitor

Agents/Abbreviation	Tradename	Formulation/Dosing
Daclatasvir (DCV)	Daklinza	60 mg tab po once daily. Note: decrease dose to 30 mg/d when co-administered with a strong CYP3A inhibitor, e.g., several ARV drugs; increase dose to 90 mg/d when co-administered with a mild-moderate CYP3A inducer. Contraindicated when co-administered with a strong CYP3A inducer.
Elbasvir + Grazoprevir	Zepatier	Fixed dose combination (Elbasvir 50 mg + Grazoprevir 100 mg) 1 tab po once daily
Glecaprevir + Pibrentasvir	Mavyret	Fixed dose combination (Glecaprevir 100 mg + Pibrentasvir 40 mg) 3 tabs once daily with food
Paritaprevir/Ritonavir + Ombitasvir (PrO)	Technivie	Fixed dose combination (Paritaprevir 150 mg/ritonavir 100 mg + Ombitasvir 25 mg) 1 tab once daily
Paritaprevir/Ritonavir + Ombitasvir + Dasabuvir (PrOD)	Viekira Pak	Fixed dose combination [(Paritaprevir 150 mg/ritonavir 100 mg + Ombitasvir 25 mg) 1 tab once daily + Dasabuvir 250 mg] 1 tab twice daily with food
	Viekira XR	Extended release fixed dose combination [(Dasabuvir 200 mg + Paritaprevir 50 mg/ritonavir 33.3 mg + Ombitasvir 8.33 mg) 3 tabs once daily with food
Simeprevir (SMV)	Olysio	150 mg tab po once daily with food
Sofosbuvir (SOF)	Sovaldi	400 mg tab po once daily

TABLE 3E (2)

Agents/Abbreviation	Tradename	Formulation/Dosing
DAAs for Initial Treatment *(continued)*		
Sofosbuvir + Ledipasvir	Harvoni	Fixed dose combination (Sofosbuvir 400 mg + Ledipasvir 90 mg) 1 tab po once daily
Sofosbuvir + Velpatasvir	Epclusa	Fixed dose combination (Sofosbuvir 400 mg + Velpatasvir 100 mg): 1 tab po once daily
Sofosbuvir + Velpatasvir + Voxilaprevir	Vosevi	Fixed dose combination (Sofosbuvir 400 mg + Velpatasvir 100 mg + Voxilaprevir 100 mg): 1 tab po once daily with food
Ribavirin	Copegus	Weight-based daily dosing: 1000 mg (Wt <75 kg) or 1200 mg (Wt >75 kg). Low dose: 600 mg/day. Taken with food.
Pegylated interferon (alfa 2a)	Roferon, Intron-A, Peg-Intron, Pegasys	180 mcg sc per week. Note: no longer a recommended regimen

Recommended Treatment Regimens

HCV Mono Infection (P = primary, A = alternative)

Genotype	P/A	Regimen	Without Cirrhosis	With Cirrhosis	Duration (Wks)	Comments
1-6	P	**Epclusa** 1 tab po once daily	X	X	12	Pan-genotypic
1-6	P	**Mavyret** 3 tabs po once daily	X		8	Pan-genotypic
				X	12	
1, 4, 5, 6	P	**Harvoni** 1 tab po once daily	X		8	If patient is non-black, HIV-uninfected, non-cirrhotic, and HCV RNA <6 million c/mL
				X	12	If patient is black, HIV-co-infected, compensated cirrhosis, or HCV RNA >6 million c/mL
1, 4	P	**Zepatier** 1 tab po once daily	X	X	12	If no baseline high-fold NS5A resistance associated mutations
1	A	**Viekira Pak** (as directed) +/- *****RBV** (if 1a)	X (only)		12	RBV dosing is wt-based (only use RBV if 1a; no RBV if 1b)
1, 2, 3	A	(**DCV** + **SOF**) po once daily	X (only)		12	
				X	24	+/- RBV (wt based dosing) for GT3
1	A	(**SOF** + **SMV** ± **RBV**) po divided twice	X (only)		12	RBV dosing is wt-based
3	A	**Vosevi** 1 tab po once daily		X	12	Use when RAS Y93H is present
4	A	**Technivie** once daily	X		12	
4	A	**Technivie** once daily + **RBV** twice daily		X	12	RBV dosing is wt-based

TABLE 3E (3)

HCV-HIV Co-infection

- Genotypes 1, 2 , 3
    - Same as for HCV mono-infection
    - Treat for 8-12 weeks. 8 weeks ONLY in HCV treatment naive co-infected patients receiving Mavyret; otherwise, minimum 12 weeks with any other regimen
    - Watch for drug-drug interactions. *See https://www.hep-druginteractions.org/*
- Genotypes 4, 5, 6
    - Not enough experience; if treatment required, use same as for HCV mono infection
- **General Comments / Warnings:**
    - **Ledipasvir/sofosbuvir should NOT be used with cobicistat when given with tenofovir disoproxil fumarate.**
    - **Dose adjustments of PPI therapy is required when either ledipasvir, glecaprevir, or velpatasvir is co-administered Paritaprevir/ritonavir/ombitasvir plus dasabuvir should NOT be used with darunavir, efavirenz, ritonavir-boosted lopinavir, or rilpivirine.**
    - **Simeprevir:** can ONLY be used with select antiretrovirals: raltegravir, rilpivirine, maraviroc, tenofovir, emtricitabine, lamivudine, and abacavir
    - **RBV should NOT be used with didanosine, stavudine, or zidovudine**

Decompensated Cirrhosis

Genotype	Regimen	Duration (Wks)	Comments
1-6	**Epclusa** 1 tab po once daily + **RBV**	12	RBV dosing is low dose (600 mg daily). If RBV-intolerant, treat without RBV for 24 weeks. If prior SOF or NS5A treatment experience, Use with low dose RBV for 24 weeks.
1, 4, 5, 6	**Harvoni** 1 tab po once daily + low dose (600 mg daily) **RBV**	12	If RBV-intolerant, treat without RBV for 24 weeks. If prior SOF or NS5A treatment experience, use with low dose RBV for 24 weeks.
2, 3	(**DCV** + **SOF**) po once daily + low dose 600 mg daily) **RBV**	12	If RBV-intolerant, 24 weeks without RBV

Post Liver Transplant (P = primary; A = alternative)

Genotype	P/A	Regimen	Cirrhosis	Duration (Wks)	Comments
1-6	P	**Mavyret** 3 tabs po once daily	Without	12	Alternative if compensated cirrhosis
1, 4, 5, 6	P	**Harvoni** 1 tab po once daily + **RBV**	With or without	12	RBV dosing is wt-based. Dose as tolerated.
2, 3	P	(**DCV** + **SOF**) po once daily + low dose **RBV**	With	12	Compensated or decompensated
1, 4, 5, 6	A	(**DCV** + **SOF**) po once daily + low dose **RBV**	Without	12	
2, 3	A	**Epclusa** 1 tab po once daily + **RBV**	With	12	Compensated or decompensated. RBV dosing is wt- based
2,3	A	**Mavyret** 3 tabs po once daily	With	12	Compensated
2, 3	A	**SOF** + **RBV** po daily		24	RBV initial dose 600 mg/day, increased monthly by 200 mg/day as tolerated up to max wt-based dose

TABLE 3E (4)

Clinically Significant NS5A resistance-Associated Variants (RAVs)

Wild-type Amino Acid (sensitive)	Position	Variant Amino Acid (reduced EBR activity)
M	28	A/G/T
Q	30	D/E/H/G/K/L/R
L	31	F/M/V
Y	93	C/H/N/S

Monitoring Response to Therapy

- Monitoring schedule is based on 12-week duration of therapy.
- If more than 12 weeks, continue monitoring every 4 weeks until end of therapy (EOT), then repeat labs per week 24 schedule.

	Before Starting Treatment	Baseline	At 2 Weeks (only if taking RBV)	At 4 Weeks	At 8 Weeks	At 12 weeks (EOT)	At 24 weeks	Every 6 months
CBC	X	X	X	X		X	Only if abnormal at EOT	
HCV RNA*				X		X	X[+]	
HIV RNA/ CD4 count (if HIV-HCV co-infection)	X	X					X	X
Abd US (if cirrhosis – F3/F4)	X						X	X
Clinic Visit	X	X		X (or telephone contact)	X (or telephone contact)	X	X	

CBC = complete blood count (watch for anemia in initial 2 weeks of therapy);
CMP = comprehensive metabolic pane.

* HCV Genotype, and when indicated, an HCV resistance assay (RAV testing recommended for Rx of pts with prior DAA therapy failure with an NS5a inhibitor).

[+] Virologic relapse is rare at 12 weeks or more post-Rx; nonetheless, some experts recommend repeat HCV RNA testing at 24-48 weeks post-EOT to confirm.

A 10-fold increase in alanine aminotransferase (ALT) activity at week 4 should prompt discontinuation of therapy. Any increase in ALT of less than 10-fold at week 4 and accompanied by any weakness, nausea, vomiting, jaundice, or significantly increased bilirubin, alkaline phosphatase, or international normalized ratio should also prompt discontinuation of therapy. Asymptomatic increases in ALT of less than 10-fold elevated at week 4 should be closely monitored and repeated at week 6 and week 8. If levels remain persistently elevated, consideration should be given to discontinuation of therapy.

TABLE 3F: HEPATITIS C DRUGS IN DEVELOPMENT

New Drugs In Development: Site of Action

- New drugs target several regions within the HCV genome:
- NS3-4a: HCV Serine Protease gene (NS3); Serine Protease Co-factor (NS4a)
- NS5a: Inhibition of viral particle assembly
- NS5b: RNA-Dependent/RNA Polymerase (Nucleosides/tides and Non-Nucleosides)
- Some new drugs enhance activity of Interferon (e.g., cyclophilin inhibitors).

Genetic Structure Map

- Hepatitis C Virus with Targets for Novel anti-HCV Agents:

TABLE 3F (2)

FIGURE 8   HCV Drug Development Targets

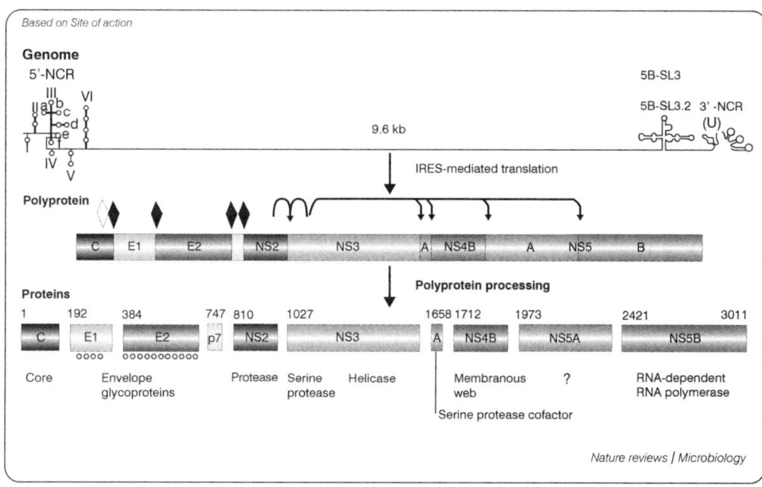

Ref: Nature Rev Microbiol 5:453, 2007.

FIGURE 9   Potential Therapeutic Targets in the HCV Replication Cycle

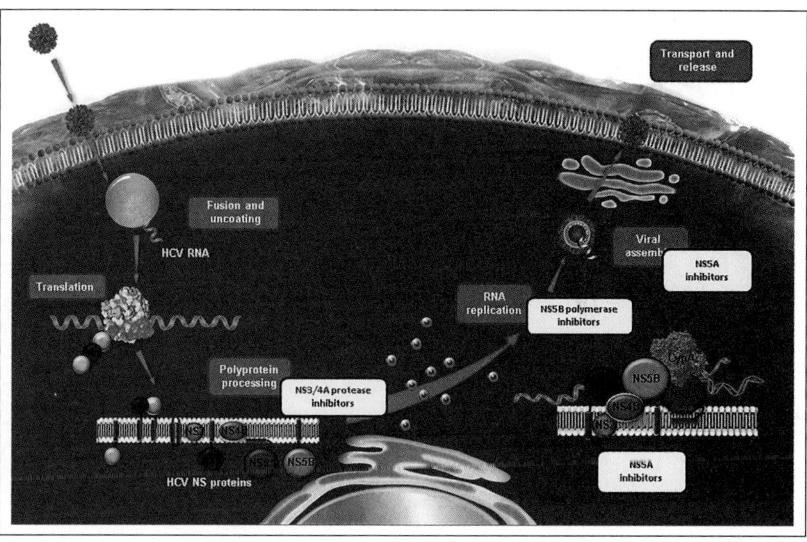

Ref: Curr HIV/AIDS Rep 12:68, 2015

TABLE 3F (3)

Selected direct acting agents in development

Site (Class)	Drug	Development Phase	Mfgr
NS3/4 (Protease Inhibitor) **First Generation** (all genotypes except genotype 3; low barrier to resistance)	Simeprevir	**Approved Dec 2013**	Janssen
	Faldaprevir (BI 1335)	II	Trek Pharma
	Vaniprevir (MK-7009)	III	Merck
	Narlaprevir (SCH 900518)	IIa	Merck
	Danoprevir/r	III	Roche
	Asunaprevir (BMS-650032)	III	Bristol Myers Squibb
	Sovaprevir (ACH-1625)	III	Achillion
	GS 9526	II	Gilead
	Paritaprevir/ritonavir	**Approved Dec 2014**	AbbVie
	IDX 320	II	Merck Idenix
	Vedroprevir (GS-9451)	III	Gilead
Second Generation PI (pan-genotypic; high barrier to resistance)	Glecaprevir (ABT-493)	**Approved Aug 2017**	Abbvie and Enanta
	ACH-2684	I	Achillion
	Grazoprevir (MK-5172)	**Approved Jan 2016**	Merck
	Voxilaprevir (GS-9857)	**Approved Jul 2017**	Gilead
NS5B (Nucleosides/tides)	Sofosbuvir	**Approved Dec 2013**	Gilead
	GS-938	IIb	Gilead
	VX-135	II	Vertex
	MK-3682 IDX-437	II	Merck Idenix
	IDX-459	II	Merck Idenix
	ACH-3422	I	Achillion
	Mericitabine	IIb/III	Roche
	AL-335	II	Janssen-Alios
	AL-516	I	Janssen-Alios
	MIV-802	I	Trek Pharma
NS5B (Non-nucleosides) Thumb domain I inhibitors	Beclabuvir (BMS-325)	III	BMS
	TMC-7055	II	Janssen
Thumb domain II inhibitors	GS-9669	II	Gilead
	Lomibuvir (VX 222)	IIb	Vertex
	CC-31244	Ia	Cocrystal Pharm
Palm domain I inhibitors	Dasabuvir (ABT-333)	**Approved Dec 2014**	AbbVie
	ABT-072	II	AbbVie
	Setrobuvir (ANA-598)	II	Roche
NS5A Inhibitors First Generation (most active vs Genotype 1 and 4)	Daclatasvir (BMS-052)	**Approved July 2015**	Bristol Myers Squibb
Genotype 1	Ledipasvir	**Approved Oct 2014**	Gilead
	Ombitasvir (ABT 267)	**Approved Dec 2014**	AbbVie
	(PPI-668)	II	Presidio
	PPI-461	II	Presidio
	ACH-2928	II	Achillion
	GSK 805	II	GSK
	BMS-393	II	Bristol Myers Squibb
	Samatasvir (IDX-719)	II	Merck Idenix
Second Generation (pan-genotypic)	Pibrentasvir (ABT 530)	**Approved Aug 2017**	Abbvie
	Odalasvir (ACH-3102)	III	Achillion-Janssen
	Velpatasvir (GS-5816)	**Approved June 2016**	Gilead
	Elbasvir (MK-8742)	**Approved Jan 2016**	Merck
	MK 8408	II	Merck
	CC-2069	IND	Cocrystal Phama
	TD-6450	I	Trek Pharma
Cyclophilin Inhibitor	Alisporivir	2b (FDA hold) Pancreatitis	Debiopharm
Peg-IFN	Peg-Lambda	III	BMS
Toll-like Receptor 7 Inhibitor	GS 9620	II	Gilead
MicroRNA (anti-miR-122)	Miravirsen	Ib / II	Santaris

TABLE 4: HEPATITIS E VIRUS

Hepatitis E Virus

- Hepatitis E virus (HEV) is a major cause of enterically-transmitted non-A, non-B viral hepatitis.
    - Caliciviridae family; but HEV has a substantially different genome than other members of this family of viruses
- Small spherical, non-enveloped, single stranded RNA virus
- Transmitted by exposure to fecally-contaminated water; typically in developing countries. Sporadic cases seen in developed countries; swine are thought to be reservoirs *(CID 36: 29-33, 2003)*
- Person-to-person infection rarely occurs
- Incubation period ~40 days post-exposure
- Usually acute hepatitis; chronic infection typically does not occur in Genotype 1, 2, or 4 HEV infection, but sporadic cases of chronic HEV infection is seen among immunocompromised Genotype 3 infected transplant patients in the developed world. The chronic HEV infection may lead to cirrhosis
- Acute infection in pregnant women can lead to fulminant hepatitis and death (similar to Hepatitis A)

Diagnosis: Antibody tests. Anti-HEV IgM and IgG antibody tests. IgM declines rapidly during early convalescence; IgG persists and provides some immunity

Treatment: Supportive care. No antiviral therapy currently available; some success (up to 78% SVR) to low dose (600 mg/d) ribavirin for 3 months among HEV chronically infected immunocompromized transplant patients *(NEJM 2014; 370:1111-1120)*. Reduction in the level of immunosuppression is advised in those developing chronic HEV infection.

Prevention: Provision of clean water supplies. Prudent hygienic practices, avoiding: drinking water or using ice of unknown purity, eating uncooked shellfish, eating uncooked fruits or vegetables that are not peeled or prepared by the traveler

Vaccine Development: A 3-dose (0, 1, 6 mos) recombinant HEV vaccine developed and currently licensed in China is efficacious and protective for up to 4.5 years *(NEJM 372:914, 2015)*.

TABLE 5: ANTI-HBV, -HCV DRUG DOSING & ADVERSE EFFECTS

DRUG NAME(S) GENERIC	DRUG TRADE NAME(S)	DOSAGE/ROUTE IN ADULTS*	COMMENTS/ADVERSE EFFECTS
Hepatitis B			
Adefovir dipivoxil	Hepsera	10 mg po q24h (with normal CrCl) 10 mg tab	It is an acyclic nucleotide analog with activity against hepatitis B (HBV) at 0.2-2.5 mM (IC_{50}). Active against lamivudine-resistant HBV strains and in vitro vs. entecavir- resistant strains. To minimize resistance, use in combination with lamivudine for lamivudine-resistant virus; consider alternative therapy if viral load remains >1,000 copies/mL with treatment. Primarily renal excretion-adjust dose. No food interactions. Generally few side effects, but **Black Box warning** regarding lactic acidosis/hepatic steatosis with nucleoside analogs. At 10 mg per day potential for delayed nephrotoxicity. Monitor renal function, esp. with pts with pre-existing or other risks for renal impairment. Pregnancy Category C. **Hepatitis may exacerbate when treatment discontinued;** Up to 25% of pts developed ALT ↑ 10 times normal within 12 wks; usually responds to re-treatment or self-limited, but hepatic decompensation has occurred. **Do not use adefovir in HIV infected patients.**
Interferon alfa	*See Table 5, page 25.*		
Entecavir	Baraclude	0.5 mg q24h. If refractory or resistant to lamivudine or telbivudine: 1 mg per day Tabs: 0.5 mg & 1 mg Oral solution: 0.05 mg/mL Administer on an empty stomach	A nucleoside analog active against HBV including lamivudine-resistant mutants. Minimal adverse effects reported: headache, fatigue, dizziness, & nausea reported in 22% of pts. Alopecia, anaphylactoid reactions reported. Potential for lactic acidosis and exacerbation of hepB at discontinuation (**Black Box warning**). Do not use as single anti-retroviral agent in HIV co-infected pts; M134 mutation can emerge *(NEJM 356:2614, 2007)*. Adjust dosage in renal impairment.
Lamivudine (3TC)	Epivir-HBV	**HBV** dose: 100 mg po q24h Dosage adjustment with renal dysfunction *(see label)* Tabs: 100 mg and oral solution 5 mg/mL	**Black Box warnings:** caution, dose is lower than HIV dose, so must exclude co-infection with HIV before using this formulation; lactic acidosis/hepatic steatosis; severe exacerbation of liver disease can occur on dc. YMDD- mutants resistant to lamivudine may emerge on treatment.
Telbivudine	Tyzeka	**HBV**: 600 mg orally q24h, without regard to food Dosage adjustment with renal dysfunction, Ccr <50 mL/min *(see label)* 600 mg tabs; 100 mg per 5 mL solution.	An oral nucleoside analog approved for Rx of Hep B. It has ↑ rates of response and superior viral suppression than lamivudine *(NEJM357:2576, 2007)*. **Black Box warnings** regarding lactic acidosis/hepatic steatosis with nucleosides and potential for severe exacerbation of HepB on dc. Generally well-tolerated with ↓ mitochondrial toxicity vs other nucleosides and no dose limiting toxicity observed *(MedicalLetter49:11, 2007)*. Myalgias, myopathy and rhabdomyolysis reported. Peripheral neuropathy. Genotypic resistance rate was 4.4% by one yr, ↑ to 21.5% by 2 yrs of rx of eAg+ pts. Selects for YMDD mutation like lamivudine. Combination with lamivudine was inferior to monotherapy *(Hepatology 45:507, 2007)*.

NOTE: All dosage recommendations are for adults (unless otherwise indicated) and assume normal renal function.

DRUG NAME(S) GENERIC	DRUG TRADE NAME(S)	DOSAGE/ROUTE IN ADULTS*	COMMENTS/ADVERSE EFFECTS
Tenofovir disoproxil fumarate (TDF); Tenofovir alafenamide fumarate (TAF)	Viread (TDF) Vemlidy (TAF)	TDF: 300 mg po q24h TAF: 25 mg po q24h	Diarrhea 11%, nausea 8%, vomiting 5%, flatulence 4% (generally well tolerated). **Black Box Warning:** Severe exacerbations of hepatitis B reported in pts who stop tenofovir. Monitor carefully if drug is stopped; anti-HBV rx may be warranted if TDF stopped. Reports of renal injury from TDF, including Fanconi syndrome (*CID 37:e174, 2003; J AIDS 35:269,204; CID 42:283, 2006*). Fanconi syndrome and diabetes insipidus reported with TDF + ddI (*AIDS Reader 19:114, 2009*). Modest decline in renal function appears greater with TDF than with NRTIs (*CID 51:296, 2010*) or TAF and may be greater in those receiving TDF with a PI instead of an NNRTI (*JID 197:102, 2008; AIDS 26:567, 2012*). In a VA study that followed >10,000 HIV-infected individuals. TDF exposure was significantly associated with increased risk of proteinuria, a more rapid decline in renal function and chronic kidney disease (*AIDS 26:867, 2012*). Monitor Ccr, serum phosphate and urinalysis, especially carefully in those with pre-existing renal dysfunction or nephrotoxic medications. TDF, but not TAF, also appears to be associated with increased risk of bone loss. In a substudy of an ACTG comparative treatment trial, those randomized to TDF-FTC experienced greater decreases in spine and hip bone mineral density (BMD) at 96 weeks compared with those treated with ABC-3TC (*JID 203:1791, 2011*). Consider monitoring BMD in those with history of pathologic fractures, or who have risks for osteoporosis or bone loss.

Hepatitis C - (For all HCV direct acting agents (DAA) a **Black Box warning** exists regarding potential flare of HBV when HCV is cured among those coinfected with HBV and HCV)

Direct Acting Agents (DAA):

DRUG NAME(S) GENERIC	DRUG TRADE NAME(S)	DOSAGE/ROUTE IN ADULTS*	COMMENTS/ADVERSE EFFECTS
Daclatasvir	Daklirza	60 mg 1 tab po once daily (dose adjustment when used with CYP 3A4 inhibitors/inducers)	Contraindicated with strong CYP3A inducers, e.g., phenytoin, carbamazepine, Rifampin, St. John's wort. Most common AE: headache and fatigue. Bradycardia when administered in combination with Sofosbuvir and Amiodarone. **Co-administration with Amiodarone not recommended.** If used, cardiac monitoring advised.
Elbasvir + Grazoprevir	Zepatie	Combination formulation (Elbasvir 50 mg + Grazoprevir 100 mg) 1 tab po once daily	NS5A and NS3-4a PI inhibitors with activity against genotypes 1 and 4. Contraindicated in patients with moderate or severe hepatic impairment (Child-Pugh Class B or C). Also contraindicated with concomitant use of organic ion transporter polypeptide 1B (OATP1B) inhibitors, strong inducers of cytochrome P450 3A (CYP3A), and efavirenz.
Glecaprevir + Pibrentasvir	Mavyret	Combination formulation (Glecaprevir 100 mg + Pibrentasvir 40 mg) 3 tabs po once daily with food	Contraindicated if severe hepatic impairment (Child-Pugh C). **Do not co-administer with Atazanavir or Rifampin.** Most common AEs: headache and fatigue.

NOTE: All dosage recommendations are for adults (unless otherwise indicated) and assume normal renal function.

TABLE 5 (3)

DRUG NAME(S) GENERIC	DRUG TRADE NAME(S)	DOSAGE/ROUTE IN ADULTS*	COMMENTS/ADVERSE EFFECTS
Ledipasvir + Sofosbuvir **Velpatasvir + Sofosbuvir** **Voxilaprevir +** **Velpatasvir + Sofosbuvir**	Harvoni Epclusa Vosevi	Combination formulations: (Ledipasvir 90 mg + Sofosbuvir 400 mg) 1 tab po once daily; (Velpatasvir 100 mg + Sofosbuvir 400 mg) 1 tab po daily; Voxilaprevir 100 mg + Velpatasvir 100 mg + Sofosbuvir 400 mg) 1 tab po once daily with food	NS5A/NS5B inhibitor combination for Genotype 1 HCV. First agent for HCV treatment without Ribavirin or Interferon. No adjustment for mile/moderate renal or hepatic impairment. Most common AEs: fatigue (16%), headache (14%), nausea (7%), diarrhea (3%), insomnia (5%). Antacids and H2 blockers interfere with absorption of ledipasvir. The drug solubility decreases as pH increases. Recommended to separate administration of ledipasvir and antacid Rx by at least 4 hours.
Paritaprevir + Ritonavir + Ombitasvir + Dasabuvir **Paritaprevir + Ritonavir + Ombitasvir**	PrOD Viekira P Technivie	Ombitasvir 12.5 mg, Paritaprevir 75 mg, and Ritonavir 50 mg co-packaged with tablets of Dasabuvir 250 mg (Viekira Pak); or without Dasabuvir (Technivie)	Do not co-administer with drugs that are highly dependent on CYP3A for clearance; strong inducers of CYP3A and CYP2C8; and strong inhibitors of CYP2C8. Do not use if known hypersensitivity to Ritonavir (e.g., toxic epidermal necrolysis, Stevens-Johnson syndrome). If used with Ribavirin: fatigue, nausea, pruritus, other skin reactions, insomnia and asthenia. When used without Ribavirin: nausea, pruritus and insomnia. **Warning: Hepatic decompensation and hepatic failure, including liver transplantation or fatal outcomes, have been reported mostly in patients with advanced cirrhosis.**
Simeprevir	Olysio	150 mg 1 cap po once daily with food + both Ribavirin and Interferon	NS3/4A inhibitor. Need to screen patients with HCV genotype 1a for the Q80K polymorphism; if present consider alternative therapy. Contraindicated in pregnancy and in men whose female partners are pregnant (risk category C); concern is combination with ribavirin (risk category X). No dose adjustment required in patients with mild, moderate or severe renal impairment; no dose adjustment for mild hepatic impairment. Most common AEs (in combination with Ribavirin, Interferon): rash, pruritus, nausea. CYP3A inhibitors affect plasma concentration of Simeprevir.
Sofosbuvir	Sovaldi	400 mg 1 tab po once daily with food + both Pegylated Interferon and Ribavirin. For combination formulation, *see Ledipasvir.*	NS5B inhibitor for Genotypes 1, 2, 3, 4 HCV. Efficacy established in patients awaiting liver transplant and in patients with HIV-1/HCV co-infection. No adjustment needed for mild to moderate renal impairment. No dose adjustment for mild, moderate, or severe hepatic impairment. Most common AEs (in combination with interferon and ribavirin): fatigue, headache, nausea, insomnia, anemia. Rifampin and St. John's wort may alter concentrations of Sofosbuvir.

NOTE: All dosage recommendations are for adults (unless otherwise indicated) and assume normal renal function.

TABLE 5 (4)

DRUG NAME(S) GENERIC	DRUG TRADE NAME(S)	DOSAGE/ROUTE IN ADULTS*	COMMENTS/ADVERSE EFFECTS
Other:			
Note: Interferon-based regimens for treatment of HCV are no longer recommended. Interferon alpha remains relevant to HBV treatment.			
Interferon alfa is available as: alfa-2a; alfa-2b	Roferon-A; Intron-A Intron-A	For HCV combination therapy, usual Roferon-A and Intron-A doses are 3 million international units 3x weekly subQ.	Depending on agent, available in pre-filled syringes, vials of solution, or powder. **Black Box warnings:** can cause/aggravate psychiatric illness, autoimmune disorders, ischemic events, infection. Withdraw therapy if any of these suspected. **Adverse effects: Flu-like syndrome** is common, esp. during 1st wk of rx: fever 98%, fatigue 89%, myalgia 73%, headache 71%. **GI:** anorexia 46%, diarrhea 29%. CNS: dizziness 21%. Hemorrhagic or ischemic stroke. Rash 18%, may progress to Stevens Johnson or exfoliative dermatitis. Alopecia. ↑ TSH, autoimmune thyroid disorders with T ↓- or ↑- thyroidism. **Hematol:** ↓ WBC 49%, ↓ Hgb 27%, ↓ platelets 35%. Post-marketing reports of antibody-mediated pure red cell aplasia in patients receiving interferon/ribavirin with erythropoiesis- stimulating agents. Acute reversible hearing loss &/or tinnitus in up to 1/3 *(Ln 343:1134, 1994)*. Optic neuropathy (retinal hemorrhage, cotton wool spots, ↓ in color vision) reported *(AIDS 18:1805, 2004)*. Doses may require adjustment (or dc) based on individual response or adverse events, and can vary by product, indication (eg, HCV or HBV) and mode of use (mono- or combination-rx). (Refer to labels of individual products and to ribavirin if used in combination for details of use).
PEG interferon alfa-2b (PEG-Intron)	PEG-Intron	0.5-1.5 mcg/kg subQ q wk	
Pegylated-40k interferon alfa-2a	Pegasys	180 mcg subQ q wk	
Ribavirin	Rebetol, Copegus	For use with an interferon for hepatitis C. Available as 200 mg caps and 40 mg/mL oral solution (Rebetol) or 200 mg and 400 mg tabs (Copegus) *See Comments regarding dosage*	**Black Box warnings:** ribavirin monotherapy of HCV is ineffective; hemolytic anemia may precipitate cardiac events; teratogenic/ embryocidal **(Preg Category X).** Drug may persist for 6 mos, avoid pregnancy for at least 6 mos after end of rx of women or their partners. Only approved for pts with Ccr >50 mL/min. Do not use in pts with severe heart disease or hemoglobinopathies. ARDS reported *(Chest 124:406, 2003)*. **Adverse effects:** hemolytic anemia (may require dose reduction or dc), dental/periodontal disorders, and all adverse effects of concomitant interferon used *(see above)*. Postmarketing: retinal detachment, ↓ hearing, hypersensitivity reactions. Dosing depends on: weight, HCV genotype, and is modified (or dc) based on side effects (especially degree of hemolysis, with different criteria in those with/without cardiac disease). **Initial Rebetrol dose with Intron A (interferon alfa-2b) is wt-based:** 400 mg am & 600 mg pm for ≤75 kg, and 600 mg am & 600 mg pm for wt >75 kg, but with Pegintron approved dose is 400 mg am & 400 mg pm with meals. Doses and duration of Copegus with peg-interferon alfa-2a are less in pts with genotype 2 or 3 (800 mg per day divided into 2 doses, for 24 wks) than with genotypes 1 or 4 (1000 mg per day divided into 2 doses for wt >>75 kg and 1200 mg per day divided into 2 doses for ≥75 kg for 48 wks); in HIV/HCV co-infected pts, dose is 800 mg per day regardless of genotype. *See individual labels for details, including initial dosing and criteria for dose modification in those with/without cardiac disease.*

NOTE: All dosage recommendations are for adults (unless otherwise indicated) and assume normal renal function.

TABLE 6: PHARMACOLOGY AND INTERACTIONS

For Drug-Drug Interactions, *see The Sanford Guide to Antimicrobial Therapy 2019, Table 22A* and *http://hep-druginteractions.org*

TABLE 6A: PHARMACOLOGY, PHARMACODYNAMICS OF ANTI-HEPATITIS DRUGS

DRUG	REFERENCE DOSE (SINGLE OR MULTIPLE)	PREG RISK	FOOD REC (PO)[1]	ORAL ABS (%)	PEAK SERUM CONC[2] (µg/mL)	PROTEIN BINDING (%)	VOLUME OF DISTRIBUTION (Vd)[3]	AVG SERUM T½ (hr)[4]	INTRACELL T½ (HR)	CPE[5]	AUC[6] (µg*hr/mL)	Tmax (hr)
HEPATITIS B												
Adefovir	10 mg po	C	Tab ± food	59	0.02 (SD)	≤4	0.37 L/kg Vss	7.5			0.22	1.75
Emtricitabine (FTC)	200 mg po q24h	B	Cap/soln ± food	cap 93, soln 75	1.8 (SS)	<4	ND	10	39	3	10 (24 hr)	1-2
Entecavir	0.5 mg po q24h	C	Tab/soln no food	100	4.2 ng/mL (SS)	13	>0.6 L/kg V/F	128-149			0.14	0.5-1.5
Lamivudine (3TC)	300 mg po q24h	C	Tab/soln ± food	86	2.6 (SS)	<36	1.3 L/kg	5-7	18	2	11 (300 mg x1)	ND
Telbivudine	600 mg po q24h	B	Tab/soln ± food		3.7 (SS)	3.3	>0.6 L/kg V/F	40-49			26.1 (24 hr)	2
Tenofovir alafenamide fumarate (TAF)	25 mg po q24h	No human data	Tab + food	ND	0.27 (SS)	80	ND	0.51	No data	No data	0.27 (24 hr)	0.48
Tenofovir disoproxil fumarate (TDF)	300 mg po q24h	B	Tab ± food	39 w/food	0.3 (300 mg x1)	<7	1.2-1.3 L/kg Vss	17	>60	1	2.3 (300 mg x1)	1

[1] Refers to adult oral preparations unless otherwise noted; + food = take with food, no food = take without food, ± food = take with or without food

[2] SD = after a single dose, SS = at steady state

[3] V/F = Vd/oral bioavailability; Vss = Vd at steady state; Vss/F = Vd at steady state/oral bioavailability

[4] Assumes CrCl >80 mL/min

[5] CPE (CNS Penetration Effectiveness) value: 1=low penetration, 2-3=intermediate penetration, 4=highest penetration (Letendre et al, CROI 2010, abs #430)

[6] AUC = area under serum concentration vs. time curve; 12 hr = AUC 0-12, 24 hr = AUC 0-24

TABLE 6A (2)

DRUG	REFERENCE DOSE (SINGLE OR MULTIPLE)	PREG RISK	FOOD REC (PO)[1]	ORAL ABS (%)	PEAK SERUM CONC[2] (μg/mL)	PROTEIN BINDING (%)	VOLUME OF DISTRIBUTION (Vd)[3]	AVG SERUM T½ (hr)[4]	AUC[5] (μg·hr/mL)	Tmax (hr)
HEPATITIS C										
Dasabuvir	250 mg po q12h	B	Tab + food	ND	0.03-3.1 (10-1200 mg SD)	ND	ND	5-8	ND	3
Daclatasvir	60 mg po q24h	ND	Tab ± food	67	0.18 (Cmin, SS)	99	47 Vss	12-15	ND	ND
Elbasvir	50 mg + 100 mg Grazoprevir	ND	Tab ± food	ND	0.121 (SS)	>99.9	680L	24	1.92 (24 hr)	3
Glecaprevir/ Pibrentasvir	Gle 300 mg + Pib 120 mg q24h	ND	Tab + food	ND	Gle 0.6, Pib 0.11 (SS)	Gle 97.5, Pib >99.9	ND	Gle 6, Pib 13	Gle 4.8, Pib 1.43 (24 hr)	Gle 5, Pib 5
Grazoprevir	100 mg – 50 mg Elbasvir	ND	Tab ± food	ND	0.165 (SS)	>98.8	1250L	31	1.42 (24 hr)	2
Ledipasvir/ Sofosbuvir	(90 mg + 400 mg) po q24h	B	Tab ± food	ND	**LDV**: 0.3 (SS)	**LDV**: >99.8	ND	**LDV**: 47	**LDV**: 7.3 (24 hr)	**LDV**: 4-4.5
Ombitasvir (with Paritaprevir/RTV)	25 mg po q24h	B	Tab + food	ND	0.56 (SS)	ND	ND	28-34	0.53 (24 hr)	4-5
Paritaprevir/RTV (with Ombitasvir)	150 mg (+ RTV 100 mg) po q24h	B	Tab + food	ND	ND	ND	ND	5.8	ND	4.3
Ribavirin	600 mg po	X	Tab/cap/ soln + food	64	0.8 (SD)	minimal	2825 L V/F	44	25.4	2
Simeprevir	150 mg po	C	Cap + food	ND	ND	>99.9	ND	41	57.5 (24 hr)	4-6
Sofosbuvir	400 mg po q24h	B	Tab ± food	ND	**SOF**: 0.6 (SS)	**SOF**: 61-65	ND	**SOF**: 0.5-0.75	**SOF**: 0.9-1.3 (24 hr)	0.5-2
Velpatasvir (+ Sofosbuvir)	(100 mg + 400 mg) po q24h	B	Tab + food	ND						
Voxilaprevir/ Velpatasvir/ Sofosbuvir	Vox 2.6, Vel 4.0, Sof 1.7 (24 hr)	ND	Tab + food	ND	Vox 0.19, Vel 0.31, Sof 0.68 (SS)	Vox >99, Vel>99, Sof 61-65	ND	Vox 33, Vel 17, Sof 0.5	Vox 2.6, Vel 4.0, Sof 1.7 (24 hr)	Vox 4, Vel 4, Sof 2

[1] Refers to adult oral preparations unless otherwise noted; + food = take with food, no food = take without food, ± food = take with or without food

[2] SD = after a single dose, SS = at steady state

[3] V/F = Vd/oral bioavailability; Vss = Vd at steady state; Vss/F = Vd at steady state/oral bioavailability

[4] Assumes CrCl >80 mL/min

[5] AUC = area under serum concentration vs. time curve; 12 hr = AUC 0-12, 24 hr = AUC 0-24

TABLE 6B: ENZYME- & TRANSPORTER-MEDIATED INTERACTIONS

DRUG	Substrate	Inhibits	Impact
Daclatasvir	3A4, PGP	PGP, OATP1B1/3, BCRP	↑
Dasabuvir	3A4, PGP, OATP1B1	2C8, UGT1A1, OATP1B1, OATP1B3	↑
Elbasvir	CYP3A4, PGP	BCRP	↑
Glecaprevir	PGP, BCRP, OATP1B1/3	1A2 (weak), 3A4 (weak), PGP, BCRP, OATP1B1/3, UGT1A1 (weak)	↑
Grazoprevir	CYP3A4, PGP, OATP1B1/3	CYP3A4 (weak), BCRP	↑
Ledipasvir	PGP, BCRP	PGP, BCRP	↑
Ombitasvir	3A4, PGP	2C8, UGT1A1	↑
Paritaprevir	2C8, 2D6, 3A4, PGP	UGT1A1, OATP1B1	↑
Pibrentasvir	PGP, BCRP	1A2 (weak), 3A4 (weak), PGP, BCRP,OATP1B1/3, UGT1A1 (weak)	↑
Simeprevir	3A4, PGP, OATP1B1/3	1A2 (weak), 3A4 (gut only), PGP, OATP1B1/3	↑
Sofosbuvir	PGP, BCRP		No effect expected
Velpatasvir	2B6, 2C8, 3A4 PGP, BCRP, OATP1B1/3	PGP, BCRP, OATP1B1/3, OATP2B1	↑

TABLE 7: DOSING ADJUSTMENTS FOR RENAL IMPAIRMENT

- Adjustments for renal failure are based on an estimate of creatinine clearance (CrCl) which reflects the glomerular filtration rate.
- **Different methods for calculating estimated CrCl are suggested for non-obese and obese patients.**
  - Calculations for ideal body weight (IBW) in kg:
    - *Men:* 50 kg plus 2.3 kg/inch over 60 inches height.
    - *Women:* 45 kg plus 2.3 kg/inch over 60 inches height.
  - Obese is defined as 20% over ideal body weight or body mass index (BMI) >30
- Calculations of estimated CrCl. For References, see *NEJM 354:2473, 2006* (non-obese); *AJM 84:1053, 1988* (obese).
  - **Non-obese patient—**
    - Calculate ideal body weight (IBW) in kg (as above)
    - Use the following formula to determine estimated CrCl

$$\frac{(140 \text{ minus age})(\text{IBW in kg})}{72 \times \text{serum creatinine}} = \text{CrCl in mL/min for men. Multiply answer by 0.85 for women (estimated)}$$

  - **Obese patient—**
    - Weight ≥20% over IBW or BMI >30
    - Use the following formulas to determine estimated CrCl

$$\frac{(137 \text{ minus age}) \times [(0.285 \times \text{wt in kg}) + (12.1 \times \text{ht in meters}^2)]}{51 \times \text{serum creatinine}} = \text{CrCl (obese male)}$$

$$\frac{(146 \text{ minus age}) \times [(0.287 \times \text{wt in kg}) + (9.74 \times \text{ht in meters}^2)]}{60 \times \text{serum creatinine}} = \text{CrCl (obese female)}$$

- What weight should be used to calculate dosage on a mg/kg basis?
  - If less than 20% over IBW, use the patient's actual weight for all drugs.
  - **For obese patients** (≥20% over IBW or BMI >30).
    - **Aminoglycosides:** (IBW plus 0.4(actual weight minus IBW) = adjusted weight.
    - **Vancomycin:** actual body weight whether non-obese or obese.
    - **All other drugs:** insufficient data *(Pharmacotherapy 27:1081, 2007).*
- For slow or sustained extended daily dialysis **(SLEDD)** over 6-12 hours, adjust does as for CRRT. For details, *see CID 49:433, 2009; CCM 39:560, 2011.*
- General reference: Drug Prescribing in Renal Failure, 5th ed., Aronoff, et al. (eds) *(Amer College Physicians, 2007 and drug package inserts).*

TABLE 7 (2)

ANTIMICROBIAL	HALF-LIFE (NORMAL/ESRD) hr	DOSE FOR NORMAL RENAL FUNCTION	ADJUSTMENT FOR RENAL FAILURE Estimated creatinine clearance (CrCl), mL/min			HEMODIALYSIS, CAPD	COMMENTS & DOSAGE FOR CRRT
			>50–90	10–50	<10		
Adefovir	7.5/15	10 mg po q24h	10 mg q24h	10 mg q48–72h	10 mg q72h	HEMO: 10 mg q week AD	CAPD: No data; CRRT: Dose?
Daclatasvir	12-⁻5/No data	60 mg q24h	No change	No change	No change	No data	No data
Emtricitabine (CAPS)	10/>10	200 mg q24h	200 mg q24h	**30–49:** 200 mg q48h **10–29:** 200 mg q72h	200 mg q96h	HEMO: Dose for CrCl <10	*See package insert for oral solution.*
Emtricitabine + TDF	See each drug	200-300 mg q24h	No change	**30–50:** 1 tab q48h	**CrCl <30:** Do not use		
Entecavir	128–149/No data	0.5 mg q24h	0.5 mg q24h	0.15–0.25 mg q24h	0.05 mg q24h	HEMO/CAPD: 0.05 mg q24h	Give after dialysis on dialysis days
Epclusa	velpat ⁻5, sofos 0.5/ No data	1 tab po q24h	1 tab po q24h	Use with caution (no data for use in patients with CrCl<30)		No data	No data
Harvoni	ledipasvir 47/No data	1 tab po q24h	1 tab q24h	Use with caution (no data for use in patients with CrCl<30)		No data	No data
Lamivudine	5–7/15–35	300 mg po q24h	300 mg po q24h	50–150 mg q24h	25–50 mg q24h	HEMO: Dose AD; CAPD: Dose for CrCl<10. CRRT: 100 mg 1st day, then 50 mg/day.
Ribavirin							
Simeprevir		(no adjustment; use with caution if CrCl <30 mL/min; RBV if CrCl <50 mL/min)					
Sofosbuvir							
Telbivudine	40-49/No data	600 mg po daily	600 mg q24h	**30-49:** 600 mg q48h **<30:** 600 mg q72h	600 mg q96h	HEMO: As for CrCl <10 AD	
TDF, po	17/?	300 mg q24h	300 mg q24h	**30-49:** 300 mg q48h **10-29:** 300 mg q72-96h	No data	HEMO: 300 mg q7d or after 12 hrs of HEMO[1]	
Technivie	omb t 28-34, parita 5.8/No data	2 tabs po q24h	2 tabs q24h	2 tabs q24h	2 tabs q24h	No data	No data
Viekira Pak	dasabuvir 5-8/No data	2 Ombit/Parita/RTV tabs q24h, Dasa 250 mg q12h	2 Ombit/Parita/ RTV tabs q24h, Dasa 250 mg q12h	2 Ombit/Parita/RTV tabs q24h,Dasa 250 mg q12h	2 Ombit/ Parita/RTV tabs q24h, Dasa 250 mg q12h	No data	No data
Zepatier	elba ≤4, grazo 31/No data	1 tab po q24h	1 tab po q24h	1 tab po q24h	1 tab po q24h	1 tab po q24h/ No data	No data

[1] Acute renal failure and Fanconi syndrome reported.

Abbreviation Key: Adjustment Method: **D** = dose adjustment, **I** = interval adjustment; **CAPD** = continuous ambulatory peritoneal dialysis; **CRRT** = continuous renal replacement therapy; **HEMO** = hemodialysis; **AD** = after dialysis; "Supplement" or "Extra" is to replace drug lost during dialysis – additional drug beyond continuation of regimen for CrCl < 10 mL/min.

TABLE 8: DOSING ADJUSTMENTS FOR HEPATIC IMPAIRMENT

Drug	Adjustment/Comments
Paritaprevir/Ritonavir + Ombitasvir + Dasabuvir	• No dosage adjustment in patients with mild hepatic impairment (Child-Pugh A). • Not recommended in patients with moderate hepatic impairment (Child-Pugh B). • Contraindicated in patients with severe hepatic impairment (Child-Pugh C).
Ledipasvir + Sofosbuvir	No adjustment
Velpatasvir + Sofosbuvir	Not recommended in patients with severe renal impairment or end stage renal disease

TABLE 9: MANAGEMENT OF EXPOSURE TO HBV, HCV

OCCUPATIONAL EXPOSURE TO BLOOD, PENILE/VAGINAL SECRETIONS OR OTHER POTENTIALLY INFECTIOUS BODY FLUIDS OR TISSUES WITH RISK OF TRANSMISSION OF HEPATITIS B/C (E.G., NEEDLESTICK INJURY)

Free consultation for occupational exposures, call (PEPline) 1-888-448-4911.

General steps in management:

1. Wash clean wounds/flush mucous membranes immediately (use of caustic agents or squeezing the wound is discouraged; data lacking regarding antiseptics).
2. Assess risk by doing the following: (a) Characterize exposure; (b) Determine/evaluate source of exposure by medical history, risk behavior, & testing for hepatitis B/C, HIV; (c) Evaluate and test exposed individual for hepatitis B/C & HIV.

Hepatitis B Occupational Exposure Prophylaxis *(MMWR 62(No.10, Suppl):1, 2013)*

Exposed Person Vaccine Status	Exposure Source		
	HBs Ag+	HBs Ag–	Status Unknown or Unavailable for Testing
Unvaccinated	Give HBIG 0.06 mL per kg IM & initiate HB vaccine	Initiate HB vaccine	Initiate HB vaccine
Vaccinated (antibody status unknown)	Do anti-HBs on exposed person: If titer ≥10 milli-International units per mL, no rx If titer <10 milli-International units per mL, give HBIG + 1 dose HB vaccine**	No rx necessary	Do anti-HBs on exposed person: If titer ≥10 milli-International units per mL, no rx[§] If titer <10 milli-International units per mL, give 1 dose of HB vaccine**

[§] Persons previously infected with HBV are immune to reinfection and do not require postexposure prophylaxis.

For known vaccine series responder (titer ≥10 milli-International units per mL), monitoring of levels or booster doses not currently recommended. Known non-responder (<10 milli-International units per mL) to 1º series HB vaccine & exposed to either HBsAg+ source or suspected high-risk source—rx with HBIG & re-initiate vaccine series **or** give 2 doses HBIG 1 month apart. For non-responders after a 2nd vaccine series, 2 doses HBIG 1 month apart is preferred approach to new exposure.

If known high risk source, treat as if source were HBsAG positive

** Follow-up to assess vaccine response or address completion of vaccine series.

Hepatitis B Non-Occupational Exposure & Reactivation of Latent Hepatitis B

Non-Occupational Exposure *(MMWR 59(RR-10):1, 2010)*

- Exposure to blood or sexual secretion of HBsAg-positive person
  - Percutaneous (bite, needlestick)
  - Sexual assault
- Initiate immunoprophylaxis within 24 hrs or sexual exposure & no more than 7 days after parenteral exposure
- Use Guidelines for occupational exposure for use of HBIG and HBV vaccine

TABLE 9 (2)

Hepatitis B Non-Occupational Exposure & Reactivation of Latent Hepatitis B *(continued)*

Reactivation of Latent HBV *(Eur J Cancer 49:3486, 2013; Seminar of Liver Dis 33:167, 2013; Crit Rev Oncol-Hematol 87:12, 2013)*

- Patients requiring administration of anti-CD 20 monoclonal antibodies as part of treatment selected malignancies, rheumatoid arthritis and vasculitis are at risk for reactivation of latent HBV
- Two FDA-approved anti-CD 20 drugs: Ofatumumab (Arzerra) & Rituximab (Rituxan)
- Prior to starting anti-CD 20 drug, test for latent HBV with test for HBsAg and Anti IgG HB core antibody

If pt has latent HBV & anti-CD 20 treatment is necessary, treatment should include an effective anti-HBV drug

Hepatitis C Exposure

Determine antibody to hepatitis C for both exposed person &, if possible, exposure source. If source + or unknown and exposed person negative, follow-up HCV testing for HCV RNA (detectable in blood in 1-3 weeks) and HCV antibody (90% who seroconvert will do so by 3 months) is advised.

No recommended prophylaxis; immune serum globulin not effective. Monitor for early infection, as therapy may ↓ risk of progression to chronic hepatitis. Persons who remain viremic 8-12 weeks after exposure should be treated with a course of DAA therapy as per treatment described above for chronic HCV infection. Case-control study suggested risk factors for occupational HCV transmission include percutaneous exposure to needle that had been in artery or vein, deep injury, male sex of HCW, & was more likely when source VL >6 log10 copies/mL.

For HCV-HIV exposure prophylaxis, see *The Sanford Guide to HIV/AIDS* Therapy and *webedition.sanfordguide.com*

TABLE 10: HEPATITIS A & B IMMUNIZATION

(http://www.cdc.gov/vaccines/schedules/hcp/imz/adult-shell.html)

Hepatitis A
- HAV vaccination is indicated for:
    - MSM and IDU
    - Persons working with HAV-infected primates or with HAV in a lab setting
    - Chronic liver disease pts and pts receiving clotting factor concentrates
    - Those infected with either Hepatitis B or Hepatitis C virus
    - Travel to or work in countries with high/moderate endemic HAV
    - Close personal contact (e.g., household or regular babysitting) with an international adoptee during the first 60 days after arrival from a country with high or intermediate endemicity. First dose of HAV vaccine series should be administered as soon as adoption is planned, ideally 2 or more weeks before arrival of adoptee
- Single-antigen vaccine 2-dose series:
    - **Havrix** (0, 6 to 12 mos)
    - **Vaqta** (0, 6 to 18 mos)
- Combined HAV/HBV vaccine 3-dose series:
    - **Twinrix** (0, 1, 6 mos), 4 dose alternative (0, 7, 21-30 days, then booster at 12 mos)

Hepatitis B
- HBV vaccination is indicated for:
    - MSM, IDU, multiple sex partners (within 6 mos)
    - Co-morbidities/risk factors: STD, diabetes (age < 60 yrs)(discretionary in age > 60 yrs based on additional risk factors, e.g., long-term care facility, end stage renal disease, hemodialysis, HIV co-infection, Hepatitis C infection, chronic liver disease
    - HCW/ public safety workers potentially exposed to blood or other infectious body fluids and/or those working in elevated risk settings
    - Household contacts and sex partners of HBs antigen–positive persons
    - International travel to high-prevalence destinations
- **Heplisav-B** (Dynavax, GSK): is a two-dose vaccine approved and recommended in the U.S. for use in adults aged 18 and older. The vaccine is administered as two doses given one month (at least 28 days) apart.
- Recombivax HB (Merck): Administer missing doses to complete a 3-dose series HBV vaccine to persons not vaccinated or not completely vaccinated (0, 1, 4 mos).
- Combined HAV/HBV vaccine 3-dose series:
    - **Twinrix** (0, 1, 6 mos), 4 dose alternative (0, 7, 21-30 days, then booster at 12 mos)
- Adult pts on hemodialysis or immunocompromised: 1 dose of 40 mcg/mL **(Recombivax HB)** administered on a 3-dose schedule at 0, 1, and 6 months or 2 doses of 20 mcg/mL (**Engerix-B**) administered simultaneously on a 4-dose schedule at 0, 1, 2, and 6 months.

TABLE 11: GENERIC AND TRADE NAMES

Generic Name	Abbreviation/Trade Name
Adefovir dipivoxil	Hepsera
Daclatasvir	Daklinza
Entecavir	Baraclude
Glecaprevir + Pibrentasvir	Mavyret
Grazoprevir + Elbasvir	Zepatier
Interferon alfa	Roferon, Intron-A, Peg-Intron, Pegasys
Lamivudine	3TC, Epivir, Epivir-HBV
Ledipasvir + Sofosbuvir	Harvoni
Ombitasvir + Paritaprevir + Ritonavir + Dasabuvir	Viekira Pak/Viekira XR
Ribavirin	Rebetol, Copegus
Simeprevir	Olysio
Sofosbuvir	Sovaldi
Tenofovir	TDF, Viread
Tenofovir Alafenamide Fumarate	TAF, Vemlidy
Tenofovir + Emtricitabine	Truvada
TAF + Emtricitabine	Descovy
Velpatasvir + Sofosbuvir	Epclusa

Abbreviation/Trade Name	Generic Name
3TC, Epivir, Epivir-HBV	Lamivudine
Daklinza	Daclatasvir
Descovy	TAF + Emtricitabine
Baraclude	Entecavir
Epclusa	Velpatasvir + Sofosbuvir
Harvoni	Ledipasvir + Sofosbuvir
Hepsera	Adefovir dipivoxil
Mavyret	Glecaprevir + Pibrentasvir
Olysio	Simeprevir
Rebetol, Copegus	Ribavirin
Roferon, Intron-A, Peg-Intron, Pegasys	Interferon alfa
Sovaldi	Sofosbuvir
TAF, Vemlidy	Tenofovir Alafenamide Fumarate
TDF, Viread	Tenofovir
Truvada	Tenofovir + Emtricitabine
Viekira Pak / Viekira XR	Ombitasvir + Paritaprevir + Ritonavir + Dasabuvir
Zepatier	Grazoprevir + Elbasvir

NOTES

NOTES